Ocular Rigidity, Biomechanics and Hydrodynamics
of the Eye

Ioannis Pallikaris • Miltiadis K. Tsilimbaris
Anna I. Dastiridou

Editors

Ocular Rigidity, Biomechanics and Hydrodynamics of the Eye

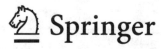 Springer

Editors
Ioannis Pallikaris
Department of Ophthalmology
University of Crete
Heraklion, Crete
Greece

Miltiadis K. Tsilimbaris
Department of Ophthalmology
University of Crete
Heraklion, Crete
Greece

Anna I. Dastiridou
2nd Ophthalmology Department
Aristotle University of Thessaloniki
Thessaloniki
Greece

School of Medicine
University of Thessalia
Larissa
Greece

ISBN 978-3-030-64424-6   ISBN 978-3-030-64422-2   (eBook)
https://doi.org/10.1007/978-3-030-64422-2

This Springer imprint is published by the registered company Springer Nature Switzerland AG
The registered company address is: Gewerbestrasse 11, 6330 Cham, Switzerland

Preface

What do we mean by the term ocular rigidity? Is it a concept that is relevant in 2020? What is the interplay between ocular biomechanics and hydro- and hemodynamics?

These are some of the questions this book is trying to answer. The concept of ocular rigidity has been one of the main research interests of our team during the past few years, but ocular rigidity is a rather old concept, probably since the early 1930s. But how and why is it relevant now? The recent reappraisal of eye biomechanics in the pathophysiology of eye diseases, as well as the recent increase in the existing body of knowledge around eye biomechanics, gives us the opportunity to revisit the concept of ocular rigidity. In fact, this book tries to bridge the varying terminology. This is indeed an attempt to gather and present all the available knowledge around ocular rigidity, the factors that may affect it, and its associations with common eye conditions like glaucoma, age-related macular degeneration, high myopia, and corneal ectasias. The book also tries to give both the clinician's and the engineer's perspective on the subject. For instance, we now have new information on the properties of the cornea, and it seems that we are going to understand more on what these new parameters mean in the years to come. We also have new instruments that can help us characterize tissue properties in vivo, and these may provide new important disease biomarkers. In many chapters, some basic terminology is repeated in order for the reader to follow the fundamental principles and in a way that each chapter can be read separately and appreciated individually. There are chapters focusing specifically on the local biomechanical properties of the different structures: the lens, the cornea, the sclera, and the choroid. And because the shape, structure, and function of most components of the eye are affected from the hydrodynamics of the blood and aqueous flow, we have added a chapter discussing aqueous fluidics. The perception of the eye as a dynamic structure and the understanding of ocular hydrodynamics are crucial in this book.

We sincerely thank all the authors for their valuable contribution to this book.

Heraklion, Crete, Greece   Ioannis Pallikaris
Heraklion, Crete, Greece   Miltiadis K. Tsilimbaris
Larissa, Greece   Anna I. Dastiridou

Contents

Chapter 1
Basic Engineering Concepts and Terminology Underlying Ocular Rigidity

Elizabeth M. Boazak and C. Ross Ethier

An Introduction to Stress and Strain

Much of tissue mechanics seeks to understand forces within tissues, the resulting deformations of the tissue, and how the forces are related to the deformations. To understand these concepts, an understanding of relevant terminology is essential. For introductory information regarding stress and strain beyond what is reported here, we recommend referring to the books by Fung [1], Timoshenko [2], and Wang [3]. More advanced concepts are described by Humphrey [4] and Holzapfel [5].

Stress, typically represented with the Greek letter σ, is the ratio of an applied force, F, to the cross sectional area over which it is applied, A.

$$\sigma = F / A \tag{1.1}$$

Conceptually, stress is a normalized load; the normalization by area is useful when comparing the response of differently-sized samples to mechanical loading, since it reflects what the cells and extracellular matrix "feel" at the local level as load is applied. There are important differences in the types of stress (Fig. 1.1): tensile and compressive stresses are referred to as normal stresses, as they arise from loads applied normal (perpendicular) to the area of interest, which is often the cross sectional area of the sample, as shown in Fig. 1.1. On the other hand, shear stresses arise when the force is applied parallel to the area of interest, such as the stress produced on vascular endothelium in the direction of blood flow. In the eye, a very important normal compressive stress is pressure, which, by definition, always acts normal to any surface that is exposed to the pressure.

E. M. Boazak · C. R. Ethier (✉)
Wallace H. Coulter Department of Biomedical Engineering, The Georgia Institute
of Technology & Emory University School of Medicine, Atlanta, GA, USA
e-mail: ross.ethier@bme.gatech.edu

© Springer Nature Switzerland AG 2021
I. Pallikaris et al. (eds.), *Ocular Rigidity, Biomechanics and Hydrodynamics of
the Eye*, https://doi.org/10.1007/978-3-030-64422-2_1

1

Fig. 1.1 Schematic of the forces and areas used to calculate compressive, tensile, and shear stresses. Here we have considered stresses internal to the body produced by internal forces acting on a virtual surface within the body

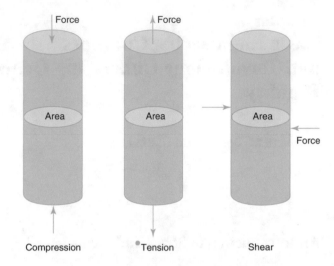

Fig. 1.2 Schematic of deformation arising from tensile loading. Change in length is normalized by the original length to give tensile strain

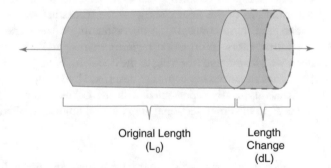

In the same way that stress is the normalized metric of load, strain is the normalized metric of deformation. Typically represented with the Greek letter ε, strain is the ratio of the change in length to the original length of the sample (or tissue region of interest; Fig. 1.2).

$$\varepsilon = dL / L_0 \qquad (1.2)$$

The normalization of the magnitude of deformation by the original length means that the value for strain is dimensionless. As such, it is common to give strains as a percentage or to state units such as mm/mm.

It is of note that the stress at a single location depends on both the orientation of the cross-sectional area, A, and the orientation of the applied force, F, acting on A. A mathematical entity that depends on two directions is called a second-order tensor [4, 5], a mathematically complex object. It is possible to extract three key quantities (in 3D) from such a tensor, termed the first, second and third principal stress. For most biological materials, the first principal stress is the largest tensile stress, while the third principal stress is the compressive stress with greatest magnitude. Often these principal stresses are reported, rather than the various components of the stress tensor. Similarly, strain is a second order tensor, and we can speak about principal strains and report the first and third principal strains, and quantities derived from them.

The aforementioned definitions are for *engineering* stress and strain, as opposed to true stress and strain. Engineering stresses and strains are calculated from the initial sample geometry, while true stresses and strains are calculated from the instantaneous sample geometry, accounting for the gradual changes in dimensions and orientations as the sample deforms. For this reason, engineering stresses and strains can include an artifactual contribution as the tissue region rotates, which in general can occur as part of an arbitrary deformation. The consideration of such effects can be very complex [5] and is beyond the scope of this chapter.

A generic graph showing stress vs. engineering and true strain is shown in Fig. 1.3. The true strain curve is the more intuitive of the two, as the stress in the material continually increases with sample deformation until the point of fracture. In contrast, the region immediately preceding material failure in the engineering stress vs. strain curve will often show decreasing stress values. In reality, the stress in the material is not decreasing. Rather, the decrease in sample cross-sectional area, which is unaccounted for in the engineering stress calculation, is marked enough to offset the small increase in force magnitude for a given change in deformation. Despite this misrepresentation of the internal state of a tested material, engineering stress and strain are significantly more straightforward to calculate and understand, and in many situations, provide adequate information about specimen material properties. Specifically, if deformations are small, then true stress and strain can be shown to be well-approximated by engineering stress and strain. The question as to whether engineering stress/strain are acceptable approximations to true stress/strain in the eye depend on the specific situation under consideration, and must be evaluated carefully.

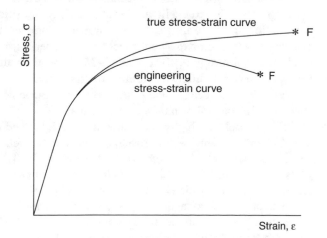

Fig. 1.3 Comparison of true and engineering stress strain curves, with the fracture point (F) indicated for each

When calculating the stress generated in a tissue under a given loading scenario, it is important to consider the shape and uniformity of a sample, as well as the uniformity of an applied load. Nonuniformities can cause stress concentration [2, 3], where some portions of the sample experience higher stresses than others. For example, in the eye, the optic nerve head concentrates stress in the peripapillary sclera [6]. Stress is also concentrated at the limbus, due to a transition in composition between cornea and sclera and slightly different curvatures of these two tissue regions.

Tissue Material Properties

The relationship between stress and strain is important, in as much as it reflects and depends on the intrinsic biomechanical properties of the loaded material/tissue. Such relationships between physical quantities that are unique to individual materials are known as constitutive relationships [1, 4]. In its simplest form, this constitutive relationship can be quantified through the elastic modulus, or Young's modulus, defined as the slope of the linear elastic portion of the stress-strain curve. Young's modulus is commonly represented with the letter E.

$$E = stress / strain = \sigma / \varepsilon \qquad (1.3)$$

The elastic portion of a stress-strain curve is comprised of the strains at which deformation is recoverable (i.e. if the load is removed, the sample will return to its original length). Beyond a certain stress and strain, termed the elastic limit or yield point, deformation is no longer recoverable. This may occur at or beyond the end of the region of linear proportionality. Much like fracture, yielding of ocular tissues is not of particular concern, even in diseased tissues. However, the elastic limit may warrant consideration in experiments subjecting tissues to large deformations.

In most soft tissues, such as the sclera and cornea, the Young's modulus is primarily governed by extracellular matrix (ECM) composition and organization. The organization of load bearing extracellular matrix components, such as collagen, can give rise to direction-dependent mechanical properties, a phenomenon known as mechanical anisotropy [4]. The Young's Modulus of an anisotropic (as opposed to isotropic) material differs according to the direction in which the material is deformed. Both cornea [7] and sclera [8] have anisotropic material properties, and anisotropy has been shown to decrease with age [9].

Collagen itself is a highly structured molecule, formed from a triple helix structure. Collagen molecules are crosslinked outside the cell to form collagen fibrils, and fibrils may further assemble into large fibers [1, 4]. This rope-like structure gives collagen its high tensile strength. Collagen fibers are observed to have an undulating structure which is known as crimp [11–15]. Collagen crimp, in combination with staggered collagen fiber engagement, gives rise to what is known as the "toe region" observed in the stress-strain curve of most biological tissues (Fig. 1.4); a phenomenon which has been directly observed in the peripapillary sclera [16]. As

Fig. 1.4 Model stress-strain curve for collagenous tissue. As collagen fibers uncrimp and begin to uniformly bear load the stress-strain relationship transitions from the toe region to the linear elastic region. Reproduced with permission from reference [10]. Copyright 2005 American Society of Mechanical Engineers

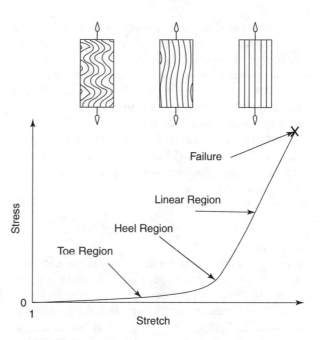

collagen uncrimps, little force is required to achieve comparatively large deformations. Resistance to deformation in this phase is provided by both the collagen crimp and the surrounding glycosaminoglycans (GAGs). Once all the collagen fibers are uncrimped, aligned, and uniformly bearing load, the tissue is observed to be much stiffer. This is the linear elastic portion of the stress train curve, in which the tensile properties of collagen fibers are primarily being measured.

It is readily apparent from the model stress-strain curve for a biological tissue (Fig. 1.4) that while there is a linear elastic *region*, a linear elastic model ($\sigma = E*\varepsilon$) does not adequately describe the data. For simple comparisons between materials, it may be useful to describe both a "toe-region modulus" as well as a Young's modulus. Hyperelastic material models, such as Neo-Hookean, Mooney-Rivlin, and others can be used to better capture these nonlinearities [4, 5].

Both the cornea and the sclera are comprised of highly organized collagen in lamellar structures [9, 17], providing strength to maintain eye shape in the presence of intraocular pressure. For even more complex description of material properties, tissues can be considered to have a fiber-reinforced structure, where crosslinked collagen fibers are interspersed with proteoglycans. Proteoglycans, comprised of glycosaminoglycan (GAG) chains attached to core proteins, are hydrophilic in nature, and retain water in the tissue. Many authors have developed microstructural constitutive models for fiber-reinforced composites which define the relationship between stress and strain based on information about isotropic matrix material properties and the characteristics of fibers. For example, Gasser & Holzapfel have created a very well-known model that includes two families of fibers [18], and other such models exist [1, 4]. Such mathematical models can be used to make predictions about three-dimensional stresses and strains, accounting for anisotropy introduced by fiber orientation.

In addition to nonlinear elastic tissue behavior, biological tissues usually exhibit some degree of viscoelasticity, i.e. they are not purely elastic but have some characteristics of a fluid [1]. This arises because the water content in tissues combines with elastic components. Importantly, this means that tissue deformation can be time-dependent, e.g. the amount of deformation that tissue experiences when it is loaded depends on how quickly the load is applied, or more generally, on the history of loading, rather than the instantaneous load alone.

Just as elastic material behavior can be simply modeled as a spring (with Eq. (1.3) paralleling Hooke's Law [2]), viscous material behavior is modeled as a dashpot. In a dashpot the stress is proportional to the strain rate multiplied by a damping coefficient (η):

$$\sigma = \eta \frac{d\varepsilon}{dt} \tag{1.4}$$

where $\frac{d\varepsilon}{dt}$ is the rate of deformation, i.e. the time derivative of strain. Springs and dashpots can be combined in series or parallel to mathematically represent the behavior of viscoelastic materials. A single spring and dashpot combined in series or in parallel are known as the Maxwell and Voight models [1], respectively. While more complex combinations of spring and dashpot elements better describe viscoelastic materials, these two simple models are useful in explaining two key features of viscoelastic behavior: stress relaxation and creep. In a stress relaxation test, a constant strain is applied, and the stress over time in the material is measured. The decrease in stress is reflected in the "relaxation time" which is characteristic for a material. In a creep test, a constant load is applied and the strain rate over time is measured.

The viscoelastic behavior of ocular tissues is relevant to ocular physiology and pathophysiology, as it determines their response to a dynamic environment. Intraocular pressure (IOP) fluctuates by 4 mmHg [19] on the order of seconds due to arterial pressure cycles ("the ocular pulse"). These IOP fluctuations correspond to 0.5% macroscopic compressive strains in the optic nerve head [20], which could be amplified ten-fold [6] to around 5% at the cellular level. IOP is also subject to large diurnal variations in some individuals, which is an independent risk factor for glaucoma [21]. Tissue viscoelasticity is of intrinsic interest, due to its potential contributions to ocular pathologies. More specifically, the viscoelastic nature of biological tissues must still be taken into account when attempting to describe them with elastic constants, or properties such as compliance; sufficiently low loading rates are required in order to reasonably neglect the viscous component of mechanical behavior.

Mechanics at the Organ Level

Both compressive and tensile strains (and compressive and tensile stresses) occur in ocular tissues as a result of IOP. Computational modeling has indicated that neural tissues in the optic nerve head primarily experience compressive strains in response to elevated IOP, although shear and tensile strains are also present [22]. However, over most of the corneoscleral shell, the IOP produces primarily tensile stresses within the wall of the eye (the so-called "hoop stresses"), which are carried by the ECM fibers of the cornea and sclera. This situation can be conceptualized as similar to that of a balloon; as the pressure inside the balloon is increased, the balloon itself is forced to stretch, accommodating the increase in pressure. Three key concepts are useful for quantifying and describing this mechanical behavior: compliance, ocular rigidity, and Laplace's Law. We also briefly discuss computational modeling of stress and strain, often necessary due to the limited applicability of Laplace's law.

Compliance

Compliance, which describes how changes in volume and pressure are related within a chamber, is a concept used extensively in cardiovascular and respiratory physiology [4]. The relationship between volume and pressure can also be used to understand the response of the whole eye to changes in IOP, and reflects the combined mechanical behavior of the cornea and sclera. Because it is, by definition, an integrated measure of mechanical behavior [4], compliance cannot reveal local variations in corneoscleral shell stiffness. Ocular compliance is calculated from the slope of the internal volume vs. intraocular pressure curve [23], giving units of volume per unit pressure, and is commonly represented by the letter ϕ:

$$\psi(P) = dV / dP \qquad (1.5)$$

Compliance should be calculated over a range of pressures, as it typically decreases nonlinearly with increasing pressure [24, 25] due to tissue stiffening with increasing deformation. Thus, in order to compare values for ocular compliance between individual samples, a reference pressure must be defined (i.e. a pressure at which to report and compare the compliance), which would typically be the normal IOP for the species or genetic strain of animal being evaluated, although individual experimental aims may imply an alternative.

Tissue viscoelasticity may contribute differently to the calculated compliance, depending on whether a volume injection or pressure clamped measurement approach is used. Volume injection approaches use a syringe pump to introduce a known volume of fluid into the eye and measure the subsequent changes in IOP [23, 26], while the pressure clamped approaches make use of an adjustable pressure reservoir to fix the IOP while the flow rate into the eye (and hence ocular volume) is measured. In the absence of aqueous humor outflow, the infusion of a bolus of fluid into an eye would result in an initial increase in IOP, followed by a gradual decay to a stable pressure between the starting IOP and the peak pressure. As outflow will result in a continuously decreasing IOP, it is not possible in practice to find this stable pressure following a bolus infusion, and this complexity must be accounted for in analysis of experimental data. The corresponding difficulty in accounting for corneosclearal relaxation in measurements of ocular compliance using volume injection methods typically results in lower reported values for compliance as compared to measurements using pressure clamped methods (personal observations).

Friedenwald's Equation and Ocular Rigidity

The ophthalmological community has long recognized the importance of understanding the mechanical behavior of ocular tissues, as reflected in the well-known Friedenwald's Equation [27] which defines the concept of ocular rigidity, K.

$$\frac{dP}{P} = k\frac{dV}{V} = KdV \tag{1.6}$$

In Friedenwald's Equation, k is a dimensionless constant representing the rigidity of the corneoscleral shell which can be used to relate changes in pressure (dP) and volume (dV) in the eye. Changes in volume are considered small relative to the initial volume, so V is considered to be approximately constant. As such, it can be incorporated with k into the ocular rigidity K, where K = k/V. This calculation results in units for ocular rigidity of reciprocal volume, which are less intuitive than the ocular compliance units of volume per unit pressure. By rearranging Eq. (1.5) to solve for dV/dP, we can directly describe the relationship between compliance and ocular rigidity: $\phi = 1/KP$.

Law of Laplace

Laplace's Law describes the tensile strain developed in the wall of a pressurized thin-walled sphere [1]. In order to be considered "thin-walled", the sphere radius (r) should be at least 10 times the wall thickness (t) [28]. At this ratio, the thin-walled approximation underestimates the peak wall stress (occurring at the inner wall) by only 0.6%. In human eyes, r/t ranges from 8.8 to 29 [29]. Laplace's law can be simply derived by considering half of a sphere, formed by virtually cutting through an internally pressurized sphere (Fig. 1.5). In order for the pressure applied to the interior surface to not move the half sphere through space, the wall tension, or stress, must counter the net force due to the internal pressure, ΔP. In the half sphere, all components of the internal pressure cancel each other, except for those in the $-x$ direction. The total force in $-x$ is the transmural pressure multiplied over the cross sectional area: $\Delta P(\pi r^2)$. This is opposed by the wall stress distributed over the wall cross sectional area: $\sigma(2\pi rt)$. Solving for wall stress, we find $\sigma = \frac{Pr}{2t}$. With known material properties for ocular tissues, we can thus connect IOP to tissue strains. As discussed in the final section of this chapter, tissue strains are detected by cells and can influence their phenotype.

Fig. 1.5 The cross-section
of a thin-walled sphere
shows how tensile wall
stress (σ) opposes an
internal pressure

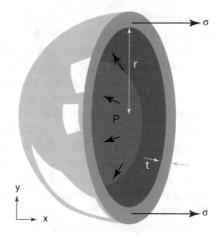

Laplace's law can describe biomechanical behavior of the eye with an attractive degree of simplicity, and may be useful for estimation. However, the eye is not a uniform, spherical, thin-walled vessel. Laplace's law is not able to accurately capture the effects of geometric and material variability in the corneoscleral shell, especially near the scleral canal. Accounting for geometrical and material factors neglected by using Laplace's law can alter the predicted ocular wall stresses by up to 456% [30].

Computational and Measurement Tools

It is possible to understand tissue mechanics by solving the equilibrium equations; using Newton's law of motion, all forces acting on a body or a portion of a body must be in equilibrium in the absence of acceleration. These equations allow for the calculation of the internal stresses in a body or tissue. However, due to the complex geometries of the eye and constitutive laws that are typical for ocular tissues, such calculations are difficult in practice. When it comes to evaluating the mechanical behavior of the whole eye (or regions of the eye) with high spatial resolution, computational approaches are thus useful.

Finite element analysis (FEA) is a particularly powerful computational approach [31]. In a finite element model, a complex geometry is broken down into a set of small elements, typically of uniform geometry. This process is called discretization or meshing. Each element is subsequently assigned material properties. Systems of equations for the stresses and strains in each element are then compiled to produce a system of equations for the whole structure. With the application of boundary conditions and loads, displacement of specific points on each element (the nodes), as well as stresses and strains in the elements, can be calculated. Downs, Girard,

Grytz, Feola, Nguyen, Sigal, and others have worked to develop models of the optic nerve head [32, 33]. An advantage of FEA is that once a model is developed it can be fairly straightforward to include patient-specific geometries. This may make it possible to predict, for example, the stains in the optic nerve head produced under a given IOP for a specific patient and to determine a target IOP to prevent glaucomatous damage for an individual. However, the utility of a finite element model for clinical or exploratory purposes is often limited by the availability of accurate values for material properties—values that typically are determined experimentally.

Material properties for individual tissues may be measured through a variety of testing methods (e.g. uniaxial and biaxial tensile testing, compression, and atomic force microscopy). Inflation testing, however, makes it possible to study the mechanical behavior of regions of the eye in more physiological conformations. Typically the eye is partially potted (glued) in a holder, and punctured. A pressure reservoir can be used to inflate the eye, and tissue deformation can be tracked via 2D projections [34] or 3-dimensional digital image correlation [35–37]. As was mentioned in the discussion of ocular compliance, the viscoelastic nature of ocular tissues will influence the strains observed and computed in response to pressure steps in inflation experiments, and must be taken into account in experimental design.

Mechanotransduction: How Do Mechanical Forces Affect Cells and Tissues?

Mechanotransduction is the process by which cells detect mechanical stimuli in their environment and turn such inputs into biochemical signals. Cell-cell adhesions, primary cilia, membrane channels and receptors, cytoskeleton, ECM, and cell nuclei are all mediators of mechanotransduction [38]. Once transduced, mechanical force can regulate ECM synthesis and maintenance, or initiate a pathological response. Physical damage is thus not required to change tissue material properties. For example, loading is required for the maintenance of bone and cartilage, and remarkably, is detected by resident cells despite them being embedded in rigid tissues that undergo relatively small macroscopic deformations. Meanwhile, the pressure waves of sound are detected and distinguished by hair cells in the ear. Disturbed flow in the vasculature, and the resultant changes in shear stress, can initiate the formation of atherosclerotic plaques due in part to pathological mechanotransduction by vascular endothelial cells.

In the eye, there are a variety of mechanosensitive cell types [39, 40]. High IOP leads to abnormal strains in the optic nerve head which may be detected by astrocytes, resulting in their transition to a reactive phenotype [41]. Prolonged astrocyte activation and the formation of a glial scar is a hallmark of glaucoma. Human scleral fibroblasts are also mechanosensitive and changes in gene expression regulating matrix components have been observed in response to tensile loading [42]. Scleral remodeling is a known to contribute to axial elongation in the development of myopia. Trabecular meshwork cells show cytoskeletal reorganization and signaling changes in response to mechanical stretch [43]. Mechanotransduction pathways are also suggested to be involved in the pathological wound healing response of corneal epithelium [44]. Increased understanding of mechanotransduction pathways may reveal novel therapeutic targets for a variety of ocular pathologies.

References

1. Fung YC. Biomechanics: mechanical properties of living tissues. 2nd ed. New York: Springer; 1993. p. xviii.
2. Timoshenko S, Goodier JN. Theory of elasticity. 3rd ed. New York: McGraw-Hill; 1969. p. xxiv.
3. Wang C-T. Applied elasticity. New York: McGraw-Hill; 1953. p. 357.
4. Humphrey JD. Cardiovascular solid mechanics: cells, tissues, and organs. New York: Springer; 2002. p. xvi.
5. Holzapfel GA. Nonlinear solid mechanics: a continuum approach for engineering. Chichester; New York: Wiley; 2000. p. xiv.
6. Downs JC, Roberts MD, Burgoyne CF. Mechanical environment of the optic nerve head in glaucoma. Optom Vis Sci. 2008;85(6):425–35. https://doi.org/10.1097/OPX.0b013e31817841cb.
7. Kling S, Remon L, Perez-Escudero A, Merayo-Lloves J, Marcos S. Corneal biomechanical changes after collagen cross-linking from porcine eye inflation experiments. Invest Ophthalmol Vis Sci. 2010;51(8):3961–8. https://doi.org/10.1167/iovs.09-4536.
8. Coudrillier B, Boote C, Quigley HA, Nguyen TD. Scleral anisotropy and its effects on the mechanical response of the optic nerve head. Biomech Model Mechanobiol. 2013;12(5):941–63. https://doi.org/10.1007/s10237-012-0455-y.
9. Coudrillier B, Pijanka J, Jefferys J, Sorensen T, Quigley HA, Boote C, Nguyen TD. Collagen structure and mechanical properties of the human sclera: analysis for the effects of age. J Biomech Eng. 2015;137(4):041006. https://doi.org/10.1115/1.4029430.
10. Freed AD, Doehring TC. Elastic model for crimped collagen fibrils. J Biomech Eng. 2005;127(4):587–93.
11. Ho LC, Sigal IA, Jan NJ, Squires A, Tse Z, Wu EX, Kim SG, Schuman JS, Chan KC. Magic angle-enhanced MRI of fibrous microstructures in sclera and cornea with and without intraocular pressure loading. Invest Ophthalmol Vis Sci. 2014;55(9):5662–72. https://doi.org/10.1167/iovs.14-14561.
12. Jan NJ, Gomez C, Moed S, Voorhees AP, Schuman JS, Bilonick RA, Sigal IA. Microstructural crimp of the lamina cribrosa and peripapillary sclera collagen fibers. Invest Ophthalmol Vis Sci. 2017;58(9):3378–88. https://doi.org/10.1167/iovs.17-21811.
13. Jan NJ, Grimm JL, Tran H, Lathrop KL, Wollstein G, Bilonick RA, Ishikawa H, Kagemann L, Schuman JS, Sigal IA. Polarization microscopy for characterizing fiber orientation of ocular tissues. Biomed Opt Express. 2015;6(12):4705–18. https://doi.org/10.1364/BOE.6.004705.
14. Jan NJ, Lathrop K, Sigal IA. Collagen architecture of the posterior pole: high-resolution wide field of view visualization and analysis using polarized light microscopy. Invest Ophthalmol Vis Sci. 2017;58(2):735–44. https://doi.org/10.1167/iovs.16-20772.
15. Grytz R, Meschke G, Jonas JB. The collagen fibril architecture in the lamina cribrosa and peripapillary sclera predicted by a computational remodeling approach. Biomech Model Mechanobiol. 2011;10(3):371–82. https://doi.org/10.1007/s10237-010-0240-8.
16. Jan NJ, Sigal IA. Collagen fiber recruitment: a microstructural basis for the nonlinear response of the posterior pole of the eye to increases in intraocular pressure. Acta Biomater. 2018;72:295–305. https://doi.org/10.1016/j.actbio.2018.03.026.
17. Meek KM. The cornea and sclera. In: Fratzl P, editor. Collagen: structure and mechanics. Boston, MA: Springer; 2008. p. 359–96. https://doi.org/10.1007/978-0-387-73906-9_13.

18. Holzapfel GA, Gasser TC. A viscoelastic model for fiber-reinforced composites at finite strains: continuum basis, computational aspects and applications. Comput Methods Appl Mech Eng. 2001;190(34):4379–403. https://doi.org/10.1016/S0045-7825(00)00323-6.
19. Avila MY, Carre DA, Stone RA, Civan MM. Reliable measurement of mouse intraocular pressure by a servo-null micropipette system. Invest Ophthalmol Vis Sci. 2001;42(8):1841–6.
20. Coudrillier B, Geraldes DM, Vo NT, Atwood R, Reinhard C, Campbell IC, Raji Y, Albon J, Abel RL, Ethier CR. Phase-contrast micro-computed tomography measurements of the intraocular pressure-induced deformation of the porcine Lamina Cribrosa. IEEE Trans Med Imaging. 2016;35(4):988–99. https://doi.org/10.1109/TMI.2015.2504440.
21. Asrani S, Zeimer R, Wilensky J, Gieser D, Vitale S, Lindenmuth K. Large diurnal fluctuations in intraocular pressure are an independent risk factor in patients with glaucoma. J Glaucoma. 2000;9(2):134–42.
22. Sigal IA, Flanagan JG, Tertinegg I, Ethier CR. Predicted extension, compression and shearing of optic nerve head tissues. Exp Eye Res. 2007;85(3):312–22. https://doi.org/10.1016/j.exer.2007.05.005.
23. Stockslager MA, Samuels BC, Allingham RR, Klesmith ZA, Schwaner SA, Forest CR, Ethier CR. System for rapid, precise modulation of intraocular pressure, toward minimally-invasive in vivo measurement of intracranial pressure. PLoS One. 2016;11(1):e0147020. https://doi.org/10.1371/journal.pone.0147020.
24. Schwaner SA, Sherwood JM, Snider E, Geisert EE, Overby DR, Ethier CR. Ocular compliance in mice. Invest Ophth Vis Sci. 2015;56(7):6143.
25. Madekurozwa M, Reina-Torres E, Overby DR, Sherwood JM. Direct measurement of pressure-independent aqueous humour flow using iPerfusion. Exp Eye Res. 2017;162:129–38. https://doi.org/10.1016/j.exer.2017.07.008.
26. Lei Y, Overby DR, Boussommier-Calleja A, Stamer WD, Ethier CR. Outflow physiology of the mouse eye: pressure dependence and washout. Invest Ophthalmol Vis Sci. 2011;52(3):1865–71. https://doi.org/10.1167/iovs.10-6019.
27. Friedenwald JS. Contribution to the theory and practice of tonometry. Am J Ophthalmol. 1937;20(10):985–1024. https://doi.org/10.1016/S0002-9394(37)90425-2.
28. Roark RJ, Young WC, Budynas RG, Sadegh AM. Roark's formulas for stress and strain. 8th ed. New York: McGraw-Hill; 2012. p. xviii.
29. Norman RE, Flanagan JG, Sigal IA, Rausch SM, Tertinegg I, Ethier CR. Finite element modeling of the human sclera: influence on optic nerve head biomechanics and connections with glaucoma. Exp Eye Res. 2011;93(1):4–12. https://doi.org/10.1016/j.exer.2010.09.014.
30. Chung CW, Girard MJ, Jan NJ, Sigal IA. Use and misuse of Laplace's law in ophthalmology. Invest Ophthalmol Vis Sci. 2016;57(1):236–45. https://doi.org/10.1167/iovs.15-18053.
31. Zienkiewicz OC, Taylor RL, Zhu JZ. The finite element method: its basis and fundamentals. 7th ed. Amsterdam: Elsevier, Butterworth-Heinemann; 2013. p. xxxviii.
32. Sigal IA, Ethier CR. Biomechanics of the optic nerve head. Exp Eye Res. 2009;88(4):799–807. https://doi.org/10.1016/j.exer.2009.02.003.
33. Nguyen TD, Ethier CR. Biomechanical assessment in models of glaucomatous optic neuropathy. Exp Eye Res. 2015;141:125–38. https://doi.org/10.1016/j.exer.2015.05.024.
34. Myers KM, Cone FE, Quigley HA, Gelman S, Pease ME, Nguyen TD. The in vitro inflation response of mouse sclera. Exp Eye Res. 2010;91(6):866–75. https://doi.org/10.1016/j.exer.2010.09.009.
35. Boyce BL, Grazier JM, Jones RE, Nguyen TD. Full-field deformation of bovine cornea under constrained inflation conditions. Biomaterials. 2008;29(28):3896–904. https://doi.org/10.1016/j.biomaterials.2008.06.011.
36. Coudrillier B, Tian J, Alexander S, Myers KM, Quigley HA, Nguyen TD. Biomechanics of the human posterior sclera: age- and glaucoma-related changes measured using inflation testing. Invest Ophth Vis Sci. 2012;53(4):1714–28. https://doi.org/10.1167/iovs.11-8009.
37. Campbell IC, Hannon BG, Read AT, Sherwood JM, Schwaner SA, Ethier CR. Correction to 'Quantification of the efficacy of collagen cross-linking agents to induce stiffening of rat sclera'. J R Soc Interface. 2017;14(130) https://doi.org/10.1098/rsif.2017.0312.

38. Ingber DE. Cellular mechanotransduction: putting all the pieces together again. FASEB J. 2006;20(7):811–27. https://doi.org/10.1096/fj.05-5424rev.
39. Morgan JT, Murphy CJ, Russell P. What do mechanotransduction, Hippo, Wnt, and TGFbeta have in common? YAP and TAZ as key orchestrating molecules in ocular health and disease. Exp Eye Res. 2013;115:1–12. https://doi.org/10.1016/j.exer.2013.06.012.
40. Jaalouk DE, Lammerding J. Mechanotransduction gone awry. Nat Rev Mol Cell Biol. 2009;10(1):63–73. https://doi.org/10.1038/nrm2597.
41. Hernandez MR. The optic nerve head in glaucoma: role of astrocytes in tissue remodeling. Prog Retin Eye Res. 2000;19(3):297–321. https://doi.org/10.1016/S1350-9462(99)00017-8.
42. Cui W, Bryant MR, Sweet PM, McDonnell PJ. Changes in gene expression in response to mechanical strain in human scleral fibroblasts. Exp Eye Res. 2004;78(2):275–84.
43. Tumminia SJ, Mitton KP, Arora J, Zelenka P, Epstein DL, Russell P. Mechanical stretch alters the actin cytoskeletal network and signal transduction in human trabecular meshwork cells. Invest Ophthalmol Vis Sci. 1998;39(8):1361–71.
44. Nowell CS, Odermatt PD, Azzolin L, Hohnel S, Wagner EF, Fantner GE, Lutolf MP, Barrandon Y, Piccolo S, Radtke F. Chronic inflammation imposes aberrant cell fate in regenerating epithelia through mechanotransduction. Nat Cell Biol. 2016;18(2):168–80. https://doi.org/10.1038/ncb3290.

Chapter 2
Ocular Rigidity: Clinical Approach

Konstantin Kotliar

"One of the Most Confusing Areas in Ophthalmology": An Attempt to Give a Definition

Ocular rigidity in ophthalmology is usually understood as a certain measurable parameter related to biomechanical properties of the entire eyeball [1]. A numerical parameter describing ocular rigidity is usually called as the coefficient of ocular rigidity. It represents a clinical measure connecting a change in intraocular pressure (IOP) with the corresponding change of intraocular volume. The entire concept of ocular rigidity adressing the question: "how soft/hard is the eyeball by touch?" might be even a quintessence of the concept "ocular biomechanics" for a layman (Fig. 2.1).

Despite the wide use of ocular rigidity concept by various researchers, it becomes evident that there is still no consence in understanding what exactly ocular rigidity is. As pointed out by White: " …ocular rigidity is an empirical concept with no physical basis and one of the most confusing areas in ophthalmology" [2, 3]. When speaking about ocular rigidity diverse researchers have in mind different parameters and properties of the eyeball or its structures and tissues. Here are for instance a few attempts to define ocular rigidity:

- Friedenwald [4]: «the resistance which the ocular tissues exert to a general increase in intraocular volume.» and «…in order not to confuse this measure with the true coefficient of elasticity (which varies in each eye with the pressure) we shall call this new measure the coefficient of rigidity.»;

K. Kotliar (✉)
Department of Medical Engineering and Technomathematics, FH Aachen University of Applied Sciences, Jülich, Germany
e-mail: kotliar@fh-aachen.de

© Springer Nature Switzerland AG 2021
I. Pallikaris et al. (eds.), *Ocular Rigidity, Biomechanics and Hydrodynamics of the Eye*, https://doi.org/10.1007/978-3-030-64422-2_2

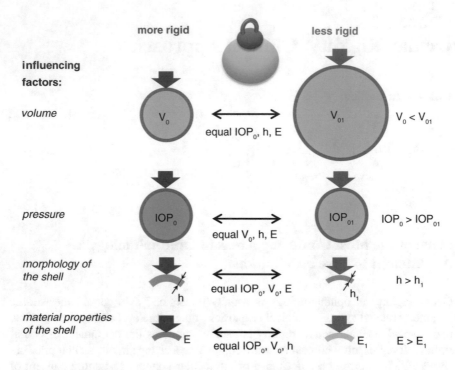

Fig. 2.1 What mechanical factors do influence ocular rigidity? A mental experiment: rigidity of thin elastic spherical shell filled with a fluid: a simplified model of the eyeball. The objects in the left column would, ceteris paribus, seem less rigid to the touch, than the objects to the right. V_0 = internal volume; IOP_0 = internal pressure; h = thickness of the shell; E = Young's (elastic) modulus of the shell

- van der Werff [5]: «The ocular rigidity function relates pressure changes to volume changes within the eye and is a measure of the elasticity of the corneoscleral shell.»;
- Moses [6]: «…ocular rigidity refers to the stretch behavior of the ocular coats.»;
- Strakhov [7]: «Under rigidity of the corneo-scleral shell one understands its ability to resist to external and internal stresses. The concept of elasticity of the sclera is directly opposite in its sense.»;
- Beaton et al. [8]: «…ocular rigidity, accounting for the combined mechanical properties of the retina, choroid and sclera».

Now let us get all this straightened out and try to clarify, where we are with ocular rigidity. It is believed that it is the ocular rigidity that ensures the maintenance of a stable shape of the eyeball to enable the functioning of its optical system (eye turgor). It compensates for internal pressure fluctuations (IOP, arterial and venous pressures) and ensures the exchange of the aqueous humor. Moreover the concept of ocular rigidity represents a basis of several clinical methods including clinical tonometry and tonography [9], methods measuring the pulse amplitude [10, 11], pulsatile blood flow [12, 13], measurements of biomechanical parameters with Ocular Response Analyser (ORA) [14] and Dynamic Scheimpflug Analyzer (Corvis ST) [15].

As a whole, most researchers agree that the concept of ocular rigidity serves to relate biomechanical properties of the corneo-scleral shell to the IOP level and IOP fluctuations, and also to connect these aspects with the etiology and pathology of certain eye disorders, e.g. glaucoma, myopia and diabetic retinopathy. Although it has been experimentally established that a clear negative correlation exists between the coefficient of ocular rigidity and the volume of the eye [16], the correlation between the coefficient of ocular rigidity and elastic characteristics of the cornea and the sclera appeared surprisingly weak and statistically insignificant, presumably due to the high measurement errors. Another quite sensible explanation of this fact: additionally to material properties of the corneo-scleral shell the ocular rigidity depends definitely on the size of the eyeball, IOP-level, corneal and scleral thickness [16–21], as well as on the ocular blood flow, especially on the reactivity of the eye microvasculature [17, 19], that affects intraocular volume and the IOP.

Let us clarify some of those aspects performing a mental experiment. How soft by touch is a thin elastic spherical shell filled with a fluid: a simplified model of the eyeball? It is easy to see that all the factors mentioned in Fig. 2.1 do contribute in the object's response to the touch.

Despite limitations regarding the understanding and the interpretation of results on ocular rigidity, its measurement has remained for a long time more or less the only, albeit indirect, method for studying biomechanical properties of the corneo-scleral shell in clinical settings. Particularly because of this reason the concept of ocular rigidity has been widely used in studies on the pathogenesis of myopia [16, 19, 21].

Further to the previous chapter this section aims to describe ocular rigidity from the clinical point of view with the intention to straighten out this concept and to show its various clinical applications. Being an engineer I am going to argue from the engineering perspective, and thus perhaps some points of the Chap. 1 will be reflected. I believe that this approach will contribute to mutual understanding of ocular rigidity by specialists from various research fields and enables them to speak the same language. The chapter follows my previous publications on this topic together with I.N. Koshitz, E.N. Iomdina, S.M. Bauer [1, 22] and benefits from fruitful inspirations of Special Interest Groups on Ocular Rigidity at EVER (European Association for Vision and Eye Research) Meetings several years ago.

First of all I am going to discuss, why clinical conception of ocular rigidity is sometimes so confusing.

Why Can We Get Confused with Ocular Rigidity?

Rigidity and Elasticity: Tell Tother from Which

One of the common profound misconceptions: rigidity is the reciprocal of mechanical elasticity. Applying to the ophthalmology this means: ocular rigidity, simplified to rigidity of the corneo-scleral shell, represents the reciprocal of elasticity of the corneo-scleral shell, in particular, the reciprocal of elasticity of the sclera: e.g.: [23]. There is some apparent logic and clinical evidence in that misconception. Judge for yourself: both the Young's modulus of the sclera [23], which characterizes its elasticity, and ocular rigidity [24, 25] increase with age; both the Young's modulus of the sclera [21] and ocular rigidity [24] decrease with increasing anterio-posterior axis of the eyeball. Finally, both the Young's modulus of the sclera [26] and ocular rigidity [7, 11, 27] increase pathologically in glaucoma. However, the misconception lies in the completely different physical meaning of the concepts of rigidity (stiffness) and elasticity.

Since we speak about mechanical interactions and biomechanics, let us take advantage of terminology from classical mechanics. Rigidity or stiffness of a body describes here the resistance of the body to elastic deformation through a force (remember Fig. 2.1) or a torque. Rigidity characterizes the ability of the body to deform (change its shape) under external load without significant change in geometric dimensions. Thus rigidity or stiffness of a body represents a structural mechanical parameter depending both on its material properties and its geometry. In contrast elasticity reflects only material properties of a body. The complementary concept to rigidity (stiffness) is flexibility, not elasticity.

Imagine two different objects made from the same material, let's say, from rubber: a ring and a thick disk (Fig. 2.2). Understanding the rigidity of a body as its ability to resist to an external mechanical load, let's try to compress both those

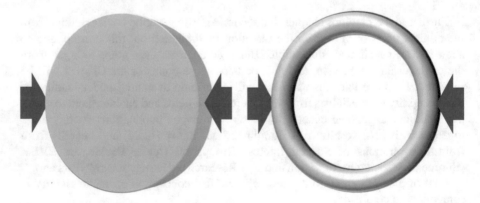

Fig. 2.2 Under the same external load a ring and a disk of the same outer diameter made of the same material will be deformed in different ways. Both objects possess different rigidity (structural stiffness), while the material, they are made of, has the same elasticity. Rigidity is a property of an object; elasticity is a material property of an object. Rigidity represents a function of material properties and morphology of an object

objects along their diameters and then compare the expended efforts: obviously the ring can be compressed more easily: rigidity (stiffness) of both objects is different, while elasticity of their material, the rubber, is the same.

Thus rigidity represents a so-called extensive property, a property of a body or an object. Its usual physical dimension in mechanics is [N/m], while the physical dimension of an elasticity parameter, Young's modulus, is [N/m²]. Elasticity is a so-called intensive property, a material property of an object.

In the particular case of uniaxial tension (or compression) of a loose homogeneous elastic body, i.e. when its material properties, and not its shape or its dimensions are important for assessing its resistance to an external load, the rigidity can be conditionally considered as a concept reciprocal of the elasticity. For the eye, as an object of complex shape, consisting of many structural elements, the concepts of rigidity and elasticity should be distinguished with care.

Rigidity (Stiffness) of What?

Another important aspect and a source of confusion: speaking about ocular rigidity we need to clearly define, the rigidity of what object or structure is mentioned. Apparently, material properties of the sclera and the cornea forming "the exoskeleton" of the eyeball are constitutive here. However other intraocular structures are involved in the resistance of the eyeball to external mechanical load as well. Therefore, it is necessary to determine clearly whether the ocular rigidity investigated in a study stands for rigidity of the eyeball as a whole, for stiffness of the corneo-scleral shell, or for stiffness of the sclera. Speaking about ocular rigidity different researchers aim to investigate one of those aspects. Hence the comparison of their results is possible only conditionally!

Aiming to assess material properties of the sclera with a clinical measurement and falsely neglecting other factors and ocular structures involved in the ocular rigidity concept some authors speak directly about scleral rigidity [28–30] instead of ocular rigidity. Some other authors adhere to ocular rigidity, but they equate the ocular rigidity measured from pressure-volume relationship and the scleral rigidity without mentioning any limitations. And we do have limitations here! Obviously, material properties of the cornea also have a significant effect on ocular rigidity. This fact was experimentally proved in a study by Liu and He [31] on enucleated animal eyes: following a rapid change of the intraocular volume, IOP changed more after elevation of corneal rigidity due to the cross-linking. Thus rigidity of the entire eyeball increased after experimental decrease of elasticity of corneal tissue. A sophisticated report by Hommer et al. [11] provides a correct cautious interpretation of their measured parameter of ocular rigidity: "Although we believe that scleral structural stiffness is the principal component of ocular rigidity as it applies to the Friedenwald equation, … our measurements most directly relate to the combined behaviors of the sclera, choroid, Bruch's membrane, retina, and cornea, and cannot be attributed to any one of these structures alone". This is true, however now one need to be careful with the interpretation of the results …

One for All and All for One?

…Then another misconception related to ocular rigidity is that one can characterize ocular rigidity using only one parameter (or sometimes a set of 2–3 parameters (Table 2.1)) and still might easily understand and interpret the results of clinical experiments using its value. Remember: the response of the eyeball to a load, say a change of its volume, depends on material and biometric properties of its structures, on the blood flow, on the intraocular pressure. Relating to the Chap. 1 I need to mention briefly, that even speaking correctly about the elasticity and an elastic modulus describing elastic material properties of the corneo-scleral shell we simplify a lot. Underneath we need to distinguish between the cornea and the sclera and to understand, that both the cornea and the sclera are orthotropic viscoelastic materials [41]. Moreover the cornea and the sclera possess elastic limits beyond which plastic deformation occurs [41]. It has been postulated that under pathological conditions like myopia the scleral properties change and plastic deformation is possible [42, 43]. Describing alone the elasticity of the sclera we need to consider an orthotropic non-linear-elastic material with its several parameters that depend on the deformation and the location within the sclera [21, 44, 45]: one Young's modulus, all the more one coefficient of ocular rigidity, is frankly speaking not enough here.

Slow or Fast Changes?

Because of its classical definition by Friedenwald and the course of manometric measurements (the volume increases in small portions following by time delay to reach equilibrium [24]) the classic coefficient of ocular rigidity seems to represent rather a macroscopic parameter referring to pseudostatic pressure–volume changes. Pallikaris et al. [40] presume that relatively fast volume changes, for example, due to cardiac cycle or air puff indentation, may show a different pressure–volume relationship that would be rather related to viscoelastic properties of the corneo-scleral shell and needs to be characterized using a separate clinical parameter. Under similar considerations Koshitz, Svetlova et al. introduced their novel parameter "fluctuation of the sclera" additionally to the coefficient of ocular rigidity and successfully tested both parameters clinically in normal and glaucomatous eyes [27, 46]. Thus it needs to be elucidated whether novel clinical methods, like those presented by [8, 11, 47] and claiming to assess ocular rigidity based on small pressure-volume changes, measure rigidity parameters that can still be related to the classic coefficient of ocular rigidity by Friedenwald [4].

Clinical Approach to Ocular Rigidity

In general, the concept of ocular rigidity can be considered from two main positions, referring to "mechanistic" (or "engineering" [3]) and "clinical" approaches.

Table 2.1 Experimental characterization of pressure-volume relationship by several authors

Equation	Ocular rigidity function	Author(s) and reference
$\dfrac{dp}{dV} = \dfrac{E}{V}$	$\Delta p = E \cdot \ln\left(\dfrac{V_2}{V_1}\right)$	Clark, 1932 [32]
$\dfrac{dp}{dV} = Kp$	$\Delta V = \dfrac{1}{K} \cdot \ln\left(\dfrac{IOP_2}{IOP_1}\right)$	Friedenwald, 1937 [4]
$\dfrac{dp}{dV} = ap^n$	$\Delta V = \dfrac{1}{a(1-n)}\left(IOP_2^{1-n} - IOP_1^{1-n}\right)$	McBain, 1958 [33][a]
$\dfrac{dp}{dV} = a(p-c)^n$	$\Delta V = \dfrac{1}{a(1-n)}\left((IOP_2 - c)^{1-n} - (IOP_1 - c)^{1-n}\right)$	Holland et al., 1960 [34][b]
$\dfrac{dp}{dV} = ap + b$	$\Delta V = \dfrac{1}{a} \cdot \ln\left(\dfrac{IOP_2 + b/a}{IOP_1 + b/a}\right)$	McEwen & St Helen, 1965 [35][c]
$\dfrac{dp}{dV} = 0.02p + 0.24$	$\Delta V = 50 \cdot \ln\left(\dfrac{IOP_2 + 12.0}{IOP_1 + 12.0}\right)$	Hibbard et al., 1970 [36]
$\dfrac{dp}{dV} = 0.016p + 0.13$	$\Delta V = 62.5 \cdot \ln\left(\dfrac{IOP_2 + 8.1}{IOP_1 + 8.1}\right)$	Woo et al., 1972 [37]
$\dfrac{dp}{dV} = 3kp^{2/3}$	$\Delta V = \dfrac{1}{k} \cdot \left(IOP_2^{1/3} - IOP_1^{1/3}\right)$	van der Werff, 1981 [5][d]
	$\Delta V = V(C + C_0\,ln\,(p) + C_1 p) = -49.8 + 30.2$ $ln(p) + 0.242p$	Silver and Geyer, 2000 [38][e]
$\dfrac{dp}{dV} = 0.0126$	$\Delta V = 79.4 \cdot (IOP_2 - IOP_1)$	Pallikaris et al., 2005 [24]
$\dfrac{dp}{dV} = 2.3Kp$	$\Delta V - \dfrac{0.43}{K} \cdot \ln\left(\dfrac{IOP_2}{IOP_1}\right)$	Simanovskiy, 2007 [39]
$\dfrac{dp}{dV} = 0.0224p$	$\Delta V = 44.6 \cdot \ln\left(\dfrac{IOP_2}{IOP_1}\right)$	Dastiridou et al., 2009 [13]

Extended review following: [1, 3, 5, 40]. Note that the constants are related to particular formulas by their authors and do not necessarily correspond to each other in different formulas
[a]The formulation given for enucleated human eyes; mean parameter values: a = 0.096; n = 0.644 [5, 33]
[b]The formulation given for cat eyes; mean parameter values: a = 0.589; n = 0.389; c = 10.71 [5, 34]
[c]Unified formulation. For human eyes in-vivo and enucleated range of parameter values: a = 0.015 − 0.027 μl⁻¹; b = 0.03 − 0.31 mmHg·μl⁻¹. For enucleated human eyes mean parameter values: a = 0.022 μl⁻¹; b = 0.21 mmHg·μl⁻¹. The formulas below by Hibbard et al. and Woo et al. are therefore consistent with this general form by McEwen and St. Helen [3, 5, 35]
[d]For enucleated human eyes: k ≈ 0.03 mmHg$^{1/3}$/μl
[e]Numerical coefficients for C_i are set for an "average" eye by Silver and Geyer [38]

The engineering approach describes ocular rigidity in detail using common concepts from other biomedical engineering applications. Elastic material properties of ocular tissues are described for the instance with Young's moduli and Poisson coefficients as in mechanics and biomechanics. Herewith one would measure for example mechanical elasticity of the equatorial sclera in transversal direction and is able to compare its value with the value of a similar parameter of the arterial wall. Using the engineering approach we know for sure where we are. However there is a simple disadvantage in it: most of "engineering" parameters cannot be assessed directly clinically and there is almost no clinical experience on their use.

The clinical approach is based on ex-vivo or in-vivo studies of a so-called pressure-volume relation (ship). Typically, using a hydraulic system [24] or a conventional syringe [48], intraocular pressure is increased by introducing an additional volume of fluid inside the eye. A similar but more sophisticated experimental ex-vivo design in biomechanics is called inflation test [45, 49]. The dependence of intraocular pressure vs. intraocular volume: the pressure-volume relation is calculated (Fig. 2.3). Using this dependence a so-called coefficient of ocular rigidity or other related parameters are computed that implicitly characterize the pressure-volume relation. The experimental pressure-volume relation can be approximated with a mathematical equation that relates IOP changes to changes in intraocular volume [38, 51] (Table 2.1). Apart from the coefficient of ocular rigidity pressure-volume relation of the eye has been used to calculate outflow facility from tonography measurements and to assess pulsatile ocular blood flow from IOP pulsations [38]. Volume changes in tonography or pulsatile ocular blood flow can be computed from IOP changes using Friedenwald's ocular rigidity relation or a corresponding nomogram.

There is a variety of analytical formulations of experimental pressure-volume relationship curves based on investigations with manometry, tonometry and other methods in living and postmortem eyes (Table 2.1). Hence there is in fact a plenty of definitions of ocular rigidity with their different or (even worse) similar names (Table 2.2). Since the formulations of pressure-volume relationship and the definitions of ocular rigidity are different, they have been described using quite different physical parameters with their different physical dimensions (Table 2.2). The absolute numbers compared within a study can still give a cue on how the values of an ocular rigidity parameter differ in several groups or due to an intervention. However a comparison of absolute numbers of different ocular rigidity parameters with their distinct definitions and physical dimensions does not make any sense and can confuse. We may not compare apples and oranges!

The introduction is still clear. We perform a classic manometric experiment and record pressure-volume relationship in an eye within a certain range of values, (e.g. Fig. 2.3 left). We aim to describe, how the IOP changes at small increase of intraocular volume V (or perhaps vice versa: how the volume change at small IOP increase), calculating a measure of rigidity, say: $Ri = \dfrac{\Delta IOP}{\Delta V}$. We know where we are: the larger is Ri, the more changes the IOP at small increase of the intraocular volume and the more rigid is the eyeball. Such a formulation of the coefficient of ocular rigidity was proposed by Römer [50] based on experiments in cadaver eyes as a 3-D analogous of the Hook's law. The physical dimension of Ri corresponds to

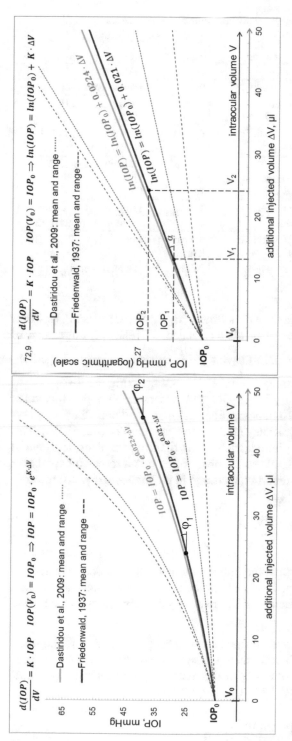

Fig. 2.3 Examples of theoretical pressure-volume relationships. One is calculated from recent results of in-vivo manometric measurements on patients undergoing cataract surgery (age 39–86 years) by Dastiridou et al. [13]: $K = 0.0224 \, \mu l^{-1}$ (range: 0.0127 to 0.0343). $IOP_0 = 15$ mmHg. Intraocular volume $V = V_0 + \Delta V$, where V_0 represents the initial volume of the eye before distension and ΔV is an additional injected volume. For the comparison in-vivo results of differential tonometry in living human eyes (age < 50 years) by Friedenwald [4] are re-computed as pressure-volume relation with his $K = 0.021 \, \mu l^{-1}$ (range: 0.006–0.037). For the Fridenwald's data the initial pressure, IOP_0 is arbitrarily set here to 15 mmHg. Note that in both examples data variation increases with the increase of additional volume fraction ΔV. *Left panel:* exponential dependence IOP vs. intraocular volume V and vs. additional volume fraction ΔV. The coefficient of ocular rigidity by Römer [50]: Ri depends on IOP level: $\tan(\varphi) = \frac{dIOP}{dV}$ increases at large IOP-values and $\varphi_2 > \varphi_1$. *Right panel:* following the classical representation by Friedenwald [4] the vertical axis is logarithmised. This results in linear dependence of $ln(IOP)$ vs. ΔV and hence vs. V. The constant slope $K = \tan(\alpha)$ in this formulation is called the coefficient of ocular rigidity by Friedenwald. Two arbitrary experimental points: $(V_1; ln(IOP_1))$ and $(V_2; ln(IOP_2))$ can be involved into the calculation of K according to Eqs. (2.5–2.7)

Table 2.2 Clinical parameters of ocular rigidity according to several authors

Parameter of ocular rigidity	Dimension	SI dimension	Author(s) and reference
Coefficient of ocular rigidity	$[Ri] = mmHg/\mu l$	Pa/m^3	Römer, 1918 [50]
Coefficient of ocular rigidity	$[K] = 1/\mu l$	$1/m^3$	Friedenwald, 1937 [4]
Distance of elasto-elevation	$[Sl] = mmHg$	Pa	Kalfa, 1927 [52]
Slope and intercept of pressure-volume relation	$[a] = 1/\mu l$ $[b] = mmHg/\mu l$	$1/m^3$ Pa/m^3	McEwen & St Helen, 1965 [35]
Proportionality constant	$[k] = mmHg^{1/3}/\mu l$	$Pa^{1/3}/m^3$	van der Werff, 1981 [5]
Small-strain modulus	$[A\alpha] = MPa$	Pa	Greene, 1985 [53]
Coefficients of pressure-volume relation	$[C,$ $C_0] = $ dimension-less $[C_1] = 1/mmHg$	dimension-less $1/Pa$	Silver and Geyer, 2000 [38]
Coefficient of ocular rigidity	$[E1] = 1/\mu m$	$1/m$	Hommer et al., 2008 [11]
Time of applanation (ORA)	$[t_A] = ms$	s	Koshitz et al., 2010 [27]
Ocular rigidity parameter	$[E_R] = 1/$arbitrary units	dimension-less	Wang et al., 2013 [47]
Ocularrigidityparameter	$[r] = mmHg \cdot Pa/\mu l$	Pa^2/m^3	Detorakis et al., 2015 [54]

Extended review following: [1, 22, 27]

our aforementioned considerations on the stiffness (rigidity): $[Ri] = Pa/m^3$. However it becomes clear that Ri is not constant when considering a relatively large range of IOP: Ri depends on the IOP level: the tangent: $\dfrac{dIOP}{dV}$ becomes steeper at large IOP-values, and the relationship "pressure-volume" is non-linear (Fig. 2.3 left).

Friedenwald found empirically that exponential fit is a suitable approximation of ex-vivo experimental pressure-volume relations in human and animal eyes by several researchers: Koster (1895); Ridley (1930) and Clark (1932), [32, 55, 56]. This observation led Friedenwald to introduction of his rigidity parameter (apparently) independent of the IOP. He formulated the observation into a research hypothesis: for an eye of a given size the proportional change in the intraocular pressure varies with the intraocular volume V [4]:

$$\frac{dIOP}{IOP} = k \frac{dV}{V} \tag{2.1},$$

where $V = V_0 + \Delta V$: V_0 represents the initial volume of the eye before distension and ΔV is an additional injected volume, which is "relatively small and finite". Because ΔV is only a small fraction of V, Friedenwald did two reasonable but not indisputable assumptions [4]:

- $V \approx V_0$: the volume V is almost constant and it is roughly the same for all eyes
- Since for an individual eye $V \approx V_0$ then: $k/V \approx k/V_0$, and it can be then replaced in Eq. (2.1) by a new constant $K = k/V_0$, the coefficient of ocular rigidity (sometimes they call it: E, k or OR). Thus from Eq. (2.1):

$$\frac{dIOP}{dV} = K \cdot IOP \tag{2.2}$$

For a given eye of the volume $V > V_0$ after distension:

$$K = \frac{\ln(IOP) - \ln(IOP_0)}{V - V_0} \qquad (2.3),$$

where IOP_0 represents the IOP-value at initial intraocular volume V_0 before distension[1]:

$$IOP_0 = IOP(V_0) \qquad (2.4)$$

and *ln* is natural logarithm. If we would logarithisc the vertical (IOP) axis of the pressure-volume relationship (Fig. 2.3 left), the curve becomes a straight line with a constant slope of K (Fig. 2.3 right): the dependence: *ln*(IOP) vs. V is linear.

According to this Friedenwald's law the slope K can be also easily calculated from two arbitrary measuring points:

$$K = \frac{\ln(IOP_2) - \ln(IOP_1)}{V_2 - V_1} \qquad (2.5),$$

where IOP_1, IOP_2; $V_1 \geq V_0$, $V_2 > V_0$ are corresponding arbitrary values of the IOP and the intraocular volume V. Other mathematically equivalent formulations of the equation (Eq. 2.5):

$$K \cdot (V_2 - V_1) = \ln\left(\frac{IOP_2}{IOP_1}\right) \qquad (2.6)$$

$$K \cdot (V_2 - V_1) = M \cdot \lg\left(\frac{IOP_2}{IOP_1}\right) \qquad (2.7),$$

where *lg* represents a logarithm to the base 10 and M = 2.303 is the conversion factor [5]. By the way one should be aware, what logarithm is used in the definition of K, since the differential equation (Eq. 2.2) is directly integrated with *ln* [4, 5, 40],

---

[1] Friedenwald explained that: "within the pressure range that is of clinical interest the fit is sufficiently good for practical purposes". Thus the solution of Friedenwald's equation should theoretically work for every initial condition $IOP(V_0) = IOP_0$ since the volume of the eye before distension V_0 is consistent and the corresponding IOP is not extremely low. Obviously for hypotonic eyes that do not maintain its shape this simplified theoretical model does not work at all. An already predistended eyeball should theoretically fit to its corresponding pressure-volume relation curve with the initial condition being shifted to the right along the volume curve (Fig. 2.3). But how small can be V_0 to fit Friedenwald's equation? At what pressure the eyeball is not hypotonic anymore but still is not yet distended? From biomechanical point of view "the eye just before distension" or stress free configuration of the eye represents an important idealized concept, which is considered in detail elsewhere, e.g. [57].

while van der Werff affirmed that "K is always calculated using logarithms to the base 10" [5].

The pressure-volume relationship described by Friedenwald can be functionally formulated as (Fig. 2.3 left):

$$IOP(V) = IOP_0 \cdot e^{K \cdot \Delta V} \qquad (2.8)$$

Thus, if one knows K (e.g. from experimental studies), initial intraocular volume V_0 of an individual eye and the corresponding IOP_0, pressure-volume relationship prediction by Friedenwald for $V > V_0$ for this eye can be easily computed.

Despite several practical and analytical advantages of Friedenwald's formulation of ocular rigidity, a physical interpretation of its results becomes more complicated than in the Römer's formulation: the dimension of K: $[K] = 1/m^3$ (Table 2.2). Besides by its definition K is inversely proportional to the individual intraocular volume V_0.

According to Friedenwald, the value of K is approximately constant in the population at IOP > 5 mmHg, and it obeys biological variability. For middle-age people of <50 years old whose axial refraction lies between +2 and −1, and whose mean corneal curvature ranges between 7.5 and 7.9 mm Friedenwald reported: $K = 0.021 \, \mu l^{-1}$ (range: 0.006–0.037 μl^{-1}).

Later on it was shown in several clinical experiments that K is not constant in the population and depends for example on the level of the IOP and individual intraocular volume [13, 19, 40, 58, 59]. Due to the mentioned disadvantages of the "classical" formulation of the coefficient of ocular rigidity K by Friedenwald, as well as because of particular problem statements and experimental designs several authors have suggested their formulae to describe pressure–volume relationship in the eye and to fit the experimental data (Table 2.1). The formula proposed by Friedenwald is still one of the most widely used. McEwen and St Helen [35] developed a more generalized two-parameter formula than Friedenwald's equation to fit the experimental data. Some other authors reported their own values for the constants in the formula by McEwen and St Helen [36, 37]. Silver and Geyer suggested an extended mathematical formulation for in-vivo measurements, based on an analysis of pressure–volume relations available in the literature on living human eyes [38].

How to Assess Pressure-Volume Relationship and to Measure Ocular Rigidity?

Referring to the next chapter a brief overview on crucial clinical measurement principles to assess ocular rigidity will introduce some definitions.

First assessments of pressure-volume relationship were conducted ex-vivo in enucleated human and animal eyes, using a manometric system and injecting the eye with known volumes of saline via cannulation of the vitreous cavity or anterior chamber [4, 32, 52, 55, 56]. Later on in-vivo measurements on the eyes scheduled to enucleation were carried out [60, 61]. Pallikaris, Dastiridou et al. presented a series of direct in-vivo manometric measurements performed before cataract surgery in human eyes under retrobulbar or topical anesthesia [13, 24, 25, 62, 63]. Even if those in-vivo series were more than successful and significant for ophthalmic research and gave fresh impact for studying ocular rigidity, the invasive nature of the proposed in-vivo manometric technique restricted its clinical use.

Friedenwald introduced in 1937 his method of differential (paired) tonometry using Schiøtz tonometer. During tonometry the eyeball is deformed, and a small amount of intraocular fluid is shifted inside the eye. It is supposed that this shift is equal to the injection of the equal fluid volume inside the eye. The coefficient of ocular rigidity is calculated in paired tonometry from two readings with two different weights (e.g. 5.5 g and 10 g). Two IOP measurements are performed resulting in IOP_1 and IOP_2. Nomograms relate IOP-values with the tonometer resting on the cornea to volumes of the indentation: V_1 and V_2 respectively [4]. Then the coefficient K can be calculated as a slope of the K-line between V_1 and V_2 using the formula (Eq. 2.3; Fig. 2.3 right). In practice they use a customized nomogram similar to one shown in [6]: from both inputted IOP-values the coefficient of ocular rigidity can be read out.

Differential tonometry had several limitations related to the application of Schiøtz technique [64]. Corneal indentation caused presumably an increase of aqueous outflow and hence distorted the measurement of ocular rigidity leading to a large variability of results of differential tonometry [65]. Pallikaris et al. [40] reported that generally coefficients of ocular rigidity measured by paired Schiøtz tonometry were higher than those measured using manometric method. This confirms the observation by Nesterov et al. [19]. Alternatively to the paired tonometry by Friedenwald with two Schiøtz devices a combination of a Goldmann and a Schiøtz tonometer has been used instead in some studies inducing even larger errors [66]. A recent pilot study on differential tonometry combining Goldmann and contour tonometry with a mathematical algorithm could potentially improve the technique [54]. Together with differential tonometry the majority of Russian ophthalmologists have used a so-called elastotonometry by Filatov-Kalfa [52] with Maklakoff's tonometers. This sophisticated method was even a precursor of Friedenwald's differential tonometry [67]. It is well elaborated, but also has several limitations and is quite difficult to implement: IOP is measured here twice using four different loads [19]. Several novel ideas on clinical non-invasive assessment of ocular rigidity picked up the basic idea from elastotonometry by Kalfa and differential tonometry by Friedenwald: two points of logarithmized pressure-volume relationship (Fig. 2.3 right) are assessed in order to calculate K using the Friedenwald's formula (Eq. 2.3).

Being quite meaningful and popular in 1950s–1970s the differential tonometry and its modifications as routine clinical measurements of ocular rigidity have almost disappeared in modern clinical ophthalmology. In fact, an important obstruction in including the ocular rigidity in the routine clinical examination has been the lack of a simple, accurate and non-invasive methodology for its quantitative assessment [54]. However a plenty of sophisticated non-invasive clinical approaches to assess ocular rigidity have been proposed in the last years, including:

- ultrasound elastography [68];
- introduction of new rigidity parameters based on ORA-assessment [27, 46, 69];
- use of pharmacological intervention, measuring the IOP with dynamic contour tonometry and eye elongation using partial coherence laser interferometry [70];
- use of intravitreal injections and measuring of the IOP alterations under a known change of the volume [48, 71];
- combination of pneumotonometry to assess IOP changes and laser interferometry to assess volumetric alterations [11, 72];
- combination of pneumotonometry with laser Doppler flowmetry to assess choroidal blood volume alterations [47];
- combination of dynamic contour tonometry to measure ocular pulse amplitude and OCT imaging to examine choroidal blood volume changes [8].

The advent of new technical modalities might enable accurate, reproducible and non-invasive assessment of ocular rigidity parameters for their successful clinical use [51]. Following the breakthrough of the ocular biomechanics in the last two decades [22, 41, 73] and a variety of recent fundamental works on ocular rigidity [24, 40, 51] the clinical importance of the ocular rigidity concept in the ophthalmology seems to approach its renaissance.

Clinical Results on Ocular Rigidity

A detailed review on ocular rigidity in ocular disorders is performed by Pallikaris and co-authors [40, 51]. In order to give a cue on absolute values of the coefficient of ocular rigidity and still not to compare apples with oranges, clinical data on ocular rigidity is reviewed below, but only values of classical Friedenwald's coefficient of ocular rigidity K [μl^{-1}] are reported. The numerical data is presented as mean value; mean ± std. deviation; mean (95% confidence interval) or range.

Normal Values and Age-Related Changes

Based on his tonometry measurements on 500 living human eyes Friedenwald reported in detail the following [4, 67]:

- K = 0.021 ± 0.007 μl^{-1} in the group of 15–50 years old people,
- K = 0.024 ± 0.007 μl^{-1} in 50–60 years old group and
- K = 0.029 ± 0.007 μl^{-1} in the group older than 60 years.

Thus the coefficient of ocular rigidity increased in his studies slightly with age, especially in elderly people, showing the famous mean value of K = 0.021 μl^{-1} in the whole cohort. Gloster and Perkins [65] reported a mean value for K = 0.025 μl^{-1} in humans, while Ytteborg measured a mean value of K = 0.0232 μl^{-1} [74]. Some other researchers including Goldmann and Schmidt [75], Drance [30], Agrawal et al. [76] and Dastiridou et al. [13] reported similar ranges of the value and the variation of Friedenwald's coefficient K, if being corrected to empirical information from clinical ocular rigidity research, which is mentioned in detail below (2.6):

- manometric measurements result in lower absolute values of the coefficient K than the results of differential tonometry
- in-vivo manometric examination may show lower values of K than ex-vivo manometric measurement

Based on literature review of different in-vivo studies using differential tonometry on a total of 6159 eyes Nesterov et al. reported $K = 0.0216 \; \mu l^{-1}$ with variation of 0.0110–$0.0400 \; \mu l^{-1}$ [19]. A clinical study by Melnik [77] on 3386 eyes (elastotonometry by Kalfa recalculated in Friedenwald's K) reports on $K = 0.0200 \; \mu l^{-1}$ with variation of 0.008–$0.038 \; \mu l^{-1}$ [19]. Recent non-invasive study on 45 eyes by Beaton et al. [8] used dynamic contour tonometry and SD-OCT to assess ocular rigidity and reported: $K = 0.028 \pm 0.022 \; \mu l^{-1}$. It seems that the values of the ocular rigidity are quite robust, although Nesterov et al. [19] admitted that the systematic measurement error of K using differential tonometry depends on the IOP level, individual volume of the eyeball, ocular blood flow and the type of tonometer. This error ranges between 20% and 100%! High rate of data scattering in the study by Beaton et al. [8] shows indirectly that modern methods to assess ocular rigidity might account to considerable systematic measurement errors presumably because of the similar aspects.

In their early in-vivo manometric studies in 79 eyes undergoing cataract surgery (age: 65.3 ± 13.9 years) under retrobulbar anesthesia the research group by Pallikaris reported $K = 0.0126 \; (0.0112$–$0.0149) \; \mu l^{-1}$ [mean (95% CI)] [24]. The ocular rigidity showed weak but significant positive correlation with age of the patients ($r = 0.27$, $p = 0.02$), which confirmed previous results of manometric experiments by Perkins [59] in cadaver eyes. Later on in a series of manometric measurements under topical anesthesia with a device capable of more accurate IOP recordings the group by Pallikaris measured in another healthy cohort of similar age: $K = 0.0224 \pm 0.0049 \; \mu l^{-1}$ [13, 40] (Fig. 2.3). Other studies performed with differential tonometry [78, 79] and manometry in enucleated eyes [59] confirm the findings of a slight increase of ocular rigidity with age. The age-related increase of ocular rigidity is definitely intriguing as it may reflect the conception of scleral aging [46, 80–82] and underlie the susceptibility to age-related ocular disorders [40, 83].

Glaucoma

The data on the ocular rigidity coefficient in glaucoma is controversial. Friedenwald affirmed that in acute congestive glaucoma ocular rigidity is very variable and shows sometimes extreme fluctuations during the course of the illness [4]. A tonometry study on 738 glaucomatous eyes by Nesterov et al. [19] did not reveal significant changes in ocular rigidity, although the data scattered a lot with standard deviation being 1.5 times higher in the subgroup with compensated glaucoma and 2 times higher in the subgroup without compensation than in healthy controls. Agrawal et al. reported a mean $K = 0.0143 \ \mu l^{-1}$ in glaucomatous eyes in comparison to the control group with $K = 0.0217 \ \mu l^{-1}$ [76]. K increased in this study following timolol 0.25% or pilocarpine 2% treatment. A recent study by Wang et al. [47] assessed choroidal blood volume alterations and confirmed significantly lower values of their ocular rigidity parameter in glaucomatous eyes.

Some other recent studies were performed in glaucoma patients using modern measuring techniques [7, 11, 27, 70]. On the contrary to the above mentioned results they reported increased values of their parameters of ocular rigidity in glaucoma patients.

Age-Related Macula Degeneration (AMD)

By using in-vivo manometric measurements Pallikaris et al. [25] examined patients with AMD. Although they did not find differences in ocular rigidity in the AMD group in comparison to the control group, the average values of the coefficient of ocular rigidity were higher in patients with neovascular AMD treated with photodynamic therapy ($K = 0.0186 \pm 0.0078 \ \mu l^{-1}$) than in control subjects ($K = 0.0125 \pm 0.0048 \ \mu l^{-1}$) and in non-treated patients with non-neovascular AMD ($K = 0.0104 \pm 0.0053 \ \mu l^{-1}$), $p < 0.05$. The authors assumed that either photodynamic therapy was able to influence ocular rigidity through its effect on choroidal circulation or different forms of AMD were associated with the increase of ocular rigidity.

Non-proliferative Diabetic Retinopathy

Since diabetes mellitus is known to affect biomechanical properties of living tissues [84], Panagiotoglou et al. [85] hypothesized that ocular rigidity measured with manometry technique is changed in diabetes patients with mild stages of diabetic retinopathy. However no statistically significant differences in ocular rigidity could be documented between patients with non-proliferative diabetic retinopathy: $K = 0.0205 \ \mu l^{-1}$ and controls: $K = 0.0202 \ \mu l^{-1}$ ($p = 0.942$). A clear trend for lower values of ocular rigidity coefficient was shown in patients with mild retinopathy compared to patients with moderate and severe diabetic retinopathy, although the difference was not statistically significant. Arora and Prasad measured ocular rigidity in diabetic patients using modified Friedenwald's nomogram [86]. They also did not find any statistically significant differences in the coefficient of ocular rigidity between patients with non-proliferative diabetic retinopathy and age-matched control subjects.

Uveitis

Friedenwald found ocular rigidity being significantly increased in uveitis patients irrespective of the IOP level. The average ocular rigidity from 38 measurements amounted to K = 0.034 μl^{-1}. Since "with the engorgement of the intraocular blood vessels, one would expect an increased compressibility of the vascular tunic and hence a decreased rigidity coefficient" Friedenwald was unable to interpret this controversial result [4]. Taniashina et al. reported no significant changes of the coefficient K in uveitis as well as in retinal detachment and in arterial hypertension [87].

Corneal Refractive Surgery

Since this type of surgery influences both the structure and the thickness of the cornea one would expect alterations of ocular rigidity after the operation. Possible changes of the ocular rigidity coefficient after photorefractive keratectomy (PRK) were assessed in-vivo in rabbits using manometric method [88]. No statistically significant difference was found in the measured ocular rigidity coefficient between eyes treated with PRK and control eyes.

In contrast laser in situ keratomileusis (LASIK) in living human eyes has been associated with a significant decrease of the coefficient of ocular rigidity measured using differential tonometry with Goldmann and Schiøtz tonometers [89], presumably due to postoperative alterations in the corneal structure and thickness. Before LASIK K = 0.0195 ± 0.0065 μl^{-1}. It decreased postoperatively to K = 0.0140 ± 0.0055 μl^{-1} after 30 days and amounted to K = 0.0120 ± 0.004 μl^{-1} after 90 days and to K = 0.0140 ± 0.0065 μl^{-1} after 720 days (p < 0.05 post- vs. preoperative) [89]. Apparently the effect of corneal thinning on ocular rigidity is proven in the study. However another possible explanation of the effect relates to the known systematic error of indentation tonometry after keratorefractive surgery.

Because of obvious limitations ocular rigidity is difficult to assess using manometric procedure or applying differential tonometry after corneal surgery. The use of novel non-invasive methods to monitor ocular rigidity in postoperative period might be promising [51].

Factors Affecting Ocular Rigidity

In the following a close structured look is taken at main factors affecting ocular rigidity and its parameters.

Intraocular Pressure

According to its correct definition ocular rigidity strongly depends on the IOP (Fig. 2.3 left). With all other factors being equal the rigidity in eyes with higher IOP is higher (Fig. 2.1). Indeed the coefficient of ocular rigidity Ri by Römer, mentioned above, depends on the IOP. However due to introduction of the logarithmic trend and the definition of his coefficient of ocular rigidity Friedenwald expected to "remove" completely the dependence of K on the IOP [4] as it can be seen in the theoretical representation of experimental data in Fig. 2.3 right. He assumed his K being independent on the IOP. Some authors also did not find any dependence of K on the IOP and herewith confirmed the hypothesis by Friedenwald [90, 91].

However some other researchers have criticized the mentioned assumption by Friedenwald. Dashevsky first reported about inversely proportional relation between IOP and K [92]. K is not truly constant, but decreases as the intraocular pressure increases [5]. Later on this relation was confirmed in other experimental studies [33, 59, 93, 94]. Perkins reported the decrease in K of approximately 25% for an increase in the IOP of 10 mmHg over the range of 10–30 mmHg in the majority of his manometric experiments on cadaver eyes, while in two eyes there was no significant change in K at different pressure levels and in one eye K even increased by 26% [59]. Kiselev and Taniashina [95] found a weak dependence of K on the IOP using differential tonometry. In their study $K = 0.0184–0.0186 \ \mu l^{-1}$ at IOP = 9–22 mmHg; $K = 0.0180–0.0184 \ \mu l^{-1}$ at IOP = 22–40 mmHg and $K = 0.0175–0.0180 \ \mu l^{-1}$ at IOP = 40–70 mmHg. The dependence of Friedenwald's ocular rigidity coefficient K on the IOP was corrected in the later formulations of ocular rigidity parameters by other authors, e.g. [5, 33, 34] (Table 2.1).

Intraocular Volume and Axial Length

According to its correct definition ocular rigidity should strongly depend on the intraocular volume (Fig. 2.3 left). With all other factors being equal the rigidity of larger eyes is lower (Fig. 2.1). Already in 1932, Clark mentioned the importance of the eye volume factor: "the value for dV/dp would differ from animal to animal owing to differences in eye volume even if the elasticity were the same" [32]. Friedenwald reported in 1937 a strong inverse proportionality of K on the intraocular volume V as well [4]. However, as mentioned above, he considered that in humans intraindividual variations in volume are neglectable. Hence the constant K in Friedenwald's formula (Eqs. 2.2–2.3) includes the total intraocular volume being assumed to be the same for all eyes. Perkins studied the relation of ocular rigidity to intraocular volume in cadaver eyes and suggested that if ocular rigidity were corrected for the volume of the individual eye, then the correlation with intraocular volume disappeared [59]. Hence he concluded that the lower ocular rigidity of myopic eyes was rather due to their greater volume than due to a presumably abnormal distensibility of the sclera. Thus a more fundamental constant $k = K \cdot V_0$, a coefficient of ocular rigidity incorporating intraocular volume, even enables to compare eyes of differing volume using this adjusted Friedenwald's formulation [4, 38, 59]. His pressure-volume relation for $V = V_0 + \Delta V$ (Eq. 2.8) can be then re-formulated as:

$$IOP(V) = IOP_0 \cdot e^{k \cdot \Delta V / V0} \qquad (2.9),$$

where k is dimensionless.

Under a rational assumption that the volume of the eye may be estimated from "its axial refraction without regard to the variations in corneal and lenticular refraction or to the deviations of the actual shape of the eye from that of a sphere" Friedenwald found a good agreement between the observed and calculated values for all states of refraction except that of extreme myopic eyes over 20 dpt. Those eyes were much less distensible than their large volume would predict. Friedenwald assume for a good reason that "these eyes have been stretched to their elastic limit or at least that their coats are no longer capable of yielding easily to increments of pressure" [4]. Consistent with this finding Goldmann [96] reported on a higher scleral rigidity in one −25 D eye than in another of only −20 D. This abrupt increase of scleral distensibility in high myopia needs to be elucidated in thorough future studies. Phillips and Quick [97] gave at least two quite reasonable alternative explanations of the mentioned effect: the sclera of largest eyes may have received support from the bony orbit. Besides more myopic eyes with higher rigidity might have shorter axial lengths and smaller volume than less myopic ones.

Phillips and Quick [97] examined physical models of the eye: thin-walled spherical rubber balls filled with water. Throughout the stress range of the examination the sclera and the rubber chosen behaved elastically and possessed almost equal values of Young's moduli. Even small volume changes of the balls influenced the value of their rigidity. This aspect could explain high values of the coefficient of ocular rigidity in newborns, despite presumably higher elasticity of their corneo-scleral shells [98].

Ocular Blood Flow and Blood Pressure: We Are Dealing with a Living Object

In clinical applications ocular rigidity will be useful especially if this parameter could be assessed in-vivo. However a variety of results obtained in ex-vivo experiments cannot be directly used to approximate in-vivo ocular rigidity. According to Nesterov et al. this aspect relates mainly to the active and passive reaction of intraocular vessels in living eyes [19]. Some fluid is passively squeezed from the venous system as IOP increases. Arterial vessels react actively, changing their caliber due to mechanisms of IOP-regulation [99].

A comparison of experimental in-vivo and ex-vivo measurements of ocular rigidity reveals significant differences: at the same level of the IOP ocular rigidity measured in-vivo is lower than the rigidity measured in enucleated eyes [40, 60]. Summarizing experimental data available to that time Silver and Geyer [38] conclude also on larger volume increment for a given increment of pressure in pressure-volume relations of living human eyes in comparison to measurements in cadaver eyes, particularly in comparison to Friedenwald's data with his logarithmic approximation based on ex-vivo measurements [4]. In rabbits, when the IOP exceeded the blood pressure (and the blood flow was interrupted therewith) the coefficient of ocular rigidity approached closely the value found in the dead eye at similar pressures [60]. In animal experiments with blockage of the carotid artery, ocular rigidity increased as the blood supply to the eyeball was reduced [98, 100]. These results indicate that ocular blood flow along with other factors can affect ocular rigidity.

Kiel studied in rabbits, whether an alteration of blood pressure would influence ocular rigidity [101]. Systemic blood pressure in these experiments changed the blood filling and choroidal blood flow, affecting therewith ocular rigidity. The initial part of the pressure-volume curve depended on the rate of choroidal autoregulation [102], which in turn depended on the blood pressure. At high IOP-level and low perfusion pressures (right-hand part of the pressure-volume curve), the blood outflow from the eye represented main source of discrepancies between the curves in living and in enucleated eyes [40]. Indeed, because of the complete absence of blood filling in enucleated eye, the dependence of ocular rigidity curve on blood pressure should disappear. Thus ocular rigidity depends on the level of arterial blood pressure and blood filling of intraocular vessels, primarily of choroidal vessels. Although, in the experimental study by Dastiridou et al. [13], the coefficient of ocular rigidity measured in-vivo in healthy people did not significantly correlate with the level of blood pressure within the normal blood pressure range, we believe that this result can be easily explained by a narrow range of values of arterial pressure in healthy participants of that study.

Subtile Question About Thickness

As it can be deduced from the definition of rigidity (Fig. 2.1), the thickness of the cornea and the sclera is an important factor affecting ocular rigidity. Nevertheless, as noted in the review by Pallikaris et al. [40], a few studies on this issue did not find any significant dependence of ocular rigidity on either central corneal thickness [24] or thickness of the sclera [59]. The question about the effect of corneal thinning after refractive surgery on ocular rigidity remains open as mentioned above [89].

From the biomechanical point of view, the thickness of the cornea and the sclera will inevitably affect ocular rigidity. Most probably the influence of this factor is small in comparison to other factors: IOP, volume, material properties, ocular blood flow. Anyways the general problem of ocular rigidity associated with pressure-volume relationship still awaits a serious parametric engineering analysis on how (to what extent) various factors influence ocular rigidity, similar to an analytical study by Sigal et al. [103] on factors influencing optic nerve head biomechanics.

Measurement Error

To complete the picture it should be mentioned here again that systematic errors related to measurement techniques have been playing an important role in clinical assessment of ocular rigidity [8, 19, 89]. In clinical studies implying quantitative assessment of ocular rigidity they should take in account that systematic error of the corresponding measurement method at least does not prevail over the net effect one expects to reveal.

Material Properties of the Corneo-Scleral Shell

They represent actually the key issue of ocular rigidity measurement. However the previous analysis of all other factors influencing ocular rigidity does not allow to assess this aspect directly in clinical application using a reasonable quantitative parameter. We know that ocular rigidity depends on material properties of the corneo-scleral shell (Fig. 2.1) and that equation (Eq. 2.3) is consistent with the mechanical properties of collagen, which is "responsible" for the elastic moduli of the sclera and the cornea [5, 35, 41]. However what does remain as a "retort residue" after strong assumptions for the ocular rigidity parameter and after accounting its value to all other influencing factors? And how can one distinguish material properties of the sclera from those of the cornea and of other ocular coats within only one parameter K? An extended engineering approach together with novel sophisticated clinical and experimental studies focused on material properties of the corneo-scleral shell, like the mentioned study by Liu and He [31], would probably elucidate these questions in the future.

It seems so far that the influence of inter- and intraindividual alterations of material properties of the corneo-scleral shell on the value of coefficient of ocular rigidity by Friedenwald in the normal population and even in ocular pathology is small in comparison to the influence of other factors like measurement error or changes of the intraocular volume and the IOP [59, 104]. Supposing age-related stiffening of the corneo-scleral envelope being mostly responsible for age-related alterations of the value of K one can indirectly and roughly estimate its relative influence from Friedenwald's data mentioned above [4]: K ranged in his whole cohort: 0.006–0.037 μl^{-1}, while the difference between mean K-values in his oldest and his youngest subgroups amounted to only 0.008 μl^{-1}.

Concluding Remarks

Advantages/Disadvantages of the Clinical Approach

The main advantage of the clinical approach to ocular rigidity is the possibility of direct clinical measurement of ocular rigidity and the conceptual correctness of the approach in terms of the definition: the mechanical reaction of the entire eyeball to the external forces is measured. The simplification of a unified clinical parameter reflecting the stiffness of the whole eyeball and, with a lot of limitations, the elasticity of the corneo-scleral shell, seems to be an advantage for clinicians. The coefficient of ocular rigidity by Friedenwald with its pros and cons has been widely accepted in the clinical ophthalmology for ages. Similar to the differential tonometry Goldmann applanation tonometry is known to have several limitations in clinical applications, and it still represents the gold standard for IOP-measurements.

One of the drawbacks of the clinical approach is the impossibility of an explicit separation of material properties of the corneo-scleral shell and morphological factors. Thus, the findings of studies based on clinical measurements of ocular rigidity lose their applied significance: the conclusions are quite limited and rise more questions. For example, as noted above, some researchers report a decrease of ocular rigidity in myopia [21]. But what does this mean? Are material properties of the cornea or the sclera or rather their thickness changed? Is this simply a reflection of eye elongation and hence the increased intraocular volume in myopic eyes? Is the IOP decreased? Is the blood circulation impaired? Most likely we are dealing with a combination of these factors, which is difficult to interpret using only one parameter.

Experimental pressure-volume relationship and similar in-vivo assessments of mechanical response of the eye globe to alterations in IOP and volume might contain a lot of additional information on viscoelastic behaviour of the corneo-scleral shell. A clinical approach would definitely benefit from analytical research on clinical parameters related to material properties of the cornea and the sclera. For example some clinical parameters measured with ORA, like corneal hysteresis and corneal resistance factor do contain not only information on the corneal biomechanic response but generally speaking reflect ocular rigidity with all its aspects mentioned above [27, 69]. However the relation of these parameters to the classic parameters of ocular rigidity has not yet been elucidated [40].

With clinical formulation of ocular rigidity a unified scientific approach to the description of physical characteristics of an object is missing. Hence the relation to similar concepts from biomedical engineering, medicine, and physics is difficult. Any comparison of results of different studies with different formulations of ocular rigidity is almost impossible.

Several biometric parameters of the eyeball can be accurately measured with modern diagnostic devices. For example, the corneal thickness is determined using pachymetry, the thickness of the sclera can be assessed using ultrasound or

OCT. The length of the anterior-posterior axis can be measured with laser biometry. At the same time, there is a lack of reliable clinical methods, allowing for a direct assessment of material properties of the corneo-scleral shell, especially those of the sclera. Further development of such clinical methods would be very crucial, as they could substantially advance both researchers and clinicians in solving several ophthalmological problems associated with eye biomechanics [21, 105, 106]. Clinical assessment of the coefficient of ocular rigidity using tonometry or direct manometry is not the best method to obtain this information. A promising alternative way has been recently shown by Detorakis et al. [68]: modern shear-wave ultrasound elastography was able to detect selectively in-vivo rigidity changes in several structures of the anterior segment in the rabbit eye model and might be potentially applied in human eyes, providing useful clinical information.

Synergy with the Engineering Approach

Referring to the Chap. 1 I agree with a fundamental idea by White [2] and Kalenak [107], that future experimental and analytical projects on ocular rigidity and pressure-volume relationship "should be conducted using fundamental engineering terms to bring both rigor and clarity to the subject." The obvious value of engineering analysis is that it can explicitly separate material properties of ocular structures and morphologic factors contributing to pressure-volume relationship. It brings advantages of common ground with concepts used in other biomedical engineering applications and is therefore essential for the research. However as predicted by Purslow and Karwatowki [3] the engineering approach will bring clarity but not necessarily simplicity "as far as for many practicians may be concerned".

The most promising solution in the future is the attempt to combine both approaches introducing a unified definition of ocular rigidity, which could be applicable both in clinical practice and in experimental studies. We do not have another sensible way since the clinical approach to ocular rigidity seems neither simple nor rigorous or consistent and even leads sometimes to contradictive results that one can usually explain from engineering point of view. First attempts to link both approaches, taking advantage of each, have been already done. Purslow and Karwatowki [3] developed a simplified mathematical model of the pressure-volume relationship with the aim to separate elastic material properties of the corneo-scleral shell from biometric parameters of the eye. They derived a formula for the pressure-volume relation depending on the Young's modulus of the uniform isotropic corneo-scleral material instead of the coefficient of rigidity. Similar to this synergetic approach one can develop a more sophisticated biomechanical model of the eye based on experimental data on morphology and material properties of ocular tissues and verify this model in a clinical experiment. This combined approach would enable an explicit definition of ocular rigidity as a biomechanical response of the eyeball via biomechanical parameters of ocular tissues, particularly those of the sclera and the cornea. Recent studies have shown promising outlook of such an approach [48, 71, 108].

Definition

At conclusion the following unified definition of ocular rigidity is proposed. Ocular rigidity is a concept, which implies the resistance of the whole eyeball to a deformation due to external or internal forces. It is dependent on biomechanical material properties and on the morphology of eye structures (the sclera, the cornea, the choroid, the retina, the Bruch's membrane, etc.) as well as on the intraocular volume and the intraocular pressure, the blood pressure and ocular blood flow. Other related concepts should be defined separately and should be accurately distinguished from the concept of ocular rigidity: e.g. the rigidity of the corneo-scleral shell, the elasticity of the sclera and of the cornea.

Take Home Messages

- Ocular rigidity is a widely used concept in ophthalmology. It implies a combined measure of material and morphological properties of the eyeball. The concept is involved in the pathogenesis of various eye disorders, including glaucoma and myopia. It represents a basis for tonometry, tonography and pulsatile ocular blood flow measurements. In clinical applications ocular rigidity is described by several parameters and is interpreted differently. Technical difficulties in obtaining accurate in-vivo measurements of ocular rigidity have limited its clinical importance.
- When discussing clinical findings and comparing the data of various studies it is crucial to have clue on what is really meant under ocular rigidity: the rigidity or material parameters of the corneo-scleral shell or the elasticity of the sclera; material properties and/or the morphology of the tissues; properties in-vivo or ex-vivo, etc.
- Ocular rigidity gives an indirect insight into the material properties of the corneo-scleral shell. The estimation of these parameters using available clinical measures of ocular rigidity is inaccurate and sometimes erroneous.
- Most common clinical measure of ocular rigidity, the coefficient of ocular rigidity by Friedenwald is based on a logarithmic pressure–volume relation. It is assumed to be independent of IOP and it possesses relatively low variability in healthy population.
- The pressure–volume relation differs in living and enucleated eyes. This indicates that blood flow and tissue necrosis affect ocular rigidity. For clinical applications in-vivo ocular rigidity parameters need to be used. The results of ex-vivo experiments should be adjusted.

- Ocular rigidity is reported to be altered in glaucoma, myopia, presbyopia and age-related macular degeneration as well as after refractive corneal surgery.
- Combination of clinical and engineering approaches to ocular rigidity seems to be promising for the development of reliable non-invasive in-vivo clinical methods assessing material properties of ocular tissues, particularly those of the cornea and the sclera.
- Future analysis of pressure-volume relationship in the eye should be done in fundamental biomechanical terms in order to bring rigor and clarity to the subject; to separate structural material properties from morphologic contributions; to have common ground with concepts and parameters used in other biomedical engineering applications.

Acknowledgement I would like to acknowledge my teacher Ivan Koshitz for inspiring me and granting me the astounding world of ocular biomechanics.

References

1. Kotliar KE, Koshitz IN. Ocular rigidity: biomechanical and clinical aspects. Proceedings of international scientific-practical conference "eye biomechanics"; November 26,Moscow R&D Helmholtz Institute for Eye Diseases. 2009;121–126.
2. White OW. Ocular elasticity? Ophthalmology. 1990 Sep;97(9):1092–4.
3. Purslow PP, Karwatowski WS. Ocular elasticity. Is engineering stiffness a more useful characterization parameter than ocular rigidity? Ophthalmology. 1996 Oct;103(10):1686–92.
4. Friedenwald J. Contribution to the theory and praxis of the tonometry. Am J Ophthalmol. 1937;20:985–1024.
5. van der Werff TJ. A new single-parameter ocular rigidity function. Am J Ophthalmol. 1981 Sep;92(3):391–5.
6. Moses RA. Intraocular pressure. In: Hart WM, editor. Adler's physiology of the eye. Washington, Toronto: Mosby; 1987. p. 223–45.
7. Strakhov VV. Essential ocular hypertension and primary glaucoma. Doctoral Thesis: Dr.Sc. (in Russian). Yaroslavl Yaroslavl State Medical Institute; 1997.
8. Beaton L, Mazzaferri J, Lalonde F, Hidalgo-Aguirre M, Descovich D, Lesk MR, et al. Non-invasive measurement of choroidal volume change and ocular rigidity through automated segmentation of high-speed OCT imaging. Biomed Opt Express. 2015 May 1;6(5):1694–706.
9. Bunin AY. Hemodynamics of the eye and methods of its investigation. (in Russian). Moscow: Medicina; 1971.
10. Grieshaber MC, Katamay R, Gugleta K, Kochkorov A, Flammer J, Orgul S. Relationship between ocular pulse amplitude and systemic blood pressure measurements. Acta Ophthalmol. 2009 May;87(3):329–34.
11. Hommer A, Fuchsjager-Mayrl G, Resch H, Vass C, Garhofer G, Schmetterer L. Estimation of ocular rigidity based on measurement of pulse amplitude using pneumotonometry and fundus pulse using laser interferometry in glaucoma. Invest Ophthalmol Vis Sci. 2008 Sep;49(9):4046–50.
12. Ravalico G, Toffoli G, Pastori G, Croce M, Calderini S. Age-related ocular blood flow changes. Invest Ophthalmol Vis Sci. 1996 Dec;37(13):2645–50.
13. Dastiridou AI, Ginis HS, De Brouwere D, Tsilimbaris MK, Pallikaris IG. Ocular rigidity, ocular pulse amplitude, and pulsatile ocular blood flow: the effect of intraocular pressure. Invest Ophthalmol Vis Sci. 2009 Dec;50(12):5718–22.

14. Shah S, Laiquzzaman M, Bhojwani R, Mantry S, Cunliffe I. Assessment of the biomechanical properties of the cornea with the ocular response analyzer in normal and keratoconic eyes. Invest Ophthalmol Vis Sci. 2007 Jul;48(7):3026–31.
15. Herber R, Terai N, Pillunat KR, Raiskup F, Pillunat LE, Sporl E. Dynamic Scheimpflug analyzer (Corvis ST) for measurement of corneal biomechanical parameters: a praxis-related overview. Ophthalmologe. 2018 May 16.
16. Akpatrov AI. Experimental interrelation between the coefficient of rigidity, eye volume and scleral modulus of elasticity. (in Russian). Vestnik oftalmologii. 1981 July–Aug;4:5–7.
17. Edmund C. Corneal elasticity and ocular rigidity in normal and keratoconic eyes. Acta Ophthalmol. 1988 Apr;66(2):134–40.
18. Duke-Elder S. The physiology of the eye and vision. St. Louis: C.V. Mosby; 1968.
19. Nesterov AP, Bunin AY, Katsnelson LA. Intraocular pressure. (in Russian). Moscow: Nauka; 1974.
20. Pinter L. Active and passive components of the eye rigidity. (in Russian). Vestnik oftalmologii. 1978 May–June;3:9–10.
21. Iomdina EN. Biomechanics of scleral eye shell in myopia: diagnostic of disturbances and its experimental correction. Doctoral Thesis: Dr.Sc. (in Russian). Moscow: Moscow Helmholtz R&D Institute for Eye Diseases; 2000.
22. Iomdina EN, Bauer SM, Kotliar KE. Eye biomechanics: theoretical aspects and clinical applications. (in Russian). Moscow: Real Time; 2015.
23. Friberg TR, Lace JW. A comparison of the elastic properties of human choroid and sclera. Exp Eye Res. 1988 Sep;47(3):429–36.
24. Pallikaris IG, Kymionis GD, Ginis HS, Kounis GA, Tsilimbaris MK. Ocular rigidity in living human eyes. Invest Ophthalmol Vis Sci. 2005 Feb;46(2):409–14.
25. Pallikaris IG, Kymionis GD, Ginis HS, Kounis GA, Christodoulakis E, Tsilimbaris MK. Ocular rigidity in patients with age-related macular degeneration. Am J Ophthalmol. 2006 Apr;141(4):611–5.
26. Ethier CR. Scleral biomechanics and glaucoma: a connection? Can J Ophthalmol. 2006 Feb;41(1):9–12.
27. Koshitz IN, Svetlova OV, Ryabtseva AA, Makarov FN, Zaseeva MV, Mustyatsa VF. Role of rigidity of the corneo-scleral shell and scleral fluctuations in the early diagnostics of open-angle glaucoma. (in Russian). Ophthalmol J. 2010;(6).
28. Leydhecker G, Leydhecker W. Measurement of scleral rigidity and the 1954 Schiotz tonometric curve. Klin Monbl Augenheilkd Augenarztl Fortbild. 1956;129(1):61–7.
29. Shih YF, Horng IH, Yang CH, Lin LL, Peng Y, Hung PT. Ocular pulse amplitude in myopia. J Ocular Pharmacol. 1991;7(1):83–7.
30. Drance SM. The coefficient of scleral rigidity in normal and glaucomatous eyes. Arch Ophthalmol. 1960 Apr;63:668–74.
31. Liu J, He X. Corneal stiffness affects IOP elevation during rapid volume change in the eye. Invest Ophthalmol Vis Sci. 2009 May;50(5):2224–9.
32. Clark J. A method for measuring elasticity in-vivo and results obtained on the eyeball at different intraocular pressures. Am J Physiol. 1932;101(3):474–81.
33. McBain E. Tonometer calibration. II. Ocular rigidity. AMA. 1958 Dec;60(6):1080–91.
34. Holland MG, Madison J, Bean W. The ocular rigidity function. Am J Ophthalmol. 1960;50:958–74.
35. McEwen WK, St Helen R. Rheology of the human sclera. Unifying formulation of ocular rigidity. Int J Ophthalmol. 1965;150(5):321–46.
36. Hibbard RR, Lyon CS, Shepherd MD, McBain EH, McEwen WK. Immediate rigidity of an eye. I. Whole, segments and strips. Exp Eye Res. 1970 Jan;9(1):137–43.
37. Woo SL, Kobayashi AS, Schlegel WA, Lawrence C. Nonlinear material properties of intact cornea and sclera. Exp Eye Res. 1972 Jul;14(1):29–39.
38. Silver DM, Geyer O. Pressure-volume relation for the living human eye. Curr Eye Res. 2000 Feb;20(2):115–20.

39. Simanovskiy AI. Fundamentals of the theory of applanation tonometry and improvement of interpretation of the results of elastotonometry and tonography. (in Russian). Glaukoma. 2007;(3):42–8.
40. Pallikaris IG, Dastiridou AI, Tsilimbaris MK, Karyotakis N, Ginis HS. Ocular rigidity. Expert Rev Ophthalmol. 2010 Apr;3(5):343–51.
41. Ethier CR, Johnson M, Ruberti J. Ocular biomechanics and biotransport. Annu Rev Biomed Eng. 2004;6:249–73.
42. Greene PR. Mechanical considerations in myopia: relative effects of accommodation, convergence, intraocular pressure, and the extraocular muscles. Am J Optometry Physiol Optics. 1980 Dec;57(12):902–14.
43. Greene PR, McMahon TA. Scleral creep vs. temperature and pressure in vitro. Exp Eye Res. 1979 Nov;29(5):527–37.
44. Iomdina EN, Petrov SY, Antonov AA, Novikov IA, Pahomova IA. The Corneoscleral shell of the eye: an age-related analysis of structural biomechanical properties. Literature review (in Russian). Ophthalmol Russia. 2016;13(1):10–9.
45. Whitford C, Joda A, Jones S, Bao F, Rama P, Elsheikh A. Ex vivo testing of intact eye globes under inflation conditions to determine regional variation of mechanical stiffness. Eye Vision (London, England). 2016;3:21.
46. Svetlova OV, Balashevitsch LI, Zaseeva MV, Drozdova GA, Makarov FN, Koshitz IN. Physiological role of the scleral rigidity in the formation of the intraocular pressure in normal and glaucomatous eyes. (in Russian). Glaukoma. 2009;4:46–54.
47. Wang J, Freeman EE, Descovich D, Harasymowycz PJ, Kamdeu Fansi A, Li G, et al. Estimation of ocular rigidity in glaucoma using ocular pulse amplitude and pulsatile choroidal blood flow. Invest Ophthalmol Vis Sci. 2013 Mar;54(3):1706–11.
48. Kotliar K, Maier M, Bauer S, Feucht N, Lohmann C, Lanzl I. Effect of intravitreal injections and volume changes on intraocular pressure: clinical results and biomechanical model. Acta Ophthalmol Scand. 2007 Jun 16;85(7):777–81.
49. Coudrillier B, Tian J, Alexander S, Myers KM, Quigley HA, Nguyen TD. Biomechanics of the human posterior sclera: age- and glaucoma-related changes measured using inflation testing. Invest Ophthalmol Vis Sci. 2012 Apr 2;53(4):1714–28.
50. Römer P. Neues zur Tonometrie des Auges Bericht der Deutschen Ophthalmologischen Gesellschaft. 1918;62–8.
51. Detorakis ET, Pallikaris IG. Ocular rigidity: biomechanical role, in vivo measurements and clinical significance. Clin Exp Ophthalmol. 2013 Jan–Feb;41(1):73–81.
52. Kalfa SY. On the problem of the tonometry theory with applanation tonometers. (in Russian). Russ Ophthalmol J. 1927;6(10):1132–41.
53. Greene PR. Stress-strain behavior for curved exponential strips. Bull Math Biol. 1985;47(6):757–64.
54. Detorakis ET, Tsaglioti E, Kymionis G. Non-invasive ocular rigidity measurement: a differential tonometry approach. Acta Med (Hradec Kralove). 2015;58(3):92–7.
55. Koster W. Beiträge zur Tonometrie und Manometrie des Auges. Albrecht von Graefes Archiv für Ophthalmologie. 1895;41(2):113–58.
56. Ridley F. The intraocular pressure and drainage of the aqueous humor. Br J Exp Pathol. 1930;11:217–40.
57. Elsheikh A, Whitford C, Hamarashid R, Kassem W, Joda A, Buchler P. Stress free configuration of the human eye. Med Eng Phys. 2013 Feb;35(2):211–6.
58. Dashevskiy AI, Lvovskiy VM. Application of the shell theory to study the physical principles of ocular tonometry. (in Russian). Kiev: Budivelnik; 1975.
59. Perkins ES. Ocular volume and ocular rigidity. Exp Eye Res. 1981 Aug;33(2):141–5.
60. Eisenlohr JE, Langham ME, Maumenee AE. Manometric studies of the pressure-volume relationship in living and enucleated eyes of individual human subjects. Br J Ophthalmol. 1962;46:536–48.

61. Ytteborg J. Influence of bulbar compression on rigidity coefficient of human eyes, in vivo and encleated. Acta Ophthalmol. 1960;38:562–77.
62. Dastiridou AI, Ginis H, Tsilimbaris M, Karyotakis N, Detorakis E, Siganos C, et al. Ocular rigidity, ocular pulse amplitude, and pulsatile ocular blood flow: the effect of axial length. Invest Ophthalmol Vis Sci. 2013 Mar;54(3):2087–92.
63. Dastiridou AI, Tsironi EE, Tsilimbaris MK, Ginis H, Karyotakis N, Cholevas P, et al. Ocular rigidity, outflow facility, ocular pulse amplitude, and pulsatile ocular blood flow in open-angle glaucoma: a manometric study. Invest Ophthalmol Vis Sci. 2013 Jul;54(7):4571–7.
64. Jackson CR. Schiotz tonometers. An assessment of their usefulness. Br J Ophthalmol. 1965 Sep;49(9):478–84.
65. Gloster J, Perkins ES. Ocular rigidity and tonometry. Proc R Soc Med. 1957 Sep;50(9):667–74.
66. Moses RA, Grodzki WJ. Ocular rigidity in tonography. Doc Ophthalmol. 1969;26:118–29.
67. Friedenwald J. Contribution to the theory and praxis of the tonometry. II. An analysis of the work of Professor S. Kalfa with the applanation tonometer. Am J Ophthalmol. 1939;22:375–83.
68. Detorakis ET, Drakonaki EE, Ginis H, Karyotakis N, Pallikaris IG. Evaluation of iridociliary and lenticular elasticity using shear-wave elastography in rabbit eyes. Acta Med (Hradec Kralove). 2014;57(1):9–14.
69. Iomdina EN, Eremina MV, Ivashchenko ZN, Tarutta EP. Applicability of the ocular response analyzer in the evaluation of biomechanics of the corneoscleral eye shell and intraocular pressure in children and adolescents with progressive myopia. Proceedings of the International Conference Ocular Biomechanics, Moscow. 2007;46–51.
70. Ebneter A, Wagels B, Zinkernagel MS. Non-invasive biometric assessment of ocular rigidity in glaucoma patients and controls. Eye (Lond). 2009 Mar;23(3):606–11.
71. Kotliar K, Fuest M, Bauer SM, Voronkova E, Plange N. In-vivo estimation of the elasticity of corneoscleral shell after intravitreal injections. Ophthalmologe. 2016;Suppl.
72. Bayerle-Eder M, Kolodjaschna J, Wolzt M, Polska E, Gasic S, Schmetterer L. Effect of a nifedipine induced reduction in blood pressure on the association between ocular pulse amplitude and ocular fundus pulsation amplitude in systemic hypertension. Br J Ophthalmol. 2005 June;89(6):704–8.
73. Roberts CJ, Dupps WJ, Downs JC, editors. Biomechanics of the eye. Amsterdam: Kugler Publications; 2018.
74. Ytteborg J. Further investigations of factors influencing size of rigidity coefficient. Acta Ophthalmol. 1960;38:643–57.
75. Goldmann H, Schmidt T. Friedenwald's rigidity coefficient. Int J Ophthalmol. 1957 Apr–May;133(4–5):330–5; discussion 5-6.
76. Agrawal KK, Sharma DP, Bhargava G, Sanadhya DK. Scleral rigidity in glaucoma, before and during topical antiglaucoma drug therapy. Indian J Ophthalmol. 1991 July–Sep;39(3):85–6.
77. Melnik LS. On the norms of elastotonometric curves. (in Russian). J Ophthalmol. 1961;16(4):221.
78. Gaasterland D, Kupfer C, Milton R, Ross K, McCain L, MacLellan H. Studies of aqueous humour dynamics in man. VI. Effect of age upon parameters of intraocular pressure in normal human eyes. Exp Eye Res. 1978 Jun;26(6):651–6.
79. Lam AK, Chan ST, Chan H, Chan B. The effect of age on ocular blood supply determined by pulsatile ocular blood flow and color Doppler ultrasonography. Optom Vis Sci. 2003 Apr;80(4):305–11.
80. Jones HJ, Girard MJ, White N, Fautsch MP, Morgan JE, Ethier CR, et al. Quantitative analysis of three-dimensional fibrillar collagen microstructure within the normal, aged and glaucomatous human optic nerve head. J R Soc Interface. 2015 May 6;12(106)
81. Ho LC, Sigal IA, Jan NJ, Squires A, Tse Z, Wu EX, et al. Magic angle-enhanced MRI of fibrous microstructures in sclera and cornea with and without intraocular pressure loading. Invest Ophthalmol Vis Sci. 2014 Aug 7;55(9):5662–72.
82. Svetlova OV, Zaseeva MV, Surzhikov AV, Koshitz IN. Development of the theory of aqueous outflow and promising hypotensive treatment. (in Russian). Glaukoma. 2003;1:51–9.

83. Friedman E. The pathogenesis of age-related macular degeneration. Am J Ophthalmol. 2008 Sep;146(3):348–9.
84. To M, Goz A, Camenzind L, Oertle P, Candiello J, Sullivan M, et al. Diabetes-induced morphological, biomechanical, and compositional changes in ocular basement membranes. Exp Eye Res. 2013 Nov;116:298–307.
85. Panagiotoglou T, Tsilimbaris M, Ginis H, Karyotakis N, Georgiou V, Koutentakis P, et al. Ocular rigidity and outflow facility in nonproliferative diabetic retinopathy. J Diabetes Res. 2015;2015:141598.
86. Arora VK, Prasad VN. The intraocular pressure and diabetes: a correlative study. Indian J Ophthalmol. 1989 Jan–Mar;37(1):10–2.
87. Taniashina LB. Tonometry and elastotonometry in various body positions. (in Russian). Oftalmologicheskii zhurnal. 1971;26(1):44–8.
88. Kymionis GD, Diakonis VF, Kounis G, Charisis S, Bouzoukis D, Ginis H, et al. Ocular rigidity evaluation after photorefractive keratectomy: an experimental study. J Refract Surg. 2008 Feb;24(2):173–7.
89. Cronemberger S, Guimaraes CS, Calixto N, Calixto JM. Intraocular pressure and ocular rigidity after LASIK. Arq Bras Oftalmol. 2009 July–Aug;72(4):439–43.
90. Moses RA, Tarkkanen A. Tonometry; the pressure-volume relationship in the intact human eye at low pressures. Am J Ophthalmol. 1959 Jan;47(1 Part 2):557–63; discussion 63-4.
91. Draeger J. Studies on the rigidity coefficient. Doc Ophthalmol. 1959;13:431–86.
92. Dashevsky AI. Comparison between Friedenwald's tonometry and Filatov-Kalf's elastotonometry. (in Russian). Vestn oftalmol. 1949 Jan–Feb;28(1):14–21.
93. Ytteborg J. The effect of intraocular pressure on rigidity coefficient in the human eye. Acta Ophthalmol. 1960;38:548–61.
94. Castren J, Pohjola S. The measurement of scleral rigidity. Evaluation of various methods used. Acta Ophthalmol (Copenh). 1961;39:1005–10.
95. Kiselev GA, Taniashina LB. Verification of the new calibration tables for the Filatov-Kalf elastotonometer. (in Russian). Vestn oftalmol. 1972 Mar–Apr;2:25–30.
96. Goldmann H. Second conference on Glaucoma, 1956. In: Newell FW, editor. The central nervous system and behavior. Transactions of the second conference. New York: Josiah Macy, Jr. Foundation; 1957. p. 201.
97. Phillips CI, Quick MC. Impression tonometry and the effect of eye volume variation. Br J Ophthalmol. 1960 Mar;44:149–63.
98. Ytteborg J. The role of intraocular blood volume in rigidity measurements on human eyes. Acta Ophthalmol. 1960;38:410–36.
99. Nagel E, Vilser W. Autoregulative behavior of retinal arteries and veins during changes of perfusion pressure: a clinical study. Graefes Arch Clin Exp Ophthalmol. 2004 Jan;242(1):13–7.
100. Best M, Masket S, Rabinovitz AZ. Measurement of vascular rigidity in the living eye. Arch Ophthalmol. 1971 Dec;86(6):699–705.
101. Kiel JW. The effect of arterial pressure on the ocular pressure-volume relationship in the rabbit. Exp Eye Res. 1995 Mar;60(3):267–78.
102. Kiel JW. Choroidal myogenic autoregulation and intraocular pressure. Exp Eye Res. 1994 May;58(5):529–43.
103. Sigal IA, Flanagan JG, Ethier CR. Factors influencing optic nerve head biomechanics. Invest Ophthalmol Vis Sci. 2005 Nov;46(11):4189–99.
104. Nesterov AP. Hydrodynamics of the eye. (in Russian). Moscow: Medicina; 1967.
105. Curtin BJ. Pathologic myopia. Acta Ophthalmol Suppl. 1988;185:105–6.
106. Curtin BJ. Physiopathologic aspects of scleral stress-strain. Trans Am Ophthalmol Soc. 1969;67:417–61.
107. Kalenak JW. More ocular elasticity? Ophthalmology. 1991 Apr;98(4):411–2.
108. Poloz MV. Biomechanical model of the human eye. Doctoral Thesis: Ph.D. (in Russian). Moscow: Helmholtz Institute for Eye Diseases; 2011.

Chapter 3
Methods of Measuring Ocular Rigidity in the Human Eye

Anna I. Dastiridou and Ioannis Pallikaris

Introduction

Ocular rigidity refers to the relationship between volume and pressure changes inside the eye. It is an empiric measure, used to characterize the distensibility or elasticity of the eye [1]. While it is relatively easy to characterize the biomechanical properties of a tissue ex vivo, this is becoming increasingly difficult when trying to characterize its behavior in vivo (see Sects. "Introduction" and "Differential Schiotz Tonometry"). It is therefore understood that traditional objective methods do not apply to the living human eye. Therefore, the data available to date come from three different types of studies; those performed in eyes after enucleation, those using manometry and are mainly performed in the operating theatre and finally those that use surrogate measures of rigidity or adopt certain assumptions in order to employ non invasive means of pressure or volume displacement (see Sect. "Manometric Measurement of Ocular Rigidity"). The existing body of knowledge on manometric measurements of ocular rigidity stems from experiments carried out in animals [2–6]and measurements ex vivo, and less often in vivo [7–16]. It is clear that there is at the moment no method of ocular rigidity measurement that is at the same time universally approved, accurate, reproducible and non invasive. Our knowledge on ocular rigidity in the living human eye is mainly based on invasive manometric measurements or measurements performed with paired Schiotz tonometry.

A. I. Dastiridou
2nd Ophthalmology Department, Aristotle University of Thessaloniki, Thessaloniki, Greece

School of Medicine, University of Thessalia, Larissa, Greece

I. Pallikaris (✉)
Department of Ophthalmology, University of Crete, Heraklion, Crete, Greece

© Springer Nature Switzerland AG 2021
I. Pallikaris et al. (eds.), *Ocular Rigidity, Biomechanics and Hydrodynamics of the Eye*, https://doi.org/10.1007/978-3-030-64422-2_3

Differential Schiotz Tonometry

Friedenwald introduced the term ocular rigidity in 1937 [1]. He had a great interest in tonometry and at that time, calibration tables and research around precision in the then-available tonometers was gaining scientific attention. Friedenwald performed extensive studies to improve the accuracy of indentation tonometry. The initial calibration tables were later updated with his new experiments [17, 18]. Friedenwald used paired readings obtained with two different weights, usually the 5.5 and 10 g, and his nomogram to measure both IOP and ocular rigidity. The basic instrument to measure IOP then was the Schiotz tonometer, which is based on the principle of indentation tonometry and there was a great clinical need for precision. Since the indentation of the cornea has to be translated to an IOP reading, there is a requirement of an accurate nomogram. Friedenwald's studies provided the experimental data to construct a nomogram for use in Schiotz tonometer ocular rigidity (and IOP) measurements (see Sect. "Differential Schiotz Tonometry") [1, 17, 18]. Knowledge of the ocular rigidity was important in indentation tonometry since the error could be great if this would not be taken into account in an eye that was not close to an average reading [19, 20].

In clinical practice, the process of differential tonometry is probably the one most commonly used to quantify ocular rigidity. However, errors may occur, mainly because of the use of weights that alter the blood volume in the eye, and also because of the use of calibration tables [21, 22].

Manometric Measurement of Ocular Rigidity

In the first half of the twentieth century, experiments carried out in animal eyes suggested that the pressure volume relationship is not uniform across the range of intraocular pressure (IOP) [2, 3]. Interestingly, the eye is more rigid in higher IOP and becomes more elastic in low IOP. Following studies in humans further characterized the relationship in the human eye [7–9]. The initial human data available were mainly available from measurements performed post mortem or in eyes with melanoma that were scheduled for enucleation [7–9, 23]. Following studies carried out in otherwise normal, cataract eyes undergoing cataract surgery.

The measurement setup in these studies usually involves controlling the IOP by adjusting the height of the infusion bottle or controlled inflation of the eye with known volumes and recording of the pressure, after cannulating the eye in the anterior chamber, the posterior chamber or the vitreous cavity [24–26].

In order to measure ocular rigidity a measurement device was set and standardized at the University of Crete, Greece [10, 11]. This device consists of a pressure transducer, a volumetric dosing pump and a series of inextensible tubes, controlled by custom made software (see Figs. 3.1 and 3.2).

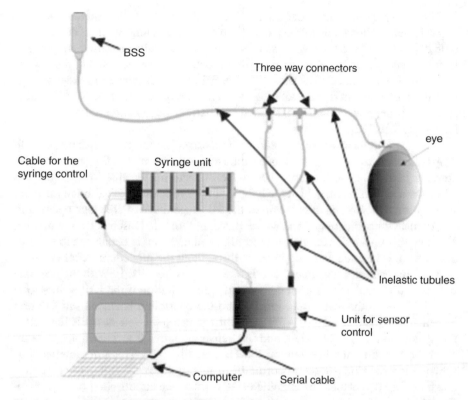

Fig. 3.1 Schematic representation of the measurement device

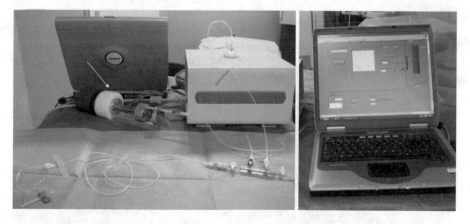

Fig. 3.2 View of the device set up ready for measurement in the operating theatre

The pressure sensor has a sensitivity threshold of 0.05 mmHg and the microdosimetric pump allows for delivery of microvolumes of saline with an accuracy of 0.08 μl per step. Custom software was designed to control the measurement process. Before each measurement, in the operating theatre, in a sterile fashion, the system of microtubes is connected as shown in Fig. 3.1. This is fashioned in order to connect the measurement device with the eye. The tubing system is filled with saline solution during preparation, and is tested extensively since the presence of air may lead to artifacts [27].

This measurement procedure can be performed under local anesthesia with drops and most measurements in our studies were performed in the operating theater, just before cataract surgery [10, 11]. Before entering the anterior chamber, the tip of the needle is being held at the height of the eye in order to calibrate the pressure sensor. The surgeon uses the tip of the 20 gauge blade to create an opening in the cornea with the tip of the knife passing through Descemet's membrane. Through this opening, a 21 gauge butterflie needle, which is connected to the tubing system, is inserted and held in place throughout the procedure. After cannulation of the anterior chamber, the initial IOP is recorded. With appropriate withdrawal of aqueous (or even delivery of saline solution if the IOP is very low) the IOP is set at the level of 10 mmHg and the controlled balanced salt solution injection in 4 μl steps begins. After each infusion step the sensor waits for 1 s for the system to reach equilibrium and the sensor acquires 2 s continuous pressure recordings with a sampling rate of 200 Hz (see Fig. 3.3). This time interval was selected in order to have the opportunity to record at least 2 full cardiac circles, and therefore two ocular pulses. When IOP reaches the cut off point of 40 mmHg, the infusion stops and the pressure sensor is set to simply record the spontaneous IOP. This can help quantify both OR in the individual eye and outflow facility [28, 29].

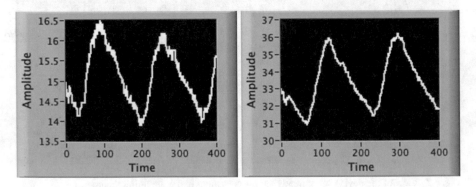

Fig. 3.3 Sample recordings of the spontaneous pressure in the eye after each infusion step

Other Approaches to Measure Ocular Rigidity

Apart from differential tonometry and manometry, other methods have also been employed as surrogate measures of ocular rigidity [30–34]. These are being discussed in the following chapter. Finally, a very promising, recently reported new optical method of measuring ocular rigidity using OCT technology has recently been validated against manometry [35].

References

1. Friedenwald JS. Contribution to the theory and practice of tonometry. Am J Ophthalmol. 1937;20:985–1024.
2. Ridley F. The intraocular pressure and drainage of the aqueous humor. Br J Exp Pathol. 1930;11:217–40.
3. Clark JH. A method for measuring elasticity in vivo and results obtained on the eyeball at different intraocular pressures. Am J Physiol. 1932;101:474–81.
4. Ytteborg J. Changes in the coefficient of rigidity from the live to the dead eye. Experiments on rabbits. Acta Ophthalmol (Copenh). 1962;40:484–91.
5. Schmerl E, Steinberg B. Determination of ocular tension and rigidity in rabbits. Am J Ophthalmol. 1946;29:1400–4.
6. Eisenlohr JE, Langham ME. The relationship between pressure and volume changes in living and dead rabbit eyes. Investig Ophthalmol. 1962;1:63–77.
7. Eisenlohr JE, Langham ME, Maumenee AE. Manometric studies of the pressure–volume relationship in living and enucleated eyes of individual human subjects. Br J Ophthalmol. 1962;46:536–48.
8. Ytteborg J. Influence of bulbar compression on rigidity coefficient of human eyes, in vivo and encleated. Acta Ophthalmol Copenh. 1960;38:562–77.
9. Ytteborg J. The role of intraocular blood volume in rigidity measurements on human eyes. Acta Ophthalmol. 1960;38:410–36.
10. Pallikaris IG, Kymionis GD, Ginis HS, Kounis GA, Tsilimbaris MK. Ocular rigidity in living human eyes. Invest Ophthalmol Vis Sci. 2005;46:409–14.
11. Dastiridou AI, Ginis HS, De Brouwere D, Tsilimbaris MK, Pallikaris IG. Ocular rigidity, ocular pulse amplitude, and pulsatile ocular blood flow: the effect of intraocular pressure. Invest Ophthalmol Vis Sci. 2009;50:5718–22.
12. Pallikaris IG, Kymionis GD, Ginis HS, Kounis GA, Christodoulakis E, Tsilimbaris MK. Ocular rigidity in patients with age-related macular degeneration. Am J Ophthalmol. 2006;141:611–5.
13. Dastiridou AI, Ginis H, Tsilimbaris M, Karyotakis N, Detorakis E, Siganos C, Cholevas P, Tsironi EE, Pallikaris IG. Ocular rigidity, ocular pulse amplitude, and pulsatile ocular blood flow: the effect of axial length. Invest Ophthalmol Vis Sci. 2013;54:2087–92.
14. Dastiridou AI, Tsironi EE, Tsilimbaris MK, Ginis H, Karyotakis N, Cholevas P, Androudi S, Pallikaris IG. Ocular rigidity, outflow facility, ocular pulse amplitude, and pulsatile ocular blood flow in open-angle glaucoma: a manometric study. Invest Ophthalmol Vis Sci. 2013;54:4571–7.
15. Karyotakis NG, Ginis HS, Dastiridou AI, Tsilimbaris MK, Pallikaris IG. Manometric measurement of the outflow facility in the living human eye and its dependence on intraocular pressure. Acta Ophthalmol. 2015;93:e343–8.
16. Panagiotoglou T, Tsilimbaris M, Ginis H, Karyotakis N, Georgiou V, Koutentakis P, Pallikaris I. Ocular rigidity and outflow facility in nonproliferative diabetic retinopathy. J Diabetes Res. 2015;2015:141598.

17. Friedenwald JS. Some problems in the calibration of tonometers. Trans Am Ophth Soc. 1947;45:355.
18. Friedenwald JS. Tonometer calibration; an attempt to remove discrepancies found in the 1954 calibration scale for Schiotz tonometers. Trans Am Acad Ophthalmol Otolaryngol. 1957;61:108–22.
19. Mc Bain E. Tonometer calibration. II. Ocular rigidity. AMA Arch Ophthalmol. 1958;60:1080–91.
20. Holland MG, Madison J, Bean W. The ocular rigidity function. Am J Ophthalmol. 1960;50:958–74.
21. Jackson CR. Schiotz tonometers. An assessment of their usefulness. Br J Ophthalmol. 1965;49:478–84.
22. Goodside V. Ocular rigidity: a clinical study. AMA Arch Ophthalmol. 1959;62:839.
23. Prijot E, Weekers R. Contribution to the study of the rigidity of the normal human eye. Ophthalmologica. 1959;138:1–9.
24. Gloster J, Perkins ES. Distensibility of the human eye. Br J Ophthalmol. 1959;43:97–101.
25. Gloster J, Perkins ES. Ocular rigidity and tonometry. Proc R Soc Med. 1957;50:667–74.
26. Gloster J, Perkins ES. Distensibility of the eye. Br J Ophthalmol. 1957;41:93–102.
27. Tsilimbaris MK, Ghinis H, Kounis G, Kimionis G, Pallikaris IG. Attenuation of ocular wall pulsation in eyes containing a gas bubble after vitrectomy. Curr Eye Res. 2002;24:202–5.
28. Moses RA, Grodzki WJ. Ocular rigidity in tonography. Doc Ophthalmol. 1969;26:118–29.
29. Grant WM, Trotter RR. Tonographic measurements in enucleated eyes. AMA Arch Ophthalmol. 1955;53:191–200.
30. Hommer A, Fuchsjäger-Mayrl G, Resch H, Vass C, Garhofer G, Schmetterer L. Estimation of ocular rigidity based on measurement of pulse amplitude using pneumotonometry and fundus pulse using laser interferometry in glaucoma. Invest Ophthalmol Vis Sci. 2008;49:4046–50.
31. Wang J, Freeman EE, Descovich D, et al. Estimation of ocular rigidity in glaucoma using ocular pulse amplitude and pulsatile choroidal blood flow. Invest Ophthalmol Vis Sci. 2013;54:1706–11.
32. Ebneter A, Wagels B, Zinkernagel MS. Non-invasive biometric assessment of ocular rigidity in glaucoma patients and controls. Eye (Lond). 2009;23:606–11.
33. Pallikaris I, Ginis HS, De Brouwere D, Tsilimbaris MK. A novel instrument for the non-invasive measurement of intraocular pressure and ocular rigidity. Invest Ophthalmol Vis Sci. 2006;47:2268.
34. Panagiotoglou TD, De Brouwere D, Ginis HS, Tsilimbaris MK, Pallikaris IG. Non-invasive measurement of ocular rigidity with a novel instrument. Invest Ophthalmol Vis Sci. 2008;49:4598.
35. Sayah DN, Mazzaferri J, Ghesquière P, Duval R, Rezende F, Costantino S, Lesk MR. Non-invasive in vivo measurement of ocular rigidity: clinical validation, repeatability and method improvement. Exp Eye Res. 2019 Oct 10;190:107831.

Chapter 4
Surrogate Non-invasive Methods of Ocular Rigidity Measurement

Efstathios T. Detorakis

Introduction

The accurate and reproducible measurement of ocular rigidity has been an elusive target for several scientific endeavors so far [1]. By definition, tissue rigidity refers to the relation between a force acting on a tissue and the induced deformation [1, 2]. This *"stress versus strain"* ratio (Young modulus) [3] is particularly applicable for linear structures defined as the ratio of the compressive stress to the longitudinal strain. Reported Young's modulus values for corneal tissue ranged between 72.4 and 102.4 kPa and 38.3–58.9 kPa for central and peripheral specimens, reflecting the complexity of *ex-vivo* corneal bio-mechanical behavior, which also includes a visco-elastic or anisotropic element, implying that that the rate at which a load is applied changes the measured value for cornea's Young's modulus [4].

However, in the case of concave spheroidal structures filled with incompressible contents (fluid), such as the eyeball, rigidity is best expressed as the mathematical relationship between the structure volume and the pressure inside it [2]. In this case, from a mechanistic point of view, rigidity reflects the elastic properties of the structure walls, namely in the case of the eyeball the anterior wall (cornea) and the posterior wall (sclera) [5]. However, the biomechanical behavior of the living eye is affected by more intrinsic factors, such as the blood circulation and the condition of the vascular element (mainly the choroid) [2, 5]. Moreover, the eyeball is not a homogeneous spheroidal structure but rather a compartmentalized one, with an anterior segment filled with aqueous humor (which is completely incompressible) and a posterior segment filled with hyaloid, which may display more complex bio-mechanical behavior, including visco-elasticity or poro-elasticity (i.e. elasticity which displays spatial variation) [2, 6]. Therefore, rigidity may have different values for different areas of the eyeball (Fig. 4.1) and it would be more appropriate to

E. T. Detorakis (✉)
Department of Ophthalmology, University Hospital of Heraklion, Heraklion, Crete, Greece

© Springer Nature Switzerland AG 2021
I. Pallikaris et al. (eds.), *Ocular Rigidity, Biomechanics and Hydrodynamics of the Eye*, https://doi.org/10.1007/978-3-030-64422-2_4

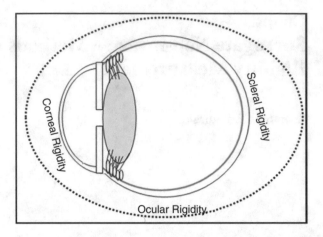

Fig. 4.1 Topographical distribution of corneal, scleral and total ocular rigidity

speak of corneal rigidity (referring exclusively to the cornea), scleral rigidity and total ocular rigidity (the last term describing the elastic behavior of the living eyeball *in toto*) [2, 7].

The involvement of ocular rigidity in serious ophthalmic morbidities such as glaucoma [8] and age-related macular degeneration [9] has been reported by several studies so far. Moreover, rigidity may be involved in important biological functions and changes, such as the accommodation ocular ageing and presbyopia [2, 10, 11]. However, despite its undeniable clinical significance, rigidity has not been equally accepted by clinicians as a parameter affecting decision making in the every-day practice [2, 12]. The main reason for this disparity is the fact that rigidity is difficult to measure with accurate, reproducible and, more importantly, non-invasive methods [2, 12] (Fig. 4.2). Historically, the first method of quantitative assessment of ocular rigidity has been the differential tonometry, described by Jonas Friedenwald in the early twentieth century [13, 14]. Several researchers have attempted to measure ocular rigidity ever since, with methodologies which were in most cases represent variations of differential tonometry (Fig. 4.3) [8, 15–17]. In this chapter, we are going to present some recently described alternative methods of ocular rigidity assessment which may be particularly useful from a practical point of view.

Historical Perspective

The need to assess differences in ocular rigidity between individuals originated from clinical observations on the accuracy of tonometry. Indeed, an early clinical observation was that intraocular pressure (IOP) measurements differed when taken with different tonometers, such as the Schiötz, Souter, McLean and Gradle tonometers from the same eyes [14, 18]. This intriguing finding led Jonas Friedenwald to suggest that such disparities may be explained by differences in bio-mechanical behavior in human eyes [13, 14]. He proposed that the calibration of tonometers was

Fig. 4.2 Advanatages and disadvantages of non-invasive ocular rigidity measurements

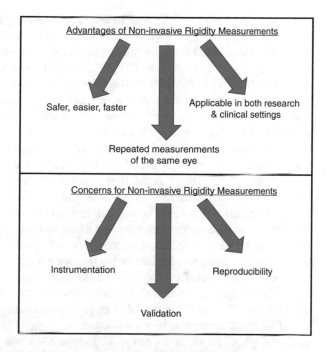

Researcher	Date	Methodology	r score
Friedenwald	1037	Differential tonometry	0.0215
Goldmann & Schmidt	1957	Differential tonometry	0.0200
Drance	1960	Differential tonometry	0.0217
Agrawal	1991	Differential tonometry	0.0217
Pallikaris	2005	Anterior chamber manometry	0.0126

Fig. 4.3 Historical overview of methodologies for ocular rigidity measurement

based on average values of ocular wall rigidity but individual eyes may deviate significantly from these mean values [13, 14]. Friedenwald then introduced the concept of "ocular rigidity coefficient" (*r*) as a metric of ocular rigidity and proposed a classic methodology (differential tonometry) based on paired measurements of IOP with 2 different weights in Schiötz indentation tonometry (or alternatively, Schiötz indentation and Goldmann applanation tonometry) to measure r [13, 14]. According to classic Friedenwald teaching, the volume change of the eye associated with the change of the IOP from IOP_0 to IOP_1 is directly proportional to the common logarithm of the ratio of IOP_0 and IOP_1 ($Log[P_1/P_0]/DV$) and r represents the proportionality constant in this equation. Moreover, although Friedenwald calculated a mean value for r of 0.0215 mmHg/mL for human eyes he also reported a wide variation in the value of r between individual eyes and developed a nomogram for the customized measurement of r [13, 14]. However, his calculations were based on observation on enucleated human eyes and this has lead to severe criticism for his method since rigidity in enucleated eyes differs significantly from that in living eyes due to several post-mortem changes [2, 16]. Such changes include, apart from the lack of blood circulation and vascular collapse, structural alterations in the ocular walls and changes in the tone of the muscular apparatus surrounding the eyeball [2, 16]. In fact, it has been reported that ocular rigidity may display characteristic variations after death, including a reduction during the first 4 h post-mortem and increase 14 h post-mortem [2]. Therefore, the quest for the accurate measurement of ocular rigidity in living eyes remained and several researchers, including Goldmann and Schmidt [15], Drance [8], Agrawal et al. [17] and Pallikaris et al. [16] attempted to revisit this important issue by measuring ocular rigidity in living eyes with similar methodologies. The Central Corneal Thickness (CCT) has also been used as a surrogate measurement of corneal biomechanics [19, 20], although it soon became evident that CCT does not completely describe corneal rigidity since it is affected by corneal hydration status, whereas corneal rigidity is also affected by qualitative differences of collagen fibers apart from the sheer thickness of tissue. More recently, the problem of ocular rigidity measurement has been addressed by interesting alternative methods, taking advantage of technological advances in ophthalmic examinations.

Axial Length (AL)-Associated OR Measurement

Previous studies have stressed the close association between axial length (AL) of the eyeball and ocular rigidity [21]. The fact that a quick reduction in IOP is followed by a reduction in AL lead Ebneter et al. [22] to propose an interesting, non-invasive method of ocular rigidity measurement. This method takes advantage of the sharp reduction of IOP induced by the oral administration of 500 mg of acetazolamide. AL and IOP are measured before acetazolamide administration as well as 2 h post-acetazolamide administration. AL is measured with partial coherence laser interferometry, a non-touch method, avoiding any mechanical stress which could cause anterio-posterior deformation of the eyeball. IOP is measured by non-applanation tonometry, which also reduces the possibility of corneal deformation and the resulting AL decrease per mmHg of IOP reduction has been used as an estimate of OR. Theoretically, the lack of mechanical forces acting on the eyeball during measurements (apart from the non-applanation tonometry) strengthens the validity of the method. On the other hand, some pharmacological actions of acetazolamide, such as effects of acetazolamide on the choroidal and retinal circulations, through vasodilator action, possibly mediated by induced extracellular acidosis or through an increased ocular perfusion pressure, raise concerns on potential induced rigidity changes during measurements.

Measurement of Pulse Amplitude and Fundus Pulse

The Ocular Pulse Amplitude (OPA) corresponds to the IOP changes during the cardiac circle (cardiac systole and diastole), presuming that the venous outflow from the eye is non-pulsatile [23, 24]. A single-mode diode laser (783 nm) has been used to measure the distance between the surfaces of cornea and retina by employing interference fringes of re-emitted waves from these surfaces. A variation of the interference order [DN(t)] during the cardiac cycle can then be evaluated by counting the fringes between inward and outward move during the cardiac circle and the fundus pulse amplitude is defined as changes in the optical distance [DL(t)], corresponding to the cornea–retina distance changes, calculated as:

$$DL(t) = DN(t).\lambda / 2$$

The highest scores of IOP during systole and diastole (IOP1 and IOP2, respectively) are also calculated and a metric (E1) of the mechanical properties of the eyeball, based on the Friedenwald's equation is calculated as:

$$E1 = (\log IOP1 \quad \log IOP2) / \text{Fundus Pulse Amplitude}$$

Interestingly, the calculated factor E1 was significantly higher in the patients with primary open angle glaucoma and findings support the concept that the biomechanical properties of ocular tissues play a role in the glaucomatous pathogenetic process [24].

Elastography

Pathological tissues often differ from normal tissues in terms of elasticity. This finding was incorporated in traditional medical thinking very early and lead to the inclusion of tissue palpation in the process of physical examination. However, the subjective nature of palpation lead to the development of more objective and reproducible methods for the evaluation of living tissue elasticity, such as elastography, which was aimed at replacing tactile feedback with imaging techniques [25–27]. In the case of ultrasound elastography, tissue elasticity is examined by 2 different methodologies, i.e. strain elastography and shear-wave elastography. In the former [28], changes in ultrasound reflectivity inflicted by the mechanical pressure exerted on the tissues by the footprint of the ultrasound probe are translated in elastographic readings. In the latter, shear-waves are evaluated [29, 30]. These are low frequency waves propagated in the tissues at a direction vertical to the direction of propagation of ultrasound waves. The production and propagation of shear waves are closely associated with tissue elasticity. Strain elastography is basically a qualitative technique limited to superficial tissue evaluation due to the inability to compress deeper tissues [31]. On the contrary, shear wave elastography may be applied in the assessment of deeper tissues and produce quantitative measurements of tissue elasticity (usually expressed in KPa) [30]. Apart from ultrasonic waves, the generation of shear waves within the tissues can also be performed by tissue vibration (usually in the range of 50–500 Hz) and changes in tissue behavior may be examined by MRI imaging (MRI elastography) [32]. Another option is the assessment of shear waves generated within the tissues by normal functions such as the respiratory movements, heart beat or blood circulation. This passive examination of such tissue "noise" and its association with tissue elasticity may also be performed by other modalities such as Optical Coherence Tomography (OCT) [33]. The latter may be particularly applicable in ophthalmic elastographic imaging and may be a promising new modality to assess elasticity in living ocular tissues in the near future.

However, both forms of classic ultrasound elastography (strain and shear-wave) have also been applied for the evaluation of ocular rigidity [30, 31]. Previous studies in both human and animal living eyes have shown that ocular elastographic imaging is feasible and may produce clinically useful findings for the evaluation of various pathologies, such as ocular tumors, intraocular hemorrhages and detachments and well as periocular conditions, such as Graves' orbitopathy [30, 31]. Color or greyscale maps of the eyeball and surrounding structures may be produced displaying differences in the elastographic signals for different areas of the eyeball and in the case of shear-wave ophthalmic elastography such maps may be combined with quantitative measurements of tissue rigidity indices [30, 31].

Evaluation of Corneal Hysteresis

Hysteresis is a metric of system behavior in response to the exertion of deforming forces [34]. Upon the action of such a force, a system may reach a point of maximum departure from its original status and then, depending on its rigidity-elasticity features (essentially the system "memory") it may return to its original status [34]. Therefore, hysteresis may be considered as the dependence of the state of a system on its history. In the case of cornea, hysteresis has been examined as a metric of the "memory" of living cornea following the exertion of deforming forces [35]. The Ocular Response Analyzer (ORA) has been designed as a system to measure corneal hysteresis in living human eyes, introduced in 2004 by Reichert Ophthalmic Instruments, Inc. (Depew, NY, USA) [35, 36]. ORA is capable of providing information on a variety of parameters associated with corneal biomechanical behavior, including the IOP, CCT, corneal hysteresis (CH) and corneal resistance factor (CRF) [35, 36]. It incorporates an eye-tracking sensor capable of mediating alignment of the eye with the system and directs a stream of air towards to central cornea. This deforms (applanates) central cornea while an infrared light detector captures light from the corneal surface. The inward movement of the corneal surface reaches of point of applanation (recorded as P1 on the ORA signal plot) and then the cornea indents and retracts to a second applanation event (recorded as P2 on the ORA signal plot). The ORA provides 2 distinct measurements of IOP: The IOP_G, which is closely related to Goldmann applanation tonometry and corresponds to the IOP value at the first applanation point in the ORA waveform (P1). And the IOP_{CC}, an estimate of IOP corrected for the biomechanical properties of the cornea. CH is also recorded as the difference in IOP between the 2 applanation events and is a metric of corneal viscous damping (the ability of corneal tissue to absorb and dissipate energy), calculated as the difference in pressure between the two corneal applanation events (P1–P2). CRF is also calculated from these two pressure values according to a complex algorithm and represents a metric estimate of the viscoelastic behavior of corneal tissue.

Although CH may be indeed be linked to corneal biomechanics its true meaning and nature may be more complex and intriguing [35]. CH has been shown to decrease during aging, when the cornea is known to stiffen, as well as to decrease after the cornea has been stiffened by cross-linking techniques [35].

Such findings may sound contradictory but may comply with models of differential participation of viscous and elastic elements in corneal bio-mechanics and certainly reflect the complexity of biomechanics in living tissues.

Applanation and Non-applanation Differential Tonometry

The idea of taking advantage of the differential tonometry process as a way to measure ocular rigidity (using 2 different weights in Schiötz tonometry or Schiötz and Goldman tonometry, according to standard Friedenwald methodology), has led to the suggestion that the same methodology may be applied by taking advantage of ΔIOP, i.e. of the difference between standard Goldmann applanation tonometry and non-applanation tonometry ("Pascal" tonometry) [37]. According to this suggestion, the applanation of the corneal apex in standard Goldmann tonometry changes the volume of the anterior segment of the eyeball whereas tonometry using the non-applanation tonometer does not induce geometric alterations in the corneal apex (since the tonometer head conforms to the anterior corneal surface) and thus does not induce significant volume changes in the anterior ocular segment [12] (Fig. 4.4). The proposed methodology can arrive to a rigidity coefficient (r) by measuring volume changes induced during applanation tonometry (ΔV) and associating them with IOP differences between the 2 tonometric methodologies (applanation and non-applanation) in a process similar to the standard Friedenwald methodology.

Fig. 4.4 Schematic representation of ocular rigidity measurement by taking advantage of the displaced volume during applanation tonometry and applying differential tonometry with non-applanation tonometry

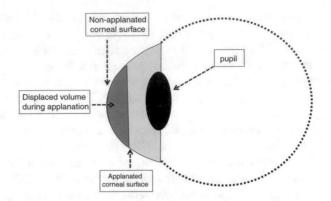

The suggested technique uses by convention the IOP readings of non-applanation tonometry as a measure of "true" IOP, but converts IOP readings of applanation tonometry according to the Orsengo-Pye algorithm, since accurate applanation tonometry readings are obtained when corneal geometry conforms to the so called "calibrated" cornea [38]. According to the previously published model of Orssengo-Pye [38], GAT IOP readings equal true IOP when corneal parameters are in agreement with the geometrical characteristics of the so-called "calibrated cornea", such as CCT of 520 μm and mean external radius of curvature of 7.8 mm. In the proposed methodology, deviations of GAT IOP from true IOP in eyes with corneas different from the "calibration cornea" were corrected by applying the Orssengo-Pye algorithm [17]: $IOP_P = \dfrac{IOP_G}{C/B}$, with the error coefficient "C/B", in which B corresponds to the IOP_G of the calibrated cornea and C corresponds to the IOP of the measured cornea [17]. B and C were calculated with the following formulas:

$$B = \frac{0,6 \cdot \pi \cdot R \cdot \left(R - \dfrac{t}{2}\right) \cdot \sqrt{1 - v^2}}{t^2}, C = \frac{\pi \cdot R \cdot \left(R - \dfrac{t}{2}\right)^2 \cdot (1 - v)}{A \cdot t.}$$

In these equations, R corresponds to the anterior corneal curvature, t corresponds to CCT, v is the corneal Poisson's index (0.49) and A corresponds to the area of applanation of the anterior corneal surface by applanation tonometry. A rigidity coefficient (r) may be calculated in this technique as:

$$r = \left[\left(IOPpascal - IOPGoldmann / \Delta V \right) * C / B \right] * E,$$

where E corresponds to the mean corneal Young's modulus.

The validity of this methodology has been tested in a group of cataract surgery candidates, not suffering from glaucoma or previous ophthalmic pathologies (including trauma, surgery or inflammation) which could potentially affects rigidity. Interestingly, the r measured (0.0174 ± 0.010 [0.0123 – 0.022] mmHg/μL) is very close to the previously reported measurements by other methodologies in living human eyes [12].

Concluding Remarks

Ocular rigidity remains an important parameter in modern clinical thinking for ophthalmologists, with potential involvement in many serious pathologies, such as glaucoma, age related macular degeneration or age-related refractive changes. The lack of an accurate and consistent methodology to measure ocular rigidity has been the main drawback for its widespread use in the every-day clinical practice. Measuring ocular rigidity by invasive methodologies is impractical and restricts its use mainly for experimental purposes. However, many interesting alternative methods for non-invasive ocular rigidity measurement in human living eyes have emerged during the previous years, providing promising options for both clinical applications and basic research in visual sciences.

References

1. Goldmann H. Applanation tonometry. In: Newell FW, editor. Glaucoma second conference. New York: J Macy Jr. Foundation; 1956. p. 167–220.
2. Detorakis ET, Pallikaris IG. Ocular rigidity: biomechanical role, in vivo measurements and clinical significance. Clin Exp Ophthalmol. 2013;41(1):73–81.
3. Kling S, Hafezi F. Biomechanical stiffening: slow low-irradiance corneal crosslinking versus the standard Dresden protocol. J Cataract Refract Surg. 2017;43:975–9.
4. Ramirez-Garcia MA, Sloan SR, Nidenberg B, Khalifa YM, Buckley MR. Depth-dependent out-of-plane Young's Modulus of the human cornea. Curr Eye Res. 2018;43:595–604.
5. Friberg TR, Lace JW. A comparison of the elastic properties of human choroid and sclera. Exp Eye Res. 1988;47:429–36.
6. Cardoso L, Cowin SC. Role of structural anisotropy of biological tissues in poroelastic wave propagation. Mech Mater. 2012 January;44:174–88.
7. Asejczyk-Widlicka M, Pierscionek BK. The elasticity and rigidity of the outer coats of the eye. Br J Ophthalmol. 2008;92(10):1415.
8. Drance SM. The coefficient of scleral rigidity in normal and glaucomatous eyes. Arch Ophthalmol. 1960;63:668–74.
9. Pallikaris IG, Kymionis GD, Ginis HS, Kounis GA, Christodoulakis E, Tsilimbaris MK. Ocular rigidity in patients with age-related macular degeneration. Am J Ophthalmol. 2006;141:611–5.
10. Tezel G, Luo C, Yang X. Accelerated aging in glaucoma: immunohistochemical assessment of advanced glycation end products in the human retina and optic nerve head. Invest Ophthalmol Vis Sci. 2007;48:1201–11.
11. Nguyen CT, Bui BV, Sinclair AJ, Vingrys AJ. Dietary omega 3 fatty acids decrease intraocular pressure with age by increasing aqueous outflow. Invest Ophthalmol Vis Sci. 2007;48:756–62.
12. Detorakis ET, Tsaglioti E, Kymionis G. Non-invasive ocular rigidity measurement: a differential tonometry approach. Acta Medica (Hradec Kralove). 2015;58(3):92–7.
13. Friedenwald JS. Clinical significance of ocular rigidity in relation to the tonometric measurement. Trans Am Acad Ophthalmol Otolaryngol. 1949;53:262–4.
14. Friedenwald JS. Tonometer calibration; an attempt to remove discrepancies found in the 1954 calibration scale for Schiotz tonometers. Trans Am Acad Ophthalmol Otolaryngol. 1957;61:108–222.
15. Goldmann H, Schmidt T. Friedenwald's rigidity coefficient. Ophthalmologica. 1957;133:330–5.
16. Pallikaris IG, Kymionis GD, Ginis HS, Kounis GA, Tsilimbaris MK. Ocular rigidity in living human eyes. Invest Ophthalmol Vis Sci. 2005;46:409–14.

17. Agrawal KK, Sharma DP, Bhargava G, Sanadhya DK. Scleral rigidity in glaucoma, before and during topical antiglaucoma drug therapy. Indian J Ophthalmol. 1991;39:85–6.
18. Eisenlohr JE, Langham ME, Maumenee AE. Manometric studies of the pressure-volume relationship in living and enucleated eyes of individual human subjects. Br J Ophthalmol. 1962;46:536–48.
19. W L, Pye D. Changes in corneal biomechanics and applanation tonometry with induced corneal swelling. Invest Ophthalmol Vis Sci. 2011 May 16;52:3207–14.
20. Kotecha A, Elsheikh A, Roberts CR, Zhu H, Garway-Heath DF. Corneal thickness- and age-related biomechanical properties of the corneameasured with the ocular response analyzer. Invest Ophthalmol Vis Sci. 2006;47:5337–47.
21. Dastiridou AI, Ginis H, Tsilimbaris M, Karyotakis N, Detorakis E, Siganos C, Cholevas P, Tsironi EE, Pallikaris IG. Ocular rigidity, ocular pulse amplitude, and pulsatile ocular blood flow: the effect of axial length. Invest Ophthalmol Vis Sci. 2013;54:2087–92.
22. Ebneter A, Wagels B, Zinkernagel MS. Non-invasive biometric assessment of ocular rigidity in glaucoma patients and controls. Eye. 2009;23:606–11.
23. Dastiridou AI, Ginis HS, De Brouwere D, Tsilimbaris MK, Pallikaris IG. Ocular rigidity, ocular pulse amplitude and pulsatile ocular blood flow: the effect of intraocular pressure. Invest Ophthalmol Vis Sci. 2009;50:5718–22.
24. Hommer A, Fuchsjäger-Mayrl G, Resch H, Vass C, Garhofer G. Schmetterer estimation of ocular rigidity based on measurement of pulse amplitude using pneumotonometry and fundus pulse using laser interferometry in glaucoma. Invest Ophthalmol Vis Sci. 2008;49:4046–50.
25. Nowicki A, Dobruch-Sobczak K. Introduction to ultrasound elastography. J Ultrason. 2016;16:113–24.
26. Low G, Kruse SA, Lomas DJ. General review of magnetic resonance elastography. World J Radiol. 2016;28(8):59–72.
27. Garra BS. Elastography: history, principles, and technique comparison. Abdom Imaging. 2015;40:680–97.
28. Dietrich CF, Barr RG, Farrokh A, Dighe M, Hocke M, Jenssen C, Dong Y, Saftoiu A, Havre RF. Strain elastography - how to do it? Ultrasound Int Open. 2017;3:E137–49.
29. Ozturk A, Grajo JR, Dhyani M, Anthony BW, Samir AE. Principles of ultrasound elastography. Abdom Radiol (NY). 2018;43:773–85.
30. Detorakis ET, Drakonaki EE, Ginis H, Karyotakis N, Pallikaris IG. Evaluation of iridociliary and lenticular elasticity using shear-wave elastography in rabbit eyes. Acta Medica (Hradec Kralove). 2014;57:9–14.
31. Detorakis ET, Drakonaki EE, Tsilimbaris MK, Pallikaris IG, Giarmenitis S. Real-time ultrasound elastographic imaging of ocular and periocular tissues: a feasibility study. Ophthalmic Surg Lasers Imaging. 2010;41:135–41.
32. Litwiller DV, Mariappan YK, Ehman RL. Magnetic resonance elastography. Curr Med Imaging Rev. 2012;8:46–55.
33. Nguyen TM, Zorgani A, Lescanne M, Boccara C, Fink M, Catheline S. Diffuse shear wave imaging: toward passive elastography using low-frame rate spectral-domain optical coherence tomography. J Biomed Opt. 2016;21:126013.
34. Piñero DP, Alcón N. Corneal biomechanics: a review. Clin Exp Optom. 2015;98:107–16.
35. Glass DH, Roberts CJ, Litsky AS, Weber PAA. Viscoelastic biomechanical model of the cornea describing the effect of viscosity and elasticity on hysteresis. Invest ophthalmol Vis Sci. 2008;49:3919–26.
36. Terai N, Raiskup F, Haustein M, Pillunat LE, Spoerl E. Identification of biomechanical properties of the cornea: the ocular response analyzer. Curr Eye Res. 2012;37:553–62.
37. Detorakis ET, Arvanitaki V, Pallikaris IG, Kymionis G, Tsilimbaris MK. Applanation tonometry versus dynamic contour tonometry in eyes treated with latanoprost. J Glaucoma. 2010;19:194–8.
38. Orssengo GJ, Pye DC. Determination of the true intraocular pressure and modulus of elasticity of the human cornea in vivo. Bull Math Biol. 1999;61:551–72.

Chapter 5
Clinical Assessment of Corneal Biomechanics

Cynthia J. Roberts

Introduction

Interest in corneal biomechanics has continually increased since the ability to measure biomechanical deformation response with a clinical instrument became possible in 2005 with the introduction of the Ocular Response Analyzer (ORA), manufactured by Reichert Technologies, Depew, NY in the United States [1]. Several years later, the Corneal Visualization Scheimpflug Technology (Corvis ST) was introduced, manufactured by Oculus Optikgeräte GmbH in Wetzlar, Germany [2]. Historically, corneal biomechanical properties have been assessed via uniaxial strip testing which required destructive loading [3–6]. A clinical device, on the other hand, requires a nondestructive load to assess corneal biomechanics. Both the ORA and the Corvis ST meet this challenge by using an air puff to deform the cornea in order to evaluate biomechanical deformation response. This does not allow measurement of classic biomechanical properties such as elastic modulus. However, it does allow quantitative analysis of deformation response and interpretation of the biomechanical parameters produced which can be correlated to viscoelasticity, change in viscoelasticity, stiffness, or change in stiffness. Although the two devices have an air puff load in common, there are important distinctions between them that affect interpretation of the parameters that each device reports. Therefore, the two systems will be discussed in detail, followed by a comparison between them.

C. J. Roberts (✉)
Martha G. and Milton Staub Chair for Research in Ophthalmology, Ohio State Havener Eye Institute, Columbus, OH, USA

Department of Ophthalmology & Visual Sciences, The Ohio State University Wexner Medical Center, Columbus, OH, USA

Department of Biomedical Engineering, The Ohio State University, Columbus, OH, USA
e-mail: roberts.8@osu.edu

© Springer Nature Switzerland AG 2021
I. Pallikaris et al. (eds.), *Ocular Rigidity, Biomechanics and Hydrodynamics of the Eye*, https://doi.org/10.1007/978-3-030-64422-2_5

The classic biomechancial properties to which the biomechanical deformation parameters can be compared include elasticity, viscosity, and viscoleasticity. Elasticity is defined as the ability of a material to return to its original state after deformation, once the load has been removed. There is no time-dependent component. The tensile elastic modulus quantifies the relationship between stress (applied force as a function of crossectional area) and strain (elongation as a percentage) [7]. The higher the elastic modulus, the greater is the resistance to deformation, and the greater is the stiffness. The elastic properties are measured during loading, and for an elastic material there is no difference between loading and unloading paths. Viscosity is defined as the resistance to permanent deformation and has a time-dependent component. As an example, honey has greater viscosity than water since honey has greater resistance to permanent deformation. Viscoelasticity defines a material that exhibits both elastic and viscous behaviors. There is a time-dependent component to the response and there is a difference between the loading and unloading paths in terms of response. This difference is called hysteresis. For a viscoelastic material like the cornea, there is a difference in response between loading with an air puff and unloading where the air pressure is reduced, and it can be quantified in multiple ways. Therefore, there must be an assessment during both loading and unloading with a comparison of the two at the same defined state or quantification of the area between the two pathways.

Only the two devices mentioned are currently commercially available, both based on response to an air puff as the nondestructive loading of the cornea. However, the responses elicited are quite distinct, since not only do the loads have different temporal profiles, but the techniques used to assess corneal biomechanical response are also distinct. Therefore, the reported parameters from the two devices should be considered complementary, rather than competitive. Details of the similarities and differences will be highlighted.

The Ocular Response Analyzer

The air pressure puff of the Ocular Response Analyzer (ORA), which is Gaussian in both spatial and temporal profiles [8], is customized to each patient such that a greater magnitude maximum air pressure is delivered to an eye with a higher intraocular pressure (IOP). This is accomplished by the device sensing the first applanation event (A1) and shutting down the signal sent to the piston in the nozzle. Inertia in the piston allows the air pressure to continue to rise after the shutdown pressure is reached. Therefore, the increasing air pressure profile prior to A1 is identical for all measurements, but the post-A1 rising pressure to maximum and subsequent decreasing pressure profile are distinct depending on the timing of A1. One consequence of this design is that each measurement will reach a different maximum magnitude of air pressure [9]. The factors that influence the timing of A1 are primarily the intraocular pressure and secondarily the stiffness of the cornea.

Corneal displacement is detected by an indirect assessment technique. The geometry of the system includes an infrared (IR) emitter that is aligned with an IR detector such that when the cornea flattens at A1, a mirror-like reflection maximizes the number of photons striking the detector. This generates a spike on the infrared signal, as illustrated in Fig. 5.1. The peak magnitude (Peak 1) of the IR signal at A1 is dependent on the number of photons striking the detector [10]. As the cornea passes through A1 at first applanation pressure (P1), it becomes concave in shape and fewer photons are aligned with the detector, reducing the IR signal. Subsequently, the cornea begins to recover, traversing the applanated state in the outward direction (A2) at the second applanation pressure, P2, generating a second peak in the IR signal. The difference between the applanation pressures at A1 and A2 is defined as corneal hysteresis (CH), and represents the viscoelastic lag in the system. In a valid measurement, P2 is always less than P1. The average of the applanation pressures is defined as Goldmann-correlated IOP (IOPg). Additional investigations were done by the manufacturer to empirically develop both Corneal Resistance Factor (CRF) and Corneal Compensated IOP (IOPcc). CRF is designed to correlate strongly with central corneal thickness (CCT), and IOPcc is designed to compensate for the

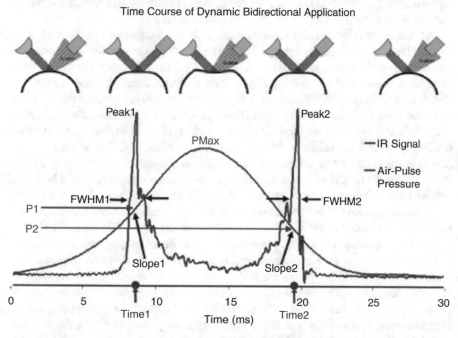

Fig. 5.1 Schematic of the signals produced by the cornea deforming under an ORA air pulse, with the infrared signal in red and the pressure signal in blue. The states of deformation are illustrated above the signals, and include pre-deformation, first applanation, concavity, second applanation, and the recovered cornea. The signals are labeled with the first and second applanation pressures (P1 and P2), the first and second applanation times (Time1 and Time2), the first and second applanation full width half maximum values (FWHM1 and FWHM2) and the maximum pressure, Pmax (Reprinted from Ref. 9)

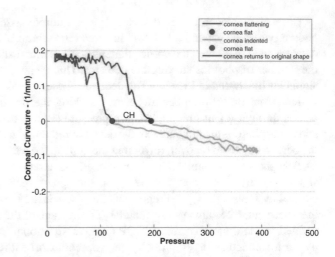

Fig. 5.2 Plot of infrared signal (y axis) vs pressure (x axis) demonstrating hysteresis in the loading and unloading paths (Reprinted from Ref. 8)

differences in biomechanics and CCT after refractive surgery in estimation of IOP [8]. The consequence of this approach is that IOPcc is more accurate than Goldmann Applanation Tonometry (GAT) in estimating IOP in corneas with reduced stiffness, such as after refractive surgery or with keratoconus [1, 11].

What is corneal hysteresis biomechanically? It is a comparison of the load at the two applanated states of the cornea, one during loading and one during unloading, and represents the viscoelastic nature of the cornea. There are other ways to evaluate hysteresis, which include plotting the loading and unloading pathways, shown in Fig. 5.2, as well as a similar concept in Hysteresis Loop Area, which actually quantifies the area circumscribed by the difference in loading vs unloading pathways [12]. Both CH and CRF are viscoelastic parameters, since both are functions of the loading (P1) and unloading pressures (P2). Unfortunately, CH is often misinterpreted in the literature as stiffness, a purely elastic parameter, which it is NOT [9]. A cornea with low CH can be a soft cornea, as in keratoconus, or it can be a stiff cornea, as in an aging eye or an eye with high IOP. The value depends on the associated viscosity, since CH is a function of both elasticity and viscosity. Different combinations of elasticity and viscosity can produce the same CH value [13]. It is necessary to examine the IR and pressure signals in detail to gain additional biomechanical information for complete interpretation of the corneal elastic response. The widths of the applanation peaks are associated with the velocity of the cornea. The faster the motion, the narrower are the peaks. The magnitudes of the applanation peaks (Peak 1 and Peak 2) are associated with corneal stiffness. The greater the magnitudes, the greater the applanated area with more photons striking the detector, and the stiffer is the cornea. This was demonstrated in small study comparing the size of the applanated area in four normal subjects and three subjects previously diagnosed with keratoconus [10]. Two high speed cameras were aligned with the ORA, providing a temporal view and an inferior view, as shown in Fig. 5.3. Typical ORA signals from a keratoconic cornea and a normal cornea are shown in Fig. 5.4. The IR signal amplitude peaks were extracted, and CH and CRF were recorded for

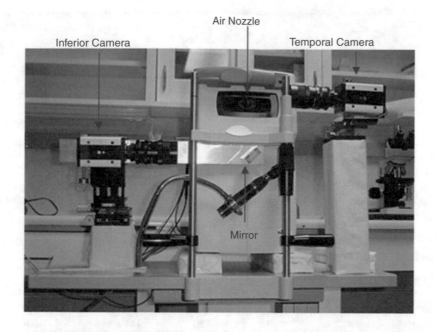

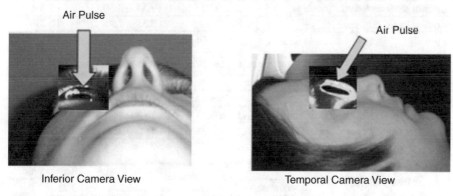

Fig. 5.3 Experimental set up of ORA with two high speed cameras aligned for a temporal view and an inferior view used to measure the deformation width (Reprinted from Ref. 10)

each group, the means of which are shown in Table 5.1. Two diameters of applanation were extracted from the two camera views of each subject, and group means are shown in Table 5.2. The correlations of Peak 1 and Peak 2 amplitudes with the applanation diameters in each group are shown in Table 5.3. These data show not only that the Peak amplitudes are significantly lower in keratoconus than normal subjects, but also strong correlations of both Peak 1 and Peak 2 with the diameters extracted from the inferior view in both normal and keratoconic subjects. The inferior view camera is aligned with the horizontal meridian of the cornea, which is the same meridian measured by the ORA. The correlations are less strong in the temporal view camera which measures the vertical meridian, and is not the same as

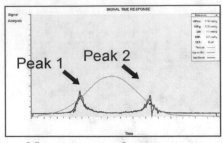
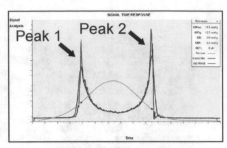

Keratoconic cornea   Normal cornea

Fig. 5.4 Infrared (red) and pressure (green) signals from ORA exams of a keratoconic patient (left) and a normal patient (right). Note that Peak 1 and Peak 2 are quite damped in the keratoconic eye (Reprinted from Ref. 10)

Table 5.1 Ocular response analyzer metrics

Normal (n = 4) vs. Keratoconic (n = 3) Corneas			
Parameter	Avg. normal	Avg. Keratoconic	P value
Infrared signal peak 1	748 ± 139	352 ± 122	0.001
Infrared signal peak 2	638 ± 150	344 ± 185	0.017
Corneal resistance factor (mmHg)	9.25 ± 0.93	7.34 ± 2.30	0.066
Corneal hysteresis (mmHg)	9.26 ± 0.68	8.55 ± 1.91	0.230

Table 5.2 Inferior and temporal camera view applanation diameter measurements

Normal (n = 4) vs. Keratoconic (n = 3) Corneas			
Parameter	Avg. normal	Avg. Keratoconic	P value
Diameter from inferior camera (mm)	4.87 ± 0.23	4.36 ± 0.44	0.029
Diameter from temporal camera (mm)	4.81 ± 0.33	4.43 ± 0.22	0.046

Table 5.3 Correlations between IR signal peak heights and deformation diameters

	Normal	Keratoconic
Diameter inferior and peak 1	0.92	0.88
Diameter inferior and peak 2	0.72	0.92
Diameter temporal and peak 1	−0.09	0.64
Diameter temporal and peak 2	−0.35	0.70

measured by the ORA. The conclusion is that normal subjects have a larger applanation diameter which aligns a larger number of photons with the detector, generating greater applanation Peak amplitudes in the IR signal. The stiffer corneas in the normal subjects are more resistant to deformation, producing a wider, shallower deformation. The softer keratoconic corneas are less resistant to deformation, and produce a narrower, deeper deformation. The differences are profound enough to reach significance, even with the small number of subjects. Interestingly, neither CH nor CRF are significantly different between normal and keratoconic subjects in this small study. This is very likely due to the low number of subjects and the low sensitivity of CH alone, without the signal parameters, to differentiate normal subjects from those with keratoconus, which is consistent with the literature [1].

There is a great body of literature on custom analysis of the IR and pressure signals of the ORA to evaluate disease processes and response to procedures such as refractive surgery and corneal crosslinking [14]. The first such paper was a case report of a patient who had refractive surgery and developed ectasia in only one eye. The magnitude of Peak 1 in the IR signal was greater in the eye without complications after refractive surgery than the lower Peak 1 in the fellow eye that developed ectasia, despite no difference in CH. This case can be interpreted that the cornea with the uncomplicated post-operative course is stiffer than the cornea that developed ectasia [15]. The Peak amplitude was also compared between post-op and pre-op myopic LASIK (n = 14) and myopic LASEK (n = 15), which is a form of surface ablation. There was a significantly greater reduction in the amplitude of Peak 1 post-operatively in the LASIK group than the LASEK group. This can be interpreted that LASIK with a flap causes a greater biomechanical impact than LASEK, which is consistent with the literature.

Interpreting the biomechanical data after corneal collagen crosslinking (CXL) requires evaluation of the IR signal data to be definitive, since it has been reported by multiple authors that there is no difference in CH after the procedure, but there are significant differences in various features of the IR and pressure signals [16–18]. CXL affects not only the stiffness of the cornea, but also the viscosity, such that changes in elasticity are masked by changes in viscosity. In a study of 26 eyes of 26 subjects who received CXL using the Dresden protocol, compared to 16 untreated fellow eyes of the same subjects, the changes in ORA parameters 6 months after the procedure are given in Table 5.4 and show that both P1 and P2 increase significantly after CXL, resulting in no difference in CH [19]. To link biomechanical changes to curvature changes, the Cone Location and Magnitude Index (CLMI) was calculated on pre and 6 months post-CXL tomographic maps [20]. Part of this calculation is to locate the 2 mm diameter circular region of the greatest curvature, called Cspot in the current analysis. There were significant negative correlations between ΔCspot and ΔIOPcc (p = 0.0020 in treated group, not significant in control) and between ΔCspot and ΔP2 (p = 0.0036 in treated group, not significant in control). However, ΔCspot was not significantly related to ΔP1 in either group. This can be interpreted that an increase in the unloading parameter, P2, is significantly correlated with reduction in curvature in the treated group, but not the loading parameter, P1. Therefore, the

Table 5.4 Pre-CXL to 6 months Post-CXL ocular response analyzer parameters

Treated eyes (n = 26) vs. Fellow control eyes (n = 16)			
Parameter	Treatment eyes	Fellow control eyes	P value
Δ IOPg (mmHg)	+1.2 ± 2.2	−1.1 ± 1.4	0.0004
Δ IOPcc (mmHg)	+1.4 ± 3.5	−1.3 ± 1.9	0.0020
Δ P1 (mmHg)	+7.5 ± 17.3	−5.8 ± 15.3	0.0155
ΔP2 (mmHg)	+10.8 ± 20.7	−8.3 ± 10.9	0.0003

significant increase in both IOPcc, and IOPg do NOT indicate an actual increase in IOP, but rather an increase in stiffness since both P1 and P2 also increased.

Correlation of the viscoelastic CH parameter with evidence of glaucomatous damage was first reported in 2006, where a low CH value was associated progressive field worsening [21]. This launched many studies of the value of CH in managing glaucoma. More recently, a prospective longitudinal study showed that CH was significantly associated with glaucomatous progression, with lower CH associated with a faster rate of visual field loss [22]. Evidence suggests that there may be a benefit in using CH to manage glaucoma, and highlights the value of a viscoelastic parameter.

The Corvis ST

The Corvis ST produces a consistent air puff for every exam, independent of the corneal properties or the IOP of the individual eye under examination [23]. Therefore, every cornea reaches its limit of displacement prior to the time point where the air puff reaches its peak magnitude. At the point where the limit of corneal displacement is achieved, but with the air pressure continuing to increase, backward motion of the whole eye becomes rapid and nonlinear in nature. Once the air pressure peaks and begins to decrease, the cornea begins to recover. However, the whole eye is still moving backwards. In other words, the cornea is moving in the forward direction while the globe is moving backwards. Once the cornea recovers its pre-deformation shape, the whole eye begins to move forward in recovery towards its original position. This process is illustrated in Fig. 5.5 which also shows the phases of deformation, plus the ingoing and outgoing applanation points. These

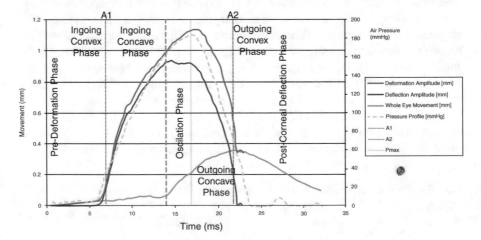

Fig. 5.5 Schematic of the nine phases of corneal deformation response to a Corvis ST air puff, superimposed over the plots of apex deformation (blue) that includes whole eye motion (green) and isolated corneal deflection (red) which is the difference between the other two. Also included in dotted gray is the air pressure profile (Reprinted from Ref. 23)

include the Pre-Deformation Phase, the Ingoing Convex Phase, First Applanation, followed by the Ingoing Concave Phase, which transitions into the Oscillation Phase at the point where maximum corneal displacement occurs. The Oscillation Phase transitions to the Outgoing Concave Phase at the point where the maximum air pressure occurs and the cornea begins to recover. Maximum whole eye motion occurs near the second applanation time point, which defines the transition to the Outgoing Convex Phase. Once the cornea is fully recovered, the final phase involves recovery of the whole eye to its pre-deformation state [23].

Corneal displacement is detected via direct assessment of motion using an ultra high-speed camera that acquires images at about 4330 frames per second for a total of 140 images over a 32 ms time frame. Selected images in various states of deformation from a single exam are shown in Fig. 5.6. A single horizontal meridian is imaged with Scheimpflug geometry to maximize depth of focus during the exam. The field of view is about 8 mm in width and 2 mm of depth into the eye, so that the

Fig. 5.6 Selected frames from a series of 140 images of the cornea deforming under a Corvis ST air puff. The top image is pre-deformation, the second and third images show the cornea deforming inward, the fourth and fifth images show the cornea recovering outward, and the bottom image shows the recovered cornea (Reprinted from Ref. 9)

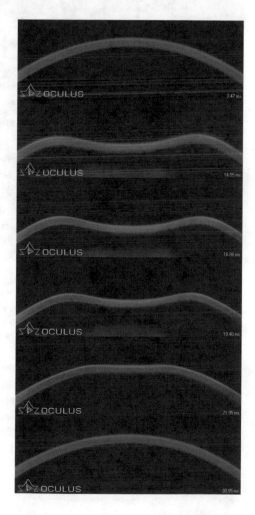

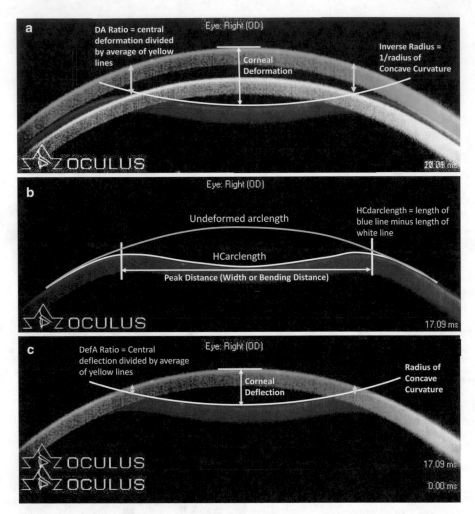

Fig. 5.7 Superimposed frames extracted from a single exam, showing (**a**) blue cornea in the pre-deformation state, red cornea in maximum cornea deflection, and a white cornea with maximum whole eye motion. Note the temporal progression of the corneal periphery at the edges of the image; (**b**) Maximum cornea deflection relative to the undeformed arc length; and (**c**) all three corneas superimposed with whole eye motion subtracted (Reprinted from Ref. 23)

entire thickness of the cornea can be captured in various states of deformation, as long as the apex of the cornea is aligned 11 mm form the nozzle, which places it in the center of the imaging window. Corneal apex displacement includes both corneal and whole eye motion. The Corvis ST differentiates between the two by defining corneal motion after subtraction of whole eye motion as corneal deflection. Therefore, "deflection" parameters refer to corneal motion only, and "deformation" parameters refer to the combination of both corneal and whole eye motion. Whole eye motion can be determined from peripheral corneal motion, outside of the region which becomes concave, as illustrated in Fig. 5.7. Many dynamic corneal response parameters (DCRs) are reported which describe the biomechanical deformation response. These include velocity parameters, timing parameters, amplitude of displacement in both deformation and deflection parameters, as well as parameters defining the shape of the deformed cornea. Specific time points include the first and second applanation events, as well as highest concavity (HC) which is the point of maximum corneal apex displacement. A stiffness parameter at first applanation (SP-A1) was developed that was defined as the load at applanation, divided by corneal displacement [23]. The load was calculated as the air pressure at applanation, adjusted for time of applanation and position within the imaging window, minus the biomechanically corrected IOP (bIOP). The displacement was calculated between the undeformed state and A1. This is more complex than the other DCR's in that the air pressure and bIOP are taken into account in the calculation.

The major factors which influence corneal deformation include IOP, corneal properties, and scleral properties. The DCRs which are sensitive to corneal biomechanical properties and relatively independent of IOP have been reported to be the shape parameters [24]. These include the radius of curvature at highest concavity (RadHC), the integrated inverse radius (IR) which is the area under the curve of concave curvature between the two applanation points, and the two ratios of deformation amplitude and deflection amplitude in the center and average deformation at a defined distance from the center (DA Ratio and DefA Ratio, respectively). Other DCRs are strongly influenced by IOP, and this should be taken into account during interpretation of individual exams. A keratoconic eye with higher IOP may exhibit stiffer behavior than a normal eye at lower IOP. Therefore, it is important to use parameters less affected by IOP in individual patient assessment, or use the Vinciguerra Display for parameters in which the individual exam values are bracketed with normative values, as shown in Fig. 5.8 [24]. It has also been shown that stiffer boundary conditions (sclera) will limit corneal deformation [25].

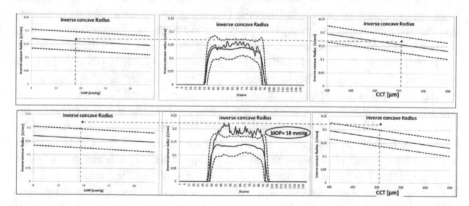

Fig. 5.8 Inverse concave radius from two exams. The top exam is from a normal subject, and the bottom exam is from a subject with keratoconus. The mean (solid line) and ±2 standard deviations lines (dotted) are shown in each side figure for bIOP (left) and CCT (right), along with an indication in red of the measured values from the specific patients. The normal patient (top) is within the normal population distribution, but the keratoconic subject (bottom) is outside of the normal range (Adapted from Ref. 24)

How can these parameters be interpreted relative to corneal stiffness? The only one that is intuitive is SP-A1, where higher values indicate greater stiffness and lower values indicate lower stiffness. For the rest, stiffness should be considered as resistance to deformation. Greater resistance to deformation is associated with greater stiffness. For the DCRs related to shape, greater DA Ratios and greater DefA Ratios indicate lower resistance to deformation and lower stiffness. Inverse radius of concave curvature is equivalent to curvature. Greater curvature (greater IR) is associated with less resistance to deformation and less stiffness. The opposite is true for radius of curvature, where a shorter radius of curvature means greater curvature. Therefore, a lower radius of concave curvature is associated with lower stiffness. The same logic can be applied to the remaining DCRs that are related to IOP.

Keratoconus is known to be a local biomechanical decompensation of the cornea, [26] and the detection of the disease is important in screening for "at risk" corneas prior to refractive surgery [27]. The Corvis Biomechanical Index (CBI) was developed as a combination index of specific DCRs and the stiffness parameter, SP-A1 [28]. This index was based on analysis of 658 patients (478 healthy and 180 diagnosed with keratoconus) from two different countries with one serving as the development database and one as the validation database. The final set of parameters that produced the best performance of CBI in separation of the two groups included DA Ratio at 1 mm, DA Ratio at 2 mm, velocity at A1, standard deviation of deformation amplitude at HC, Ambrósio's Relational Thickness to the horizontal profile (ARTh), and SP-A1. The receiver operator characteristic curve (ROC) analysis showed an area under the curve of 0.983. It was later reported that using an artificial intelligence approach called the Random Forest method produced a Tomographic and Biomechanical Index (TBI) that showed improved performance when compared to a tomographic combined index alone or the CBI alone [29]. It should be noted that the input to the random forest was basic biomechanical parameters and basic tomographic parameters, not combined indices like CBI. It is also important to remember that both CBI and TBI are designed for *detecting* keratoconus, not for monitoring progression or response to treatment.

Biomechanical changes were reported in the shape-related DCRs and SP-A1 after both transepithelial PRK (tPRK) and femtosecond LASIK (FS-LASIK), all consistent with softening. This included a significant decrease in SP-A1 and a significant increase in both DA Ratio 2 mm and Integrated Inverse Radius (IR) [30]. In comparing response between tPRK (n = 65) and FS-LASIK (n = 64) with similar myopic corrections, there was significantly greater biomechanical softening in FS-LASIK than tPRK with greater increase of both DA Ratio 2 mm and IR without a difference in mean bIOP between the two groups. This is consistent with clinical experience that LASIK alters more tissue than PRK due to the presence of a flap [31]. Similar results were reported after SMILE (n = 43), with a significant increase in the DA Ratio parameters and IR, as well as a significant reduction in SP-A1, all consistent with softening or greater compliance. Only the stiffness parameter did not correlate significantly with the change in corneal thickness due to surgery, indicating additional biomechanical changes other than the tissue removal or change in corneal volume may be involved [32].

In addition, corneal biomechanical changes have been reported in the shape-related DCR's and SP-A1 after corneal collagen crosslinking, all consistent with stiffening in the early 4–7 weeks period after the procedure [33]. A total of 34 patients were treated with 6 mW/cm², 15 min exposure, with total energy delivered of 5.4 J/cm². Corvis ST measurements pre and post-procedure showed a significant decrease in DA Ratio and IR, with a significant increase in SP-A1. This illustrates the sensitivity of these parameters to detect and quantify corneal biomechanical changes after a procedure which alters the cornea. Further studies are needed to determine changes over time. Accelerated corneal crosslinking (CXL) with short exposure times immediately after refractive surgery is a relatively new procedure intended to increase post-operative corneal stiffness after refractive surgery. Measurable changes in post-operative corneal properties were only reported recently in a study comparing tPRK (n = 35) and tPRK-CXL (n = 34) with similar corrections in each group [34]. The crosslinking procedure was performed after completion of the excimer ablation with power of 30 mW/cm², exposure of either 90 s of continuous irradiation or 180 s of pulsed irradiation for a total dose of 2.7 J/cm². Although SP-A1 was significantly reduced 6 months after both procedures, it was not different between groups. However, both DA Ratio and IR were significantly different between the 2 groups, with less increase of both parameters in the tPRK-CXL group. In other words, less biomechanical softening was shown after tPRK-CXL, with accelerated crosslinking, leaving this group stiffer than the group without crosslinking, but still significantly softer than pre-operatively.

Comparison of ORA and Corvis ST

Although the ORA and Corvis ST both rely on an air puff to deform the cornea, both generate inward and outward applanation events with a state of concavity in between them and both analyze the horizontal meridian of the cornea, the responses they measure and report are quite distinct. First, the air puff pressure profiles are different between the two devices. Since corneal biomechanical response depends on the applied load, the response would be expected to be distinct. In addition, the ORA customizes the air puff to each exam, based on the timing of A1. The Corvis ST delivers the same air pressure profile with each exam. Second, each device uses a different assessment technology with the ORA using an indirect assessment technique and the Corvis ST using direct assessment with high-speed imaging. Both devices provide a global assessment of corneal biomechanical response, without spatially resolved information.

What are the consequences of these two strategies in deforming and assessing the cornea? First, the Corvis generates the maximal corneal concavity that can be reached earlier than the maximum applied air pressure with each exam, and then generates rapid, nonlinear backward movement of the globe. Therefore, the energy in the air puff once the cornea reaches its limit of displacement is split between the cornea and the globe. In the ORA, the cornea will never reach the limit of obtainable concavity, since it is inertia in the piston that determines the maximum air pressure, which coincides with largest backward movement of the cornea during an exam. The difference in applanation pressures will not be the same between the two devices, since in the unloading recovery of the Corvis ST where A2 occurs, the air pressure is reducing relative to both the cornea and the globe. Both must be taken into account.

Can the data produced be compared between the ORA and the Corvis ST? First, each device developed a more accurate estimation of IOP than Goldmann using a different approach. The ORA used an empirical approach for IOPcc, and the Corvis ST used an analytical approach for bIOP. Both approaches have advantages and disadvantages. Second, due to the important differences in both loading and unloading the cornea, as well as the manner of assessing response, the data from both devices should be considered complimentary and not competitive. Although an analysis of both the elastic and viscoelastic corneal response is possible from both devices with additional development, it is easier clinically to obtain a measurement of viscoelastic response from the ORA and a measurement of the elastic response from the Corvis ST. To obtain information about the elastic response from the ORA would require analysis of the infrared and pressure signals produced. To obtain information about the viscoelastic response from the Corvis ST would require untangling the corneal recovery from that of the whole eye in the unloading state as the air pressure is reduced.

Disclosures Dr. Roberts is a consultant to Oculus Optikgeräte GmbH and Ziemer Ophthalmic Systems AG.

References

1. Luce DA. Determining in vivo biomechanical properties of the cornea with an ocular response analyzer. J Cataract Refract Surg. 2005;31:156–62.
2. Ambrósio R Jr, Ramos I, Luz A, Faria-Correia F, Steinmueller A, Krug M, Belin MW, Roberts C. Dynamic ultra-high-speed Scheimpflug imaging for assessing corneal biomechanical properties. Rev Bras Oftalmol. 2013;72(2):99–102.
3. Andreassen TT, Simonsen AH, Oxlund H. Biomechanical properties of keratoconus and normal corneas. Exp Eye Res. 1980;31:435–44.
4. Nash IS, Greene PR, Foster CS. Comparison of mechanical properties of keratoconus and normal corneas. Exp Eye Res. 1982;35:413–24.
5. Jue B, Maurice DM. The mechanical properties of the rabbit and human cornea. J Biomech. 1986;19:847–53.
6. Hoeltzel DA, Altman P, Buzard K, Choe K. Strip extensiometry for comparison of the mechanical response of bovine, rabbit, and human corneas. J Biomech Eng. 2002;114:202–15.
7. Palko JR, Liu J. Definitions and concepts. In: Roberts CJ, Liu J, editors. Corneal biomechanics: from theory to practice. Amsterdam: Kugler Publications; 2016. p. 1–24.
8. Luce D, Taylor D. Ocular response analyzer. In: Roberts CJ, Liu J, editors. Corneal biomechanics: from theory to practice. Amsterdam: Kugler Publications; 2016. p. 67–86.
9. Roberts CJ. Concepts and misconceptions in corneal biomechanics. J Cataract Refract Surg. 2014;40:862–9.
10. Glass DH. Characterization of the biomechanical properties of the in vivo human cornea. PhD Dissertation, The Ohio State University; 2008.

11. Pepose JS, Feigenbaum SK, Qazi MA, Sanderson JP, Roberts CJ. Changes in corneal bio-mechanics and intraocular pressure following LASIK using static, dynamic and non-contact tonometry. Am J Ophthalmol. 2007;143:39–47.
12. Hallahan KM, Sinha Roy A, Ambrósio R Jr, Salomao M, Dupps WJ Jr. Discriminant value of custom ocular response analyzer waveform derivatives in keratoconus. Ophthalmology. 2014;121:459–68.
13. Glass DH, Roberts CJ, Litsky AS, Weber PA. A viscoelastic biomechanical model of the cor-nea describing the effect of viscosity and elasticity on hysteresis. Invest Ophthalmol Vis Sci. 2008;49(9):3919–26.
14. Hallahan K, Duups WJ Jr, Roberts CJ. Deformation response to an air puff: clinical methods. In: Roberts CJ, Dupps WJ, Downs JC, editors. Biomechanics of the eye. Amsterdam: Kugler Publications; 2018. p. 199–216.
15. Kérautret J, Colin J, Touboul D, Roberts C. Biomechanical characteristics of the ectatic cor-nea. J Cataract Refract Surg. 2008;34(3):510–3.
16. Vinciguerra P, Albè E, Mahmoud AM, Trazza S, Hafezi F, Roberts CJ. Intra- and postopera-tive variation in ocular response analyzer parameters in keratoconic eyes after corneal cross-linking. J Refract Surg. 2010;26(9):669–76.
17. Spoerl E, Terai N, Scholz F, Raiskup F, Pillunat LE. Detection of biomechanical changes after corneal cross-linking using ocular response analyzer software. J Refract Surg. 2011;27:452–7.
18. Hallahan KM, Rocha K, Roy AS, Randleman JB, Stulting RD, Dupps WJ Jr. Effects of cor-neal cross-linking on ocular response analyzer waveform-derived variables in keratoconus and postrefractive surgery ectasia. Eye Contact Lens. 2014;40:339–44.
19. Roberts CJ, Mahmoud AM, Lembach RG, Mauger TF. Corneal deformation characteristics and IOP before and after collagen crosslinking. Invest Ophth Vis Sci. 2013;54:1176.
20. Mahmoud AM, Roberts CJ, Lembach RG, Twa MD, Herderick EE, McMahon TT, The CLEK study group. CLMI: the cone location and magnitude index. Cornea. 2008;27(4):480–7.
21. Congdon NG, Broman AT, Bandeen-Roche K, Grover D, Quigley HA. Central corneal thickness and corneal hysteresis associated with glaucoma damage. Am J Ophthalmol. 2006;141:868–75.
22. Medeiros FA, Meira-Freitas D, Lisboa R, Kuang T-M, Zangwill LM, Weinreb RN. Corneal hysteresis as a risk factor for glaucoma progression: a prospective longitudinal study. Ophthalmology. 2013;120:1533–40.
23. Roberts CJ, Mahmoud AM, Bons JP, Hossain A, Elsheikh A, Vinciguerra R, Vinciguerra P, Ambrósio R Jr. Introduction of two novel stiffness parameters and interpretation of air puff induced biomechanical deformation parameters with a dynamic Scheimpflug analyzer. J Refract Surg. 2017;33(4):266–73.
24. Vinciguerra R, Elsheikh A, Roberts CJ, Ambrósio R Jr, Kang DS, Lopes BT, Morenghi E, Azzolini C, Vinciguerra P. The influence of pachymetry and intraocular pressure on dynamic corneal response parameters in healthy patients. J Refract Surg. 2016;32:550–61.
25. Metzler K, Mahmoud AM, Liu J, Roberts CJ. Deformation response of paired donor cor-neas to an air puff: intact whole globe vs mounted corneoscleral rim. J Cataract Refr Surg. 2014;40(6):888–96.
26. Scarcelli G, Besner S, Pineda R, Yun SH. Biomechanical characterization of keratoconus cor-neas ex vivo with Brillouin microscopy. Invest Ophthalmol Vis Sci. 2014;55:4490–5.
27. Vinciguerra R, Ambrósio R Jr, Roberts CJ, Azzolini C, Vinciguerra P. Biomechanical char-acterization of subclinical keratoconus without topographic or tomographic abnormalities. J Refract Surg. 2017;33(6):399–407.
28. Vinciguerra R, Ambrósio R Jr, Elsheikh A, Roberts CJ, Lopes B, Morenghi E, Azzolini C, Paolo Vinciguerra P. Dectection of keratoconus with a new biomechanical index. J Refract Surg. 2016;32:803–10.
29. Ambrósio R Jr, Lopes B, Faria-Correia F, Salomão MQ, Bühren J, Roberts CJ, Vinciguerra R, Vinciguerra P. Integration of Scheimpflug-based corneal tomography and biomechanical assessments for enhancing ectasia detection. J Refract Surg. 2017;33:434–43.
30. Lee H, Roberts C, Kim T-I, Ambrosio R, Elsheikh A, Kang DSY. Changes in biomechanically-corrected intraocular pressure and dynamic corneal response parameters before and after

transepithelial photorefractive keratectomy and femtosecond laser-assisted laser in situ keratomileusis. J Cataract Refract Surg. 2017;43(12):1495–503.
31. Santhiago MR. Percent tissue altered and corneal ectasia. Curr Opin Ophthalmol. 2016;27:311–5.
32. Fernández J, Rodriguez-Vallejo M, Martinez J, Tauste A, Salvestrini P, Piñero DP. New parameters for evaluating corneal biomechanics and intraocular pressure after small-incision lenticule extraction by Scheimpflug-based dynamic tonometry. J Cataract Refract Surg. 2017;43:803–11.
33. Vinciguerra R, Romano V, Arbabi E, Brunner M, Willoughby CE, Batterbury M, Kaye SB. In-vivo early corneal biomechanical changes after collagen cross-linking in patients with progressive keratoconus. J Refract Surg. 2017;33:840–6.
34. Lee H, Roberts C, Ambrósio R, Elsheikh A, Kang DSY, Kim T-I. Effect of accelerated corneal crosslinking combined with transepithelial photorefractive keratectomy on dynamic corneal response parameters and biomechanically corrected intraocular pressure measured with a dynamic Scheimpflug analyzer in healthy myopic patients. J Cataract Refract Surg. 2017;43:937–45.

Chapter 6
Biomechanical Properties of the Sclera

Ian C. Campbell, Scott Lovald, Mariana Garcia, and Baptiste Coudrillier

Introduction

Scleral Function, Structure, and Composition

The eye is a dynamic organ that is continuously subjected to simultaneous internal and external mechanical forces. The sclera, the white part of the eye (Fig. 6.1a), comprises approximately 80% of the outer tunic of the human eye [5]. In conjunction with the cornea, the sclera forms a continuous, approximately spherical shell that bears internal and external loads. Internal forces are generated by the presence of intraocular pressure (IOP), which in turn is driven by the fluid balance of the aqueous humor. IOP distributed across the inner surface of the eye results in tensile in-plane stresses. Stresses in the sclera scale approximately with the IOP and with the ratio of the eye radius to the eye wall thickness [6]. This is known as "Laplace's Law", which represents the eye wall as a spherical pressure vessel. As shown by Chung et al., this approximation can be unreliable [6]. External forces may include tensile loads applied by the extraocular muscles, physiologically applied forces such as blinking or rubbing, and forces resulting from eye trauma (e.g., blast injury or blunt impact). Maintenance of visual acuity requires that the shape, especially the axial length, of the eye to remain unperturbed by these mechanical stimuli. The extent of deformation of the sclera under applied loads depends on its shape, thickness, and material properties.

I. C. Campbell
Exponent, Atlanta, GA, USA
e-mail: icampbell@exponent.com

S. Lovald · M. Garcia · B. Coudrillier (✉)
Exponent, Menlo Park, CA, USA
e-mail: slovald@exponent.com; mgarcia@exponent.com; bcoudrillier@exponent.com

© Springer Nature Switzerland AG 2021
I. Pallikaris et al. (eds.), *Ocular Rigidity, Biomechanics and Hydrodynamics of the Eye*, https://doi.org/10.1007/978-3-030-64422-2_6

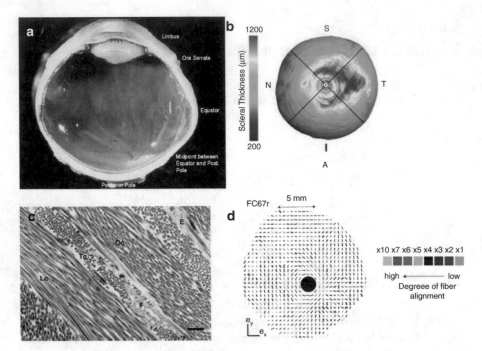

Fig. 6.1 (**a**) Transected human eye demonstrating that the sclera is thinnest at the equator and thickest at the pole. Reproduced via Creative Commons license from [1]. (**b**) Map of scleral thickness in the posterior sclera. The central point represents the location of the optic nerve head (ONH). Scleral thickness was measured using microMRI. Large scleral thickness variations were seen in the peripapillary sclera. Reproduced from [2], with permission from Elsevier. (**c**) Electron micrograph of a human sclera. The collagen fibrils are organized into lamellae. Fibrils within one lamella are unidirectional. Fibroblasts lie in the space between adjacent lamellae. Image reproduced with permission from [3]. (**d**) Maps of the preferred orientations of collagen lamellae in the posterior sclera, as measured with wide-angle X-ray scattering (WAXS). Collagen fibrils form a circumferential annulus around the ONH. In the rest of the mid-posterior sclera, the collagen fiber structure is heterogeneous. Image reproduced from [4], with permission from Springer Nature

The sclera is bounded posteriorly by the scleral canal, the opening where all of the retinal ganglion cell (RGC) axons carrying the visual information from the retina to the brain converge to form the optic nerve. Anteriorly, the sclera is bounded by the cornea at the limbus. The neural, vascular, and connective tissues that fill the scleral canal are known as the optic nerve head (ONH), and the region of the sclera located around the ONH is known as the peripapillary sclera. The scleral shell is not a perfect sphere [7]. The average inner radius of the human sclera is 12 mm [8]; however, eye size varies among individuals [9]. Spatial scleral thickness variability is also complex [2]. Olsen et al. dissected 55 human globes and reported a mean scleral thickness of 0.53 ± 0.14 mm (mean ± standard deviation) at the limbus, 0.39 ± 0.17 mm near the equator, and between 0.9 and 1.0 mm near the posterior pole [10]. These data are within 10% of another histomorphometric study of 238 human globes presented by Vurgese et al., who also noted that, immediately adjacent to the optic nerve, the peripapillary sclera thins to approximately 0.39 ± 0.09 mm [1]. Thickness is heterogeneous in the peripapillary sclera, as shown in Fig. 6.1b. The inferior-nasal quadrant is the thinnest region of the peripapillary sclera, and the superior-temporal quadrant is the thickest region [1, 2].

The external surface of the posterior sclera is covered by two vascularized fascial layers: the episclera and Tenon's capsule, and the external surface of the anterior sclera is covered by the conjunctiva and partially by Tenon's capsule. The episclera is a transitional 10-micron-thick layer connecting the sclera with Tenon's capsule, which consists of a hypocellular layer of randomly arrayed collagen bundles that run parallel to the scleral surface. Tenon's capsule is firmly attached at the limbus but becomes more loosely attached, and thus slightly mobile, about 3 mm posteriorly in human eyes, likely merging with the connective dural sheath of the optic nerve and with the fibrous bands that connect the eyeball to the orbit [11]. Furthermore, Tenon's capsule has been identified as an important site of attachment of pulleys for the extraocular muscles [11]. Other ocular tissues lining the inside of the sclera, such as the retina and choroid, are not considered load-carrying structures [12]. The average thickness of the retina is approximately 0.25 mm, while the choroid is approximately 0.2 mm thick [5]. The choroid modulus is reported to be between 300 and 600 kPa, more than an order of magnitude lower than that of the sclera [5]. The sclera is capable of tolerating a compression stress more than 50 times greater than an unperfused choroidal strip before folding [13]. The retina is even less stiff, with a modulus an order of magnitude lower than that of the choroid, approximately 18 kPa [5]. Because of the low thickness or apparent stiffness of these tissues, their biomechanical properties have not been widely characterized. The rest of this chapter, therefore, focuses on the biomechanics of the sclera.

The mechanical properties of the sclera stem from its collagen-rich extracellular matrix (ECM). Collagen accounts for approximately 50% of the human sclera's wet weight, 80–90% of which is type I collagen [14, 15]. Scleral collagen is organized into a complex hierarchical structure. Individual type I collagen fibrils are locally aligned parallel to each other and then aggregate into interwoven lamellae that are heterogeneously oriented throughout the sclera [4, 16–18] (Fig. 6.1c). For instance, the collagen fiber structure in the peripapillary sclera is highly anisotropic, with the collagen fibers forming a relatively circumferentially-aligned ring around the ONH [19] (Fig. 6.1d). Collagen fibrils also exhibit a crimped structure, forming a wave pattern axially along each fibril that imparts elasticity, similar to a spring [20, 21]. The opaque nature of the sclera is in part a product of the varying diameters of the collagen fibrils and of the anisotropic nature of the lamellae into which they are organized, causing light to scatter instead of entering the eye in an organized way, as is the case with the transparent cornea [22]. In addition to collagen, the ECM of the human sclera also contains proteoglycans [23], free glycosaminoglycans (GAGs) [15], and elastin fibers, the latter of which are predominantly located in the peripapillary sclera [24]. Proteoglycans consist of a core protein with attached negatively charged GAG side chains, which sequester water and are essential for scleral hydration [25]. Proteoglycans are also believed to play a key role in modulating the arrangement and assembly of collagen fibers [23]. The most abundant proteoglycans in the human sclera are decorin, biglycan, and aggrecan [26], while the most predominant GAGs are dermatan sulfate, chondroitin sulfate, hyaluronic acid, and heparan sulfate. Porcine sclerae become stiffer after experimental digestion of GAGs, suggesting an important contribution of the ECM component to the maintenance of scleral modulus [27]. However, the biomechanical role of GAGs is not fully understood. The primary cell type found in the sclera is fibroblasts, which synthesize and remodel the scleral ECM [23]. In healthy scleral tissue, matrix degradation is balanced by new matrix production. This balance is impaired in pathologies that impact scleral biomechanics, such as myopia and glaucoma.

Scleral Biomechanics' Role in Ocular Pathologies and Injuries

Scleral biomechanics is known to play a key role in a number of sight-threatening pathologies such as glaucoma or myopia, as well as in injuries such as ocular trauma or blast. Further quantitative study of scleral biomechanics is critical to advancing our understanding of these ocular diseases.

Glaucoma

Glaucoma is the second leading cause of blindness in the modern world; approximately 76 million people worldwide are projected to suffer from glaucoma by 2020 [28]. Glaucoma is marked by a characteristic pattern of vision loss that gradually manifests over a period of months or years and is associated with the irreversible loss of RGC axons. Population-based studies have demonstrated a strong correlation between elevated IOP and the risk to developing glaucoma [29, 30], with some concluding that elevated IOP is a causative risk factor [5]. Furthermore, IOP-lowering medication and surgical interventions to lower IOP are typically beneficial to slow the rate of disease progression [29–31]. There are several forms of glaucoma, of which open-angle glaucoma is the most common. These various forms of glaucoma are clinically distinct, but all result in an outcome of RGC axon loss. Glaucoma is a multifaceted, chronic disease, and the exact mechanisms leading to vision loss in glaucoma have not yet been fully elucidated. However, it is believed that axonal damage is initiated at least in part by excessive biomechanical stresses in the peripapillary sclera as result of IOP burden [32–35]. The stresses and resultant mechanical strains are magnified at the ONH, where soft neural tissue dominates the composition and the density of connective tissue is lower. IOP-related stresses and deformations of the ONH are believed to generate a series of biomechanical and biochemical responses that culminate with axonal degeneration. Computer modeling studies have demonstrated the importance of scleral mechanics in determining the stresses in the ONH [4, 8]. Therefore, measuring scleral biomechanics in the healthy and glaucomatous eye has been a subject of recent research to better elucidate the pathophysiology of glaucoma.

Myopia

Myopia, commonly called nearsightedness, is a condition of vision defocus wherein light entering the eye is focused anterior to the retina; it is predicted that by 2050, half of the world population will be nearsighted [36]. It is the second leading cause of preventable blindness in developing countries [37] and incurs a financial burden of more than 5 billion dollars in the United States alone [38]. As myopia develops, refractive error typically resulting from axial lengthening of the eye and/or excessive curvature of the primary refractive components of the eye (cornea and lens) moves the retina posteriorly relative to the natural focal plane of the eye, resulting in blurry vision. Myopia, especially at refractive errors larger than -6D, is also a known comorbidity for other blinding diseases such as glaucoma and retinal detachment [39]. Altered remodeling of the scleral ECM is fundamental to the changes in eye size caused by myopia. Studies in animal models have shown that scleral thinning and scleral remodeling including reductions in collagen I and GAG content, an increase in the percentage of small collagen fibrils in the scleral matrix, and disruption to the interwoven arrangement of collagen lamellae occurs during the development of myopia [23, 40]. These changes alter the viscoelastic behavior of the sclera, leading to faster creep behavior (time-dependent elongation of the eye under constant pressure) [41, 42]. Understanding how scleral biomechanics is altered with myopia is critical to understanding the mechanism by which myopia develops and progresses.

Ocular Injury

Eye injuries affect an estimated 1.9–2.5 million people in the United States every year [43, 44], of which about 40,000–50,000 result in vision loss [44, 45]. Approximately 30,000 cases result in complete blindness in one eye because of ocular trauma [46]. Because the sclera is overlaid by the conjunctiva and episcleral tissue and is mostly located within the orbit, it is not directly accessible from the outside. Scleral injury typically arises via one of two primary avenues: direct trauma or blast injury. Both are topics motivating further research to better characterize the biomechanical properties of the sclera, as the loads and loading rates on the sclera that cause injury are typically orders of magnitude greater than the physiological realm in which scleral biomechanics has traditionally been studied. The sclera itself is minimally vascularized; however, the blood vessels of the conjunctiva and episclera can rupture in cases of ocular injury, appearing as bright red pools of blood through the otherwise transparent tissue. Sometimes called "scleral petechiae," these are more accurately called subconjunctival petechiae and can indicate that direct trauma has occurred. Petechiae can also be caused by vessel rupture as a result of high blood pressure, sometimes occurring acutely from sneezing or straining [47]. Scleral/subconjunctival petechiae are frequently noted by medical examiners as forensic evidence of asphyxia [48].

Rupture of the sclera is uncommon but is nonetheless a serious injury when it does occur, as urgent medical attention is needed to prevent extrusion of ocular contents, to seal against pathogens and foreign bodies, and to maintain IOP to prevent ocular collapse. Since the sclera is a tough tissue (the etymology of its name is from the Greek word for "hard"), it can resist significant external loads before gross rupture of the eye occurs. In the absence of a laceration to a specific location, the initial site of rupture as a result of direct, general trauma to the globe is typically at the limbus or at the equator, where the sclera is thin and where deformation is expected to be high for an impact to the anterior eye [49, 50]. In the absence of a laceration, rupture from impact with a projectile has been shown experimentally to initiate from inside out [51, 52]. In high-impact automobile collisions, facial contact with the air bag has been attributed to cases of globe rupture; modern airbags that deploy at a lower power depending on crash severity have been shown to reduce the risk of such an injury [53]. Because such significant loads are required to result in globe rupture, comorbidities such as fracture of orbital bones like the lamina papyracea (which is only 200–400 μm thick) often accompany globe rupture [54]. Better understanding of the dynamic mechanical behavior of the sclera is needed to understand the stresses that can cause the eye to rupture or that can damage the internal components of the eye.

Blast injury to the eye is one of the most common types of ocular combat injuries, resulting when individuals are exposed to a shock wave, also called a primary blast injury (a secondary blast injury, wherein fragments or objects propelled by the blast might contact the eye, is a form of direct contact trauma). Blast injuries are often experienced by military personnel, particularly those in close proximity to improvised explosive devices. Fireworks, although capable of producing blast waves, have been shown by Alphonse et al. to more likely injure through direct contact of the projectiles and not via blast [55]. Blast injury is a particularly complicated phenomenon because the bones of the orbit can reflect the shock wave back and therefore increase the risk of injury compared to a free field exposure [56, 57].

The above conditions are complex; thus, a variety of investigational approaches have been used to study them, ranging from computational modeling to animal studies to clinical imaging in humans to testing of postmortem human eyes. The next section of this chapter reviews the different methods used to measure the mechanical properties of the sclera and the animal models that have been developed to better understand the role of scleral biomechanics in glaucoma and myopia.

Methods to Measure Scleral Biomechanics

General Remarks on Scleral Biomechanics

Like most collagen-rich tissue such as the cornea, tendons, or ligaments, the bulk mechanical response of the sclera is nonlinear, viscoelastic, nearly incompressible, and anisotropic [5]. The nonlinear stress/strain behavior has been attributed to the tendency of collagen fibrils to be wavy at low stresses, providing little resistance to the applied loads but becoming increasingly taut as the applied load increases [21, 58]. The sclera displays a time-dependent (viscoelastic) behavior, evidenced by creep under constant load [59], stress relaxation under constant strain [60], loading rate dependence [61], and/or hysteresis upon unloading [61]. The incompressibility of the sclera is believed to be due to the tendency of proteoglycans to conserve water within soft tissues, providing a water content of more than 70% in the sclera [25]. As mentioned earlier, the in-plane anisotropy of the sclera tangent to the ocular surface is a result of the organization of the collagen microarchitecture, which exhibits preferred orientation [17]. In addition, the mechanical properties of the sclera through its thickness differ from its planar properties. Battaglioli and Kamm conducted compression tests and determined that the through-thickness stiffness of the sclera was two orders of magnitude smaller than in the in-plane direction [58]. The authors proposed that, since collagen fibril bundles run primarily in the in-plane direction, they are better able to resist changes in circumference than changes in thickness. However, there are still very few studies in the literature on scleral elastic modulus under compressive stress in the thickness direction.

Research efforts have used a wide range of methodologies to characterize the complex mechanical properties of scleral tissue. Many published studies on scleral biomechanics have tested animal tissues. As in any animal study, one must consider the advantages, disadvantages, and human biofidelity when interpreting results. Some animal models are particularly advantageous because of ease of procurement of scleral tissue; these include porcine [62–64], rabbit [60], and bovine [59]. Other animal models are advantageous because of established procedures to induce glaucoma; these include monkey [65, 66], mouse [67], and rat [68]. Others are advantageous because of established procedures to induce myopia; such animal models include tree shrew [69, 70], mouse [59, 71], and avian [42, 72, 73]. Nonetheless, because of differences in stiffness or composition between the non-human and human sclera, the most directly relevant biomechanical information is obtained from testing human tissue, typically cadaveric [61, 74–77].

Before describing these experimental methods, it is important to review some known limitations of *in vitro* biomechanical characterization of scleral tissue.

Tissue Storage

Most experimental studies advocate testing of scleral tissue within a few days post-mortem [4, 13, 60, 63, 77–79]. Justification for this practice has primarily referenced a study by Girard et al., which concluded that sclerae can be stored up to 3 days without risking noticeable mechanical deterioration [80]. To date, there is no study that has quantified the temporal relationship between gross material properties in the sclera and mechanical deterioration. Elsheikh et al. reported no significant variation in the thickness or the tangent modulus of scleral tissue over a period of up to 16 days in Eusol-C storage media [81]. Schultz et al. tested human and porcine sclerae within 2 days postmortem and after an additional week of frozen storage and observed that differences in mechanical results were not statistically significantly distinct from fresh tissue [64]. The stability of the sclera postmortem can be explained by its low cellularity compared to other ocular tissues (e.g., retina and choroid).

Tissue Preconditioning

Preconditioning is a common experimental procedure used when testing the mechanical properties of soft biological tissues, and the sclera is no exception. Although preconditioning is required to obtain a repeatable cyclic response in uni-axial testing [70], cyclic preconditioning of scleral tissue is also thought to have two unwanted effects: [5] the reorientation of collagen lamellae toward the loading axis, resulting in an effective stiffening of the material; and [6] damage to the fibers and matrix constituents of the tissue, including breaking of collagen cross-links [67]. Damage due to preconditioning has been characterized as a Mullins effect because collagen cross-links break during repeated loading, leading to an effective softening of the stress-strain curve [67].

In most tensile testing of scleral strips, changes to the mechanical behavior after preconditioning include a shift of the load-elongation curve, a reduction in hyster-esis, and a reduction in peak stress [67]. Studies typically show a rightward shift in the force-displacement response with cycle count, indicating a gradual decrease in secant modulus, which is more apparent at higher stresses. Elsheikh and Geraghty both performed 10 loading cycles up to a stress of 1–2 MPa and observed both a rightward shift of the force-displacement response during cycling as well as increases in the tangent modulus until about the fourth cycle [76, 81]. There is no established standard for preconditioning of sclerae. Variation in preconditioning protocol parameters in published studies include the magnitude or exclusion of a pre-stress, the number of preconditioning cycles (up to 20 cycles) [69], and the stress to which the samples are cycled (up to 2 MPa) [81]. Rest periods between cycles are typically not specified.

With the limitations of *in vitro* testing in mind, we now describe the primary test approaches used to characterize the mechanical behavior of the sclera—namely, uniaxial strip tension, biaxial strip tension, inflation testing, and indentation testing.

Uniaxial Tension Testing

Uniaxial testing is a common method for characterizing the stress and strain in a material, given its relatively simple implementation for isotropic materials. However, there are many known complications associated with uniaxial testing of scleral sam-ples, particularly the limitation that cutting and clamping the tissue disrupts the native fiber structure and natural three-dimensional curvature. The sclera naturally exists in a state of primarily biaxial stress, and it has been suggested that uniaxial testing of scleral strips may not produce representative tissue behavior [63]. Of particular concern, the straightening of a naturally curved strip of sclera for testing may introduce error due to uneven straightening of fibers on the inner versus outer surface of the scleral specimen. Specimen gripping is also problematic, as it may cause stress concentrations, and sample slippage of the naturally moist sclera may occur [5, 63]. Typically, authors will aim to ensure that the specimen size is sufficient to avoid issues with gripping, edge fiber disruption, and local anisotropy of the specimens. Additionally, cutting samples may expose free collagen fibers along the sides of the strips, lowering the magnitude of the elastic response [12].

Representative stress-strain curves for various uniaxial studies are shown in Fig. 6.2. Data from Geraghty [76], Elsheikh [81], and Wollensack [82] appear relatively consistent. The comparatively lower magnitude of stiffness in the data from Friberg [13] and Chen [25] is notable, particularly because the test protocols used in these studies used a small preload without any stress preconditioning cycles.

When evaluating scleral viscoelastic properties using uniaxial tensile testing, Downs [60] observed that material properties of rabbit sclerae were largely

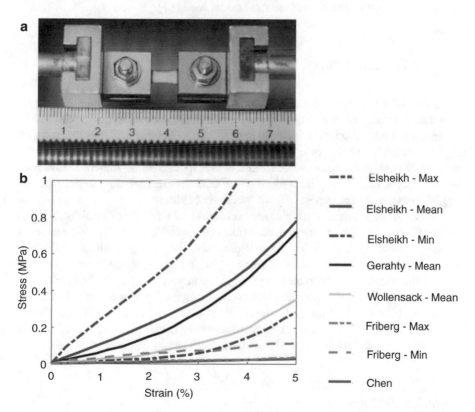

Fig. 6.2 (a) Example of a test fixture used for performing uniaxial tensile studies of scleral strip specimens. Reprinted from [82] with permission from Elsevier. (b) Stress-strain data from various studies on human scleral mechanical behavior using a uniaxial test methodology. Data were digitized from the original sources [13, 25, 76, 81, 82]

insensitive to strain rate for rates of 0.1%/s, 1%/s, and 10%/s, and at strain magnitudes below 4%. In contrast, human scleral specimens were stiffer when tested at strain rates of 3.3%/s than at 0.13%/s, indicating a greater role of viscoelasticity in human sclerae than rabbit sclerae during uniaxial testing [81]. The microstructural characteristics contributing to viscoelasticity of the sclera are not fully understood [5].

Using uniaxial tension, it has been shown that the anterior sclera has a higher stiffness than the posterior sclera [5, 76]. In fact, Friberg et al. demonstrated that the anterior sclera is about 60% stiffer than posterior sclera [13]. A more recent study found the increase in stiffness from the posterior pole of the eye to the equator was measured as 3.3%, whereas the increase in stiffness from the equator to the anterior sclera near the limbus was reported as approximately 14% [81]. It has been proposed that this increase in stiffness is due to differences in the collagen fiber alignment and microstructure between the anterior and posterior regions, with the anterior region having a more uniform weave of collagen fibers [81]. The lower mechanical stiffness in the posterior sclera is balanced by a greater wall thickness (Fig. 6.1b), providing the area surrounding the ONH with a sort of mechanical reinforcement against excessive deformation under load [81].

Biaxial Tension Testing

A number of studies have conducted biaxial testing of scleral specimens, with a goal of better matching the *in vivo* biaxial stress state of the sclera. During biaxial tensile testing, the spherical sclera is flattened and cut into a planar square specimen, which is then loaded along two orthogonal axes. This methodology is believed to more accurately capture the anisotropic mechanical response of the material. However, biaxial testing shares many limitations of uniaxial testing, including sample flattening, gripping, and fiber exposure from specimen cutting.

Results from a biaxial testing study conducted by Cruz-Perez et al. (Fig. 6.3a) indicated that the circumferential direction (i.e., parallel to the eye's equator) is significantly stiffer than the meridional direction (i.e., a line connecting the two poles of the eye) during equibiaxial loading [79]. Eilaghi subjected scleral samples from 40 human donor eyes to biaxial testing. The large variability in the mechanical behavior among different samples observed in this testing was comparable to the variability observed in uniaxial testing [77], as illustrated in Fig. 6.3b. This study found that the human sclera was nearly transversely isotropic—i.e., the stiffness in the circumferential and meridional directions were nearly identical.

Inflation Testing

Recent studies have shifted toward a preference for using inflation testing to address the limitations of uniaxial and biaxial testing. This methodology involves mounting hemispherical scleral specimens on customized inflation chambers and measuring

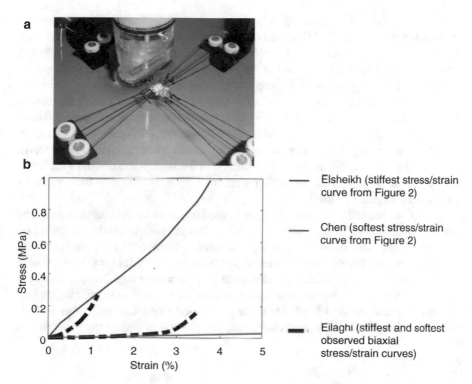

Fig. 6.3 (a) Example of a fixture used by Cruz-Perez et al. for performing biaxial tensile testing of scleral strip specimens. Reprinted from [79], with permission from Elsevier. (b) Thick black lines: Range of stress-strain curves observed in biaxial testing of the human sclera by Eilaghi et al. [77]. For comparison to uniaxial test results, only the stiffest and most compliant curves measured in the uniaxial tests shown in Fig. 6.2 have been plotted here [25, 81]

the displacement/strain response of the sclera to controlled pressurization simulating variations in IOP. Inflation testing applies loads to the sclera in a more natural state than tensile testing and therefore is believed to produce a material response of the tissue that most accurately represents the *in vivo* behavior [61]. Inflation testing further avoids issues associated with preconditioning, including fiber rearrangement and microstructural damage. In fact, preconditioning of scleral tissue has been shown to be unnecessary in inflation testing [67]. Lari et al. compared whole-globe inflation testing and uniaxial testing in matched porcine eye pairs and found that measured stiffness was approximately 2.1 times greater at 1% strain in the inflation tests [63], suggesting that material properties derived from uniaxial tensile testing may not be appropriate to extrapolate to whole-globe material properties.

Numerous imaging methods have been developed to measure the deformation of the sclera during pressure-controlled inflation testing. In the first published inflation test of human globes, performed by Woo et al. [78], the displacement of individual points of the scleral surface was monitored using a flying spot scanner. Recent inflation testing studies have used advanced optical methods to map the full-field three-dimensional displacements of the scleral surface, including 3D digital image correlation (DIC) [61, 75, 83], electronic speckle pattern interferometry (ESPI) [65, 69, 84], ultrasound speckle tracking [62, 85], and multiphoton microscopy [86]. A comparison of the strain response of the human sclera between inflation pressures of 10 and 20 mmHg observed in three studies is shown in Fig. 6.4.

One disadvantage of inflation testing compared with uniaxial testing and biaxial testing is that the stress/strain behavior of the sclera cannot be directly inferred from experimental data. Stresses in the sclera during inflation testing are complex, especially in the peripapillary sclera, where the adjacent and comparatively soft ONH, the spatially varying thickness of the sclera, and the highly anisotropic fiber structure cause the stress profile to exhibit significant spatial variations that cannot be estimated analytically [4].

Computer modeling techniques have been developed to calculate stresses and biomechanical material properties of the sclera from experimental data acquired via inflation testing [61, 65, 69, 78]. A popular method, termed "inverse finite element analysis," is used to calculate a representative constitutive model for the sclera using a combination of the finite element method and optimization algorithms, iterating to best match the model displacement to the deformation observed in an inflation test. Recent constitutive models of the sclera developed using this technique include details of the scleral ECM microstructure, such as the experimentally measured,

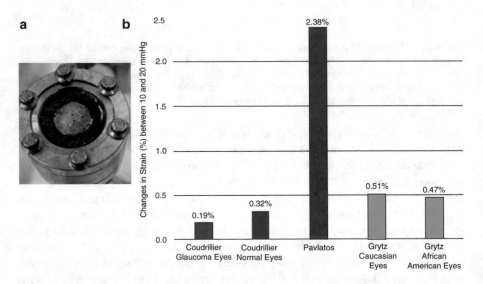

Fig. 6.4 (a) Example of a posterior human sclera placed on an inflation chamber. In this study, stereo cameras imaged the deforming sclera during controlled-pressure inflation testing, and DIC was used to calculate scleral strains. Reproduced from Coudrillier et al. with permission [61]. Image © Association for Research in Vision and Ophthalmology. (b) Since the initial pressure in inflation testing is different among studies, it is more convenient to compare the change in strains of the sclera between two inflation pressures. Represented in the bar chart is the change in strains between 10 and 20 mmHg measured by Coudrillier et al. using DIC [61], Pavlatos et al. using ultrasound speckle tracking [85], and Grytz et al. using ESPI [87]

spatially varying collagen structure [4] or a microstructural representation of the collagen fibrils [69]. These models have been used to predict the effects of scleral stiffness [8] and collagen anisotropy [4] on the biomechanics of the ONH and are important tools to better understand the role of biomechanics of the sclera in glaucoma and myopia.

Indentation Testing

Nanoindentation using atomic force microscopy (AFM) has been used to measure the local mechanical properties of the sclera [88–90]. Contrary to the methods listed above, AFM does not provide bulk properties of scleral tissue. Instead, this technique measures the compressive properties of the tissue using a very small indenter and therefore is sensitive to the composition of the sclera at the site of measurement.

High Strain Rate Testing

Measurements of the mechanical response of the sclera at high strain rates were performed by adapting experimental methods presented above. Bisplinghoff et al. used dynamic pressurization to conduct inflation testing at an average rate of 36.5 MPa/s [46]. This study showed that the sclera is significantly stiffer at high strain rates than at low strain rates, confirming the viscoelastic nature of the sclera (Fig. 6.5).

The high strain rate behavior of the sclera can also be characterized by reproducing blunt impact loading scenarios in the laboratory. Any object that impacts the eye with large amounts of energy could potentially result in globe rupture. Case studies have reported such injuries from projectiles such as airsoft pellets or BBs [51, 91], paint balls [50, 91], or sporting equipment [92, 93]; air or water jets, including fire hoses or water features [94–97]; or other blunt objects. It has been shown that a 50% injury risk of globe rupture occurs at impact energies of around 8–10 J, which, when normalized to account for the area over which the kinetic energy is applied, is approximately 24,000 kg/s^2 [50, 51, 91]. As the eye becomes compressed by an external load, IOP rises; in humans, a pressure of about 6800–7300 mmHg has been shown to cause rupture under dynamic conditions [49, 98, 99]. For comparison, blinking has been shown to raise IOP by about 10 mmHg, and squeezing the lids closed raises it by about 80 mmHg [100, 101]. The rate of loading has also been shown to affect the likelihood of rupture, as eyes that have been quasi-statically loaded have been shown to rupture at lower magnitudes of pressure [102]. Therefore, high strain rate loading of scleral tissue clearly presents a unique domain wherein material properties determined via quasi-static loading experiments may not apply well; further research is needed within this domain. As a tool to evaluate injury

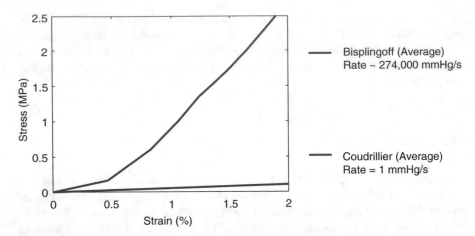

Fig. 6.5 Comparison of the stress/strain behavior of the sclera measured in a dynamic inflation test (blue curves) [46] and a quasi-static inflation test (red curves) [4]. Data were digitized from the original sources

potential from direct impact to the eye and orbit as well as to evaluate safety equipment intended to mitigate such an injury, researchers at the Virginia Tech—Wake Forest Center for Injury Biomechanics developed the Facial and Ocular CountermeasUre Safety (FOCUS) Headform as an improvement over existing anthropomorphic test devices (ATDs) [103, 104]. This headform has been used to evaluate the risk of globe rupture based on an instrumented synthetic eye and orbit, and studies suggest that a 4.5 mm-diameter BB contacting an eye with 107 N of force has a 50% likelihood of globe rupture [105, 106].

Of even greater strain rate than blunt trauma is the realm of primary blast injury from a shock wave. This domain is of great importance to the development of protective technologies (e.g., for soldiers in war zones); to date, there are limited data on the mechanical behavior of the sclera and other ocular tissues under blast conditions. Complicating the study of blast injury is the need to study ocular tissues within a bony orbit, because evidence suggests that reflected shock waves may increase the injury potential compared to a free field exposure, due to effectively multiple exposures and/or to constructive interference of the incoming and reflected waves [56, 57]. A number of physical testing methods have been developed, including detonation of explosives [56] and various designs of shock tubes [107, 108]. Documentation of injury or lack thereof after blast exposure can be used to inform injury thresholds. These methods can be used to test predictions of finite element computer models to better understand ocular risk from shock waves as well as to improve design of attenuating protective wear [57, 109–111]. It remains an experimental challenge to directly measure the properties of viscoelastic tissues in response to shock wave exposure, including ocular tissues, due to sensor limitations.

Toward in Vivo Measurement of Scleral Biomechanics

To date, the reliability of methods to measure scleral stiffness *in vivo* has been limited. Hommer et al. developed a method to measure the *in vivo* ocular expansion of the human eye induced by blood pressure pulsation, a phenomenon termed "ocular rigidity" [112]. However, this method measures the biomechanical response of the entire globe and therefore considers not only the contribution of the sclera but also that of other tissues such as the cornea and internal ocular components. This technique cannot, at present, differentiate the material properties of individual tissues of the eye. Shear wave elastography was recently adopted to measure differences in structural stiffness between the sclerae of patients with and without glaucoma [113]. This method, while still under development, offers promise to perform longitudinal measurements of scleral stiffness in the clinic.

Recently, novel imaging technologies such as optical coherence tomography (OCT) have been proposed to measure the biomechanics of the ONH and surrounding tissues *in vivo* [114]. No imaging modalities to date have been capable of visualizing the full thickness of the entire sclera at high spatial and temporal resolution in the living eye. However, we predict that novel imaging techniques and computer modeling approaches will continue to facilitate the development of methods to measure scleral mechanical properties *in vivo*.

Animal Models for Studies of Scleral Biomechanics

Animal models are widely used in biomedical research as a proxy for human subjects, and *in vivo* studies of scleral biomechanics are no exception. Although caution must be observed when interpreting and translating the results of any study employing non-human subjects to matters of human health, animal models have greatly aided our understanding of scleral anatomy and biochemical composition, pathophysiology, and development of treatments for scleral pathologies and injuries [115]. A considerable proportion of the animal models developed with regard to scleral biomechanics to date are focused on glaucoma and myopia research [116]; the advantages of various models have been reviewed at length elsewhere [72, 115, 117–123], although scleral biomechanics specifically has not often been the focus of such reviews.

Rodent models have been extremely widely studied, given their ease of availability and handling, and a number of relatively well characterized mouse and rat models of glaucoma [124–127] and myopia [71] exist. In rodents, glaucoma can be induced in a variety of methods, including the formation of transgenic animals [128]; application of steroids [129, 130]; injection of microbeads [131, 132], hypertonic saline [133, 134], or viscoelastic polymers [135]; gene modulation using viral vectors [136]; or laser photocoagulation of aqueous humor outflow pathways [137]. Rodent models have been used recently to study the potential therapeutic role of modulating scleral biomechanical properties as a treatment for glaucoma [68, 138].

Also widely used in studies of scleral biomechanics in glaucoma and myopia are model organisms such as the tree shrew [42, 70, 139–141], non-human primate [66, 142], ovine [21, 143], porcine [144, 145], rabbit [146–150], canine [151], feline [152], guinea pig [153], avian [42, 73], and zebrafish [154, 155]. Each model offers benefits and tradeoffs; the publications referenced here are in no way exhaustive of all animal studies investigating scleral biomechanics. However, it is clear that *in vivo* and *ex vivo* animal models have contributed greatly to the modern understanding of this topic.

Variations in Scleral Biomechanics

The healthy sclera is a dynamic structure. Scleral fibroblasts continuously degrade existing ECM and synthetize and organize proteins to form new scleral tissue. It is believed that this equilibrium is altered in various diseases or conditions. Using animal models or *in vitro* mechanical testing of donor eyes, researchers have shown that the structure and mechanical properties of scleral tissue change with age, glaucoma, and myopia.

Age-Related Changes in the Biomechanics of the Sclera

There is substantial evidence that the aging sclera becomes progressively stiffer. Increased stiffness was measured in older mice [59], monkeys [65], and dogs [151]. Stiffening of the human sclera has been identified using both uniaxial tension testing [13, 41, 76] and inflation testing [61, 74, 156]. In humans, older age was associated with a stiffening of the non-collagen components of the ECM (the shear stiffness) [87, 156] and a decrease in crimp angle of the collagen fibrils [87].

Increases in stiffness are accompanied with changes in the morphology of the sclera. Older age is associated with a decrease in the anisotropy of the peripapillary scleral collagen structure, as measured by wide-angle x-ray scattering (WAXS) [156]. It is unclear whether changes in scleral thickness occur with aging. Evidence demonstrating scleral thinning with age include studies by Coudrillier et al. [61] using aged human donor eyes and studies by Avetisov et al. [41]. On the other hand, Grytz et al. found no significant changes in scleral thickness when analyzing 66 eyes from human donors of European and African descents [87], and Vurgese et al. also found no correlation between scleral thickness and age in a histomorphometric study of 238 human globes [1].

Glaucoma-Related Changes in the Biomechanics of the Sclera

Alterations to the extracellular matrix composition and organization have been reported in the glaucomatous human sclera. WAXS measurements of the collagen fiber structure in eyes of donors diagnosed with glaucoma showed a decrease in fiber anisotropy (the degree of fiber alignment) in the superior-temporal and inferior-nasal quadrants of the peripapillary sclera [17]. Glaucoma-related differences in the collagen fiber structure were also identified using small angle light scattering (SALS) [157]. Thickness variation with glaucoma has been characterized with conflicting results. Coudrillier et al. found that the peripapillary sclera of diagnosed glaucomatous donor eyes with axonal damage were thicker than that of non-glaucomatous eyes [61]. In contrast, Vurgese et al. found that scleral thickness was not significantly correlated with the presence of absolute secondary angle-closure glaucoma [1]. Finally, the thickness of patients with normal-tension glaucoma measured by swept-source OCT was, on average, 174 μm thinner than that of patients with primary open-angle glaucoma [158].

Recent experimental studies have shown that the mechanical properties of the normal sclera and the glaucomatous sclera are different. General agreement among the glaucoma research community is that the glaucomatous sclera is stiffer.

Using uniaxial tensile testing, Downs et al. found that the relaxation modulus was larger for monkeys with early experimentally induced glaucoma [60]. Significant stiffening of the monkey sclera with induced chronic IOP elevation was measured by Girard et al. using inflation testing [66]. Similar scleral stiffening was also reported after induction of glaucoma in mice [67]. Inflation testing was applied to the normal and glaucomatous human sclera by Coudrillier et al., who found that mechanical strains in the peripapillary sclera at a given level of IOP were lower in eyes from donors who had glaucoma compared to eyes from non-glaucomatous donors [61]. The authors also calculated the material properties of the eyes using an inverse finite element method and found that, on average, both matrix and fiber stiffness were highest for sclerae of donors who had a diagnosis of glaucoma with axonal damage [159]. African ancestry is a known risk factor for glaucoma [160]; Grytz and colleagues measured an increased stiffness in donor eyes from African-American donors [87], confirming a correlation between increased scleral stiffness and glaucoma.

Although most studies concluded that the human glaucomatous sclera is stiffer, it remains unknown whether this biomechanical change represents an adaptive response to the disease or represents baseline structural properties that predispose one to glaucomatous axonal damage.

Myopia-Related Changes in the Biomechanics of the Sclera

The mechanical properties of the sclera are highly dependent on the nature and arrangement of its collagen fibers. The architecture of healthy sclera (collagen cross-linked into fibrils, which in turn are arranged into lamellae that are anisotropically oriented throughout the sclera) is disturbed during the development of myopia, giving rise to abnormal mechanical properties [5, 161].

Studies in animal models have provided the most insight into the scleral changes underlying myopia. The sclerae of myopic eyes exhibit greater elasticity and a more pronounced creep response (greater elongation under constant load) compared to that of normal sclerae, especially at the posterior pole [42, 162–164]. Grytz and Siegwart recently used uniaxial tensile testing and finite element modeling to show that the collagen fiber crimp angle was higher during lens-induced myopia development in a tree shrew model [70]. Scleral stiffness was also found to increase after starting and stopping negative lens treatment.

The altered mechanical behavior has been linked to scleral thinning, which goes hand-in-hand with reductions in type I collagen and GAG content; an increase in the percentage of small collagen fibrils in the scleral matrix; and disruption of the interwoven arrangement of collagen lamellae [23, 165]. Based on studies in animal models, these changes in scleral ultrastructure manifest early in myopia development [140] and are reversible. Creep experiments in tree shrews have correlated myopia recovery with a reduction in scleral creep response [162]. During the recovery process, matrix metalloprotease (MMP) activity decreases, while expression and activity of their inhibitors tissue inhibitors of metalloproteases (TIMPs), as well as proteoglycan and GAG synthesis, increase [40, 166, 167]. Such observations highlight not only the important role of the sclera in myopia development but also the dynamic remodeling process exhibited by a tissue that could be mistakenly considered an inert casing.

Taken together, all these factors paint a picture that can help us understand the chain of events behind the mechanical behavior of myopic sclerae. Synthesis of matrix components such as proteoglycans and GAGs is influenced in part by the mechanical tension within the matrix, which is transmitted to the scleral fibroblasts through mechanosensors such as integrins, a large family of transmembrane proteins composed of two main classes of subunits (termed α and β). As a result of a yet to be fully understood myopia-generating signaling cascade, the expression of integrin subunits decreases [168], diminishing the ability of scleral fibroblasts to respond to changes in eye wall stress. Resulting reductions in matrix production in conjunction with increases in matrix degradation due to higher MMP secretion ultimately lead to significant changes in tissue hydration and thickness.

Altering Scleral Biomechanics as a Potential Treatment for Glaucoma and Myopia

Computer modeling has shown that the stiffness of the sclera is a major factor controlling mechanical strains in the ONH [8]. Strains in the ONH have been shown to be higher for compliant sclerae than stiff sclerae. Further, mice with experimentally induced glaucoma with compliant sclerae were more prone to axonal damage [67], suggesting that increased scleral stiffness may be neuroprotective in glaucoma. Therefore, pharmaceutical scleral stiffening has been proposed as a potential treatment for glaucoma, motivated in part by successful clinical use of collagen cross-linking to treat corneal disorders such as keratoconus [169]. It has been shown that stiffening the peripapillary sclera of porcine eyes with glyceraldehyde reduced the strain in the LC [144], which may have a positive effect in treating glaucoma. The efficiency of different biocompatible scleral stiffening agents was recently studied by Kimball et al. [138] and Campbell et al. [68], with the former study suggesting that scleral stiffening actually increased the magnitude of damage in glaucoma. Although the finding of Kimball et al. was contrary to predictions from computer modeling studies, to date there are no successful *in vivo* studies evaluating the potential benefits of scleral stiffening to treat glaucoma. Clayson et al. have shown that stiffening the entire eye increases the magnitude of ocular pulse [145], a finding that may suggest a need for targeted peripapillary scleral stiffening rather than whole-eye scleral stiffening to treat glaucoma [144].

Scleral stiffening through cross-linking treatments has also been investigated as a treatment of myopia [82]. A recent study by Liu et al. investigated the effects of UV-riboflavin cross-linking on the biomechanics and microstructure of the guinea pig sclerae [170]. Cross-linked sclerae were stiffer and had a denser and more regularly distributed fiber structure compared to non-cross-linked sclerae. Guinea pigs that had been subjected to scleral cross-linking had a lower mean refractive error than control animals, suggesting that UV-riboflavin cross-linking of the sclera may prevent the progression of myopia. Similarly, Wang and Corpuz showed that genipin cross-linking of scleral collagen prevented the progression of myopia in guinea pigs [171]. A similar study by Chu et al. using glyceraldehyde found that stiffening did not improve outcomes in experimentally induced form deprivation myopia in guinea pigs [172]. In studies using a rabbit model of myopia, Dotan et al. demonstrated improved resistance to experimentally induced myopia using UV-riboflavin cross-linking [150, 173].

Scleral Fibroblast Biomechanics

Scleral ECM plays a central role in ocular biomechanics. Likewise, scleral fibroblasts also provide important contributions to eye growth and matrix modulation, and, consequently, to overall eye biomechanics. It is commonly discussed in the literature that the sclera has low cellularity compared to other tissues in the body [11], yet few studies have endeavored to determine scleral fibroblast density. General estimates can be gleaned from molecular biology studies of scleral matrix composition, which often normalize data to DNA content. For example, a study measuring changes in aggrecan content in chick sclerae as a result of myopia-inducing treatment reported approximately 42.5 and 23 µg of DNA in the anterior and posterior sections of the sclera of control eyes, respectively [174]. Note, however, that these data relate to the bilayered avian sclera and thus include a population of scleral chondrocytes that would not be found in mammalian eyes. Approximations can also be made by drawing parallels with the cellularity of the corneal stroma, which has been estimated at 818,000 ± 186,000 keratocytes per 7 mm central corneal button and 2,430,000 ± 551,000 keratocytes per whole cornea [175]. Despite their presumably low number, scleral fibroblasts can exert influence over large areas of tissue due to their extended cytoplasmic extensions, through which they interact with adjacent cells and with the ECM [11].

Scleral fibroblasts maintain and remodel the scleral ECM through the secretion of a variety of enzymes, including MMPs and their inhibitors, TIMPs [176]. Interactions between cells and matrix are largely mediated by integrins. Integrin subunits $\alpha 1$–6, $\alpha 9$–11, αv, $\beta 1$, $\beta 4$, $\beta 5$, and $\beta 8$ have been identified in the mammalian sclera. Besides mediating cell-matrix attachments, integrins also act as powerful intermediaries in cellular mechanotransduction pathways, allowing cells to sense and respond to mechanical cues from the environment [177]. Scleral fibroblast mechanotransduction likely plays a role in the modulation of matrix synthesis and scleral remodeling [5]. For example, integrin expression is reduced during myopia development, thereby likely decreasing the extent of cell-matrix interaction and interfering with the cell's ability to respond to mechanical cues from the ECM [177].

In vitro and *in vivo* assessments of scleral creep response suggest that contractile fibroblasts, known as myofibroblasts, are key players in the mechanical properties of the sclera [164, 178, 179]. For example, tree shrew eyes with experimentally increased IOP exhibited an initial lengthening as part of an expected viscoelastic response, followed by a shortening of axial length, effectively leading to negative creep values. Once the elevated IOP was returned to physiological values, the eyes became shorter than they were at the beginning of the study. The entire mechanical response occurred in less than an hour, making it highly unlikely that ECM remodeling could be the primary driver behind the observed phenomena. Instead, it is more probable that the shortening of the eyes was driven by a population of contractile scleral cells [180]. Myofibroblasts secrete α-smooth muscle actin (α-SMA), a highly contractile extracellular matrix protein that allows the cells to respond to and relieve imposed tissue stress [179, 180].

Myofibroblasts are usually absent from normal adult tissues throughout the body, instead differentiating from fibroblasts as needed under conditions of tissue repair, wound healing, and remodeling. However, humans, monkeys, tree shrews, and guinea pigs have been shown to possess a resident population of myofibroblasts in their sclerae. One possible explanation for the existence of this unusual resident population is that it may arise from the constant stress imparted on the sclera by intraocular pressure, as *in vitro* studies of scleral fibroblasts have demonstrated that stress imposed on collagen culture matrices can lead to increased numbers of myofibroblasts [164, 179, 180]. Myofibroblast differentiation may also occur as a result of biochemical cues, such as the cytokine transforming growth factor-beta (TGF β) [164, 181]. Recently, it has been shown that scleral fibroblasts from different regions of the eye respond differently to imposed strain [178, 182]. Scleral fibroblasts isolated from the scleral periphery exhibited increased proliferation ability when subjected to mechanical strain; this change in proliferation ability was not observed in fibroblasts isolated from the peripapillary sclera. Mechanical strain also led to increased expression of α-SMA in periphery scleral fibroblasts, but not in peripapillary fibroblasts.

Given their role as matrix modulators and their ability to respond to short- and long-term stresses imparted to the eye, scleral fibroblasts—in their native state or as differentiated myofibroblasts—play an important part in diseases involving scleral remodeling, such as myopia and glaucoma [179, 180].

References

1. Vurgese S, Panda-Jonas S, Jonas JB. Scleral thickness in human eyes. PLoS One. 2012;7(1):e29692.
2. Norman RE, Flanagan JG, Rausch SM, Sigal IA, Tertinegg I, Eilaghi A, et al. Dimensions of the human sclera: thickness measurement and regional changes with axial length. Exp Eye Res. 2010;90(2):277–84.
3. Bron AJ, Tripathi RC, Tripathi BJ. Wolff's anatomy of the eye and orbit. 8th ed. London, UK: Chapman & Hall; 1997.
4. Coudrillier B, Boote C, Quigley HA, Nguyen TD. Scleral anisotropy and its effects on the mechanical response of the optic nerve head. Biomech Model Mechanobiol. 2013;12(5):941–63.
5. Campbell IC, Coudrillier B, Ethier CR. Biomechanics of the posterior eye: a critical role in health and disease. J Biomech Eng. 2014;136(2):021005.
6. Chung CW, Girard MJ, Jan NJ, Use SIA. Misuse of Laplace's law in ophthalmology. Invest Ophthalmol Vis Sci. 2016;57(1):236–45.
7. Singh KD, Logan NS, Gilmartin B. Three-dimensional modeling of the human eye based on magnetic resonance imaging. Invest Ophthalmol Vis Sci. 2006;47(6):2272–9.
8. Sigal IA, Flanagan JG, Ethier CR. Factors influencing optic nerve head biomechanics. Invest Ophthalmol Vis Sci. 2005;46(11):4189–99.
9. Jonas JB, Holbach L. Central corneal thickness and thickness of the lamina cribrosa in human eyes. Invest Ophthalmol Vis Sci. 2005;46(4):1275–9.
10. Olsen TW, Aaberg SY, Geroski DH, Edelhauser HF. Human sclera: thickness and surface area. Am J Ophthalmol. 1998;125(2):237–41.
11. Watson PG, Young RD. Scleral structure, organisation and disease. Exp Eye Res. 2004;78(3):609–23.
12. Kobayashi AS, Woo SL, Lawrence C, Schlegel WA. Analysis of the corneo-scleral shell by the method of direct stiffness. J Biomech. 1971;4(5):323–30.
13. Friberg TR. Lace JW. A comparison of the elastic properties of human choroid and sclera. Exp Eye Res. 1988;47(3):429–36.
14. Keeley FW, Morin JD, Vesely S. Characterization of collagen from normal human sclera. Exp Eye Res. 1984;39(5):533–42.

15. Bailey AJ. Structure, function and ageing of the collagens of the eye. Eye (Lond). 1987;1(Pt 2):175–83.
16. Girard MJ, Dahlmann-Noor A, Rayapureddi S, Bechara JA, Bertin BM, Jones H, et al. Quantitative mapping of scleral fiber orientation in normal rat eyes. Invest Ophthalmol Vis Sci. 2011;52(13):9684–93.
17. Pijanka JK, Coudrillier B, Ziegler K, Sorensen T, Meek KM, Nguyen TD, et al. Quantitative mapping of collagen fiber orientation in non-glaucoma and glaucoma posterior human sclerae. Invest Ophthalmol Vis Sci. 2012;53(9):5258–70.
18. Yan D, McPheeters S, Johnson G, Utzinger U, Vande Geest JP. Microstructural differences in the human posterior sclera as a function of age and race. Invest Ophthalmol Vis Sci. 2011;52(2):821–9.
19. Jan NJ, Gomez C, Moed S, Voorhees AP, Schuman JS, Bilonick RA, et al. Microstructural crimp of the Lamina Cribrosa and Peripapillary sclera collagen fibers. Invest Ophthalmol Vis Sci. 2017;58(9):3378–88.
20. Jan NJ, Lathrop K, Sigal IA. Collagen architecture of the posterior pole: high-resolution wide field of view visualization and analysis using polarized light microscopy. Invest Ophthalmol Vis Sci. 2017;58(2):735–44.
21. Jan NJ, Sigal IA. Collagen fiber recruitment: a microstructural basis for the nonlinear response of the posterior pole of the eye to increases in intraocular pressure. Acta Biomater. 2018;72:295–305.
22. Meek KM, Fullwood NJ. Corneal and scleral collagens: a microscopist's perspective. Micron. 2001;32(3):261–72.
23. Rada JA, Shelton S, Norton TT. The sclera and myopia. Exp Eye Res. 2006;82(2):185–200.
24. Quigley EN, Quigley HA, Pease ME, Kerrigan LA. Quantitative studies of elastin in the optic nerve heads of persons with primary open-angle glaucoma. Ophthalmology. 1996;103(10):1680–5.
25. Chen K, Rowley AP, Weiland JD, Humayun MS. Elastic properties of human posterior eye. J Biomed Mater Res A. 2014;102(6):2001–7.
26. Rada JA, Achen VR, Perry CA, Fox PW. Proteoglycans in the human sclera. Evidence for the presence of aggrecan. Invest Ophthalmol Vis Sci. 1997;38(9):1740–51.
27. Murienne BJ, Chen ML, Quigley HA, Nguyen TD. The contribution of glycosamino-glycans to the mechanical behaviour of the posterior human sclera. J R Soc Interface. 2016;13(119):20160367.
28. Tham YC, Li X, Wong TY, Quigley HA, Aung T, Cheng CY. Global prevalence of glaucoma and projections of glaucoma burden through 2040: a systematic review and meta-analysis. Ophthalmology. 2014;121(11):2081–90.
29. Bengtsson B, Heijl A. A long-term prospective study of risk factors for glaucomatous visual field loss in patients with ocular hypertension. J Glaucoma. 2005;14(2):135–8.
30. Leske MC, Heijl A, Hussein M, Bengtsson B, Hyman L, Komaroff E, et al. Factors for glaucoma progression and the effect of treatment: the early manifest glaucoma trial. Arch Ophthalmol. 2003;121(1):48–56.
31. The Advanced Glaucoma Intervention Study (AGIS): 7. The relationship between control of intraocular pressure and visual field deterioration.The AGIS Investigators. Am J Ophthalmol. 2000;130(4):429–40.
32. Hernandez MR, Pena JD. The optic nerve head in glaucomatous optic neuropathy. Arch Ophthalmol. 1997;115(3):389–95.
33. Ethier CR. Scleral biomechanics and glaucoma: a connection? Can J Ophthalmol. 2006;41(1):9–12.
34. Burgoyne CF, Downs JC, Bellezza AJ, Suh JK, Hart RT. The optic nerve head as a bio-mechanical structure: a new paradigm for understanding the role of IOP-related stress and strain in the pathophysiology of glaucomatous optic nerve head damage. Prog Retin Eye Res. 2005;24(1):39–73.
35. Fechtner RD, Weinreb RN. Mechanisms of optic nerve damage in primary open angle glaucoma. Surv Ophthalmol. 1994;39(1):23–42.

36. Holden BA, Fricke TR, Wilson DA, Jong M, Naidoo KS, Sankaridurg P, et al. Global prevalence of myopia and high myopia and temporal trends from 2000 through 2050. Ophthalmology. 2016;123(5):1036–42.
37. Resnikoff S, Pascolini D, Mariotti SP, Pokharel GP. Global magnitude of visual impairment caused by uncorrected refractive errors in 2004. Bull World Health Organ. 2008;86(1):63–70.
38. Rein DB, Zhang P, Wirth KE, Lee PP, Hoerger TJ, McCall N, et al. The economic burden of major adult visual disorders in the United States. Arch Ophthalmol. 2006;124(12):1754–60.
39. Harper AR, Summers JA. The dynamic sclera: extracellular matrix remodeling in normal ocular growth and myopia development. Exp Eye Res. 2015;133:100–11.
40. McBrien NA, Gentle A. Role of the sclera in the development and pathological complications of myopia. Prog Retin Eye Res. 2003;22(3):307–38.
41. Avetisov ES, Savitskaya NF, Vinetskaya MI, Iomdina EN. A study of biochemical and bio-mechanical qualities of normal and myopic eye sclera in humans of different age groups. Metab Pediatr Syst Ophthalmol. 1983;7(4):183–8.
42. Phillips JR, Khalaj M, McBrien NA. Induced myopia associated with increased scleral creep in chick and tree shrew eyes. Invest Ophthalmol Vis Sci. 2000;41(8):2028–34.
43. McGwin G Jr, Xie A, Owsley C. Rate of eye injury in the United States. Arch Ophthalmol. 2005;123(7):970–6.
44. Kuhn F, Morris R, Witherspoon CD, Mann L. Epidemiology of blinding trauma in the United States eye injury registry. Ophthalmic Epidemiol. 2006;13(3):209–16.
45. Parver LM. Eye trauma. The neglected disorder. Arch Ophthalmol. 1986;104(10):1452–3.
46. Bisplinghoff JA, McNally C, Manoogian SJ, Duma SM. Dynamic material properties of the human sclera. J Biomech. 2009;42(10):1493–7.
47. Tarlan B, Kiratli H. Subconjunctival hemorrhage: risk factors and potential indicators. Clin Ophthalmol. 2013;7:1163–70.
48. DiMaio VJ, DiMaio D. Forensic pathology. 2nd ed. Boca Raton: CRC Press; 2001.
49. Kennedy EA, Voorhies KD, Herring IP, Rath AL, Duma SM. Prediction of severe eye injuries in automobile accidents: static and dynamic rupture pressure of the eye. Annu Proc Assoc Adv Automot Med. 2004;48:165–79.
50. Sponsel WE, Gray W, Scribbick FW, Stern AR, Weiss CE, Groth SL, et al. Blunt eye trauma: empirical histopathologic paintball impact thresholds in fresh mounted porcine eyes. Invest Ophthalmol Vis Sci. 2011;52(8):5157–66.
51. Duma SM, Ng TP, Kennedy EA, Stitzel JD, Herring IP, Kuhn F. Determination of significant parameters for eye injury risk from projectiles. J Trauma. 2005;59(4):960–4.
52. Chen X, Yao Y, Wang F, Liu T, Zhao X. A retrospective study of eyeball rupture in patients with or without orbital fracture. Medicine (Baltimore). 2017;96(24):e7109.
53. Duma SM, Rath AL, Jernigan MV, Stitzel JD, Herring IP. The effects of depowered airbags on eye injuries in frontal automobile crashes. Am J Emerg Med. 2005;23(1):13–9.
54. Joseph JM, Glavas IP. Orbital fractures: a review. Clin Ophthalmol. 2011;5:95–100.
55. Alphonse VD, Kemper AR, Strom BT, Beeman SM, Duma SM. Mechanisms of eye injuries from fireworks. JAMA. 2012;308(1):33–4.
56. Clemente C, Esposito L, Speranza D, Bonora N. Firecracker eye exposure: experimental study and simulation. Biomech Model Mechanobiol. 2017;16(4):1401–11.
57. Bhardwaj R, Ziegler K, Seo JH, Ramesh KT, Nguyen TD. A computational model of blast loading on the human eye. Biomech Model Mechanobiol. 2014;13(1):123–40.
58. Battaglioli JL, Kamm RD. Measurements of the compressive properties of scleral tissue. Invest Ophthalmol Vis Sci. 1984;25(1):59–65.
59. Myers KM, Cone FE, Quigley HA, Gelman S, Pease ME, Nguyen TD. The in vitro inflation response of mouse sclera. Exp Eye Res. 2010;91(6):866–75.
60. Downs JC, Suh JK, Thomas KA, Bellezza AJ, Burgoyne CF, Hart RT. Viscoelastic character-ization of peripapillary sclera: material properties by quadrant in rabbit and monkey eyes. J Biomech Eng. 2003;125(1):124–31.
61. Coudrillier B, Tian J, Alexander S, Myers KM, Quigley HA, Nguyen TD. Biomechanics of the human posterior sclera: age- and glaucoma-related changes measured using inflation test-ing. Invest Ophthalmol Vis Sci. 2012;53(4):1714–28.

62. Cruz-Perez B, Pavlatos E, Morris HJ, Chen H, Pan X, Hart RT, et al. Mapping 3D strains with ultrasound speckle tracking: method validation and initial results in porcine scleral inflation. Ann Biomed Eng. 2016;44(7):2302–12.
63. Lari DR, Schultz DS, Wang AS, Lee OT, Stewart JM. Scleral mechanics: comparing whole globe inflation and uniaxial testing. Exp Eye Res. 2012;94(1):128–35.
64. Schultz DS, Lotz JC, Lee SM, Trinidad ML, Stewart JM. Structural factors that mediate scleral stiffness. Invest Ophthalmol Vis Sci. 2008;49(10):4232–6.
65. Girard MJ, Suh JK, Bottlang M, Burgoyne CF, Downs JC. Scleral biomechanics in the aging monkey eye. Invest Ophthalmol Vis Sci. 2009;50(11):5226–37.
66. Girard MJ, Suh JK, Bottlang M, Burgoyne CF, Downs JC. Biomechanical changes in the sclera of monkey eyes exposed to chronic IOP elevations. Invest Ophthalmol Vis Sci. 2011;52(8):5656–69.
67. Tonge TK, Murienne BJ, Coudrillier B, Alexander S, Rothkopf W, Nguyen TD. Minimal preconditioning effects observed for inflation tests of planar tissues. J Biomech Eng. 2013;135(11):114502.
68. Campbell IC, Hannon BG, Read AT, Sherwood JM, Schwaner SA, Ethier CR. Quantification of the efficacy of collagen cross-linking agents to induce stiffening of rat sclera. J R Soc Interface. 2017;14(129):20170014.
69. Grytz R, Fazio MA, Girard MJ, Libertiaux V, Bruno L, Gardiner S, et al. Material properties of the posterior human sclera. J Mech Behav Biomed Mater. 2014;29:602–17.
70. Grytz R, Siegwart JT Jr. Changing material properties of the tree shrew sclera during minus lens compensation and recovery. Invest Ophthalmol Vis Sci. 2015;56(3):2065–78.
71. Pardue MT, Stone RA, Iuvone PM. Investigating mechanisms of myopia in mice. Exp Eye Res. 2013;114:96–105.
72. Edwards MH. Animal models of myopia. A review. Acta Ophthalmol Scand. 1996;74(3):213–9.
73. Wisely CE, Sayed JA, Tamez H, Zelinka C, Abdel-Rahman MH, Fischer AJ, et al. The chick eye in vision research: an excellent model for the study of ocular disease. Prog Retin Eye Res. 2017;61:72–97.
74. Fazio MA, Grytz R, Morris JS, Bruno L, Girkin CA, Downs JC. Human scleral structural stiffness increases more rapidly with age in donors of African descent compared to donors of European descent. Invest Ophthalmol Vis Sci. 2014;55(11):7189–98.
75. Pyne JD, Genovese K, Casaletto L, Vande Geest JP. Sequential-digital image correlation for mapping human posterior sclera and optic nerve head deformation. J Biomech Eng. 2014;136(2):021002.
76. Geraghty B, Jones SW, Rama P, Akhtar R, Elsheikh A. Age-related variations in the biomechanical properties of human sclera. J Mech Behav Biomed Mater. 2012;16:181–91.
77. Eilaghi A, Flanagan JG, Tertinegg I, Simmons CA, Wayne Brodland G, Ross Ethier C. Biaxial mechanical testing of human sclera. J Biomech. 2010;43(9):1696–701.
78. Woo SL, Kobayashi AS, Schlegel WA, Lawrence C. Nonlinear material properties of intact cornea and sclera. Exp Eye Res. 1972;14(1):29–39.
79. Cruz-Perez B, Tang J, Morris HJ, Palko JR, Pan X, Hart RT, et al. Biaxial mechanical testing of posterior sclera using high-resolution ultrasound speckle tracking for strain measurements. J Biomech. 2014;47(5):1151–6.
80. Girard M, Suh JK, Hart RT, Burgoyne CF, Downs JC. Effects of storage time on the mechanical properties of rabbit peripapillary sclera after enucleation. Curr Eye Res. 2007;32(5):465–70.
81. Elsheikh A, Geraghty B, Alhasso D, Knappett J, Campanelli M, Rama P. Regional variation in the biomechanical properties of the human sclera. Exp Eye Res. 2010;90(5):624–33.
82. Wollensak G, Spoerl E. Collagen crosslinking of human and porcine sclera. J Cataract Refract Surg. 2004;30(3):689–95.
83. Campbell IC, Sherwood JM, Overby DR, Hannon BG, Read AT, Raykin J, et al. Quantification of scleral biomechanics and collagen fiber alignment. Methods Mol Biol. 2018;1695:135–59.
84. Bruno L, Bianco G. Fazio MA. A multi-camera speckle interferometer for dynamic full-field 3D displacement measurement: validation and inflation testing of a human eye sclera. Opt Lasers Eng. 2018;107:91–101.

85. Pavlatos E, Perez BC, Morris HJ, Chen H, Palko JR, Pan X, et al. Three-dimensional strains in human posterior sclera using ultrasound speckle tracking. J Biomech Eng. 2016;138(2):021015.
86. Nguyen C, Midgett D, Kimball EC, Steinhart MR, Nguyen TD, Pease ME, et al. Measuring deformation in the mouse optic nerve head and peripapillary sclera. Invest Ophthalmol Vis Sci. 2017;58(2):721–33.
87. Grytz R, Fazio MA, Libertiaux V, Bruno L, Gardiner S, Girkin CA, et al. Age- and race-related differences in human scleral material properties. Invest Ophthalmol Vis Sci. 2014;55(12):8163–72.
88. Braunsmann C, Hammer CM, Rheinlaender J, Kruse FE, Schaffer TE, Schlotzer-Schrehardt U. Evaluation of lamina cribrosa and peripapillary sclera stiffness in pseudoexfoliation and normal eyes by atomic force microscopy. Invest Ophthalmol Vis Sci. 2012;53(6):2960–7.
89. Meller D, Peters K, Meller K. Human cornea and sclera studied by atomic force microscopy. Cell Tissue Res. 1997;288(1):111–8.
90. Choi S, Cheong Y, Lee IIJ, Lee SJ, Jin KH. Park HK. AFM study for morphological and mechanical properties of human scleral surface. J Nanosci Nanotechnol. 2011;11(7):6382–8.
91. Kennedy EA, Ng TP, McNally C, Stitzel JD, Duma SM. Risk functions for human and porcine eye rupture based on projectile characteristics of blunt objects. Stapp Car Crash J. 2006;50:651–71.
92. Rodriguez JO, Lavina AM, Agarwal A. Prevention and treatment of common eye injuries in sports. Am Fam Physician. 2003;67(7):1481–8.
93. Vinger PF, Duma SM, Crandall J. Baseball hardness as a risk factor for eye injuries. Arch Ophthalmol. 1999;117(3):354–8.
94. Georgalas I, Ladas I, Taliantzis S, Rouvas A, Koutsandrea C. Severe intraocular trauma in a fireman caused by a high-pressure water jet. Clin Exp Ophthalmol. 2011;39(4):370–1.
95. Hiraoka T, Ogami T, Okamoto F, Oshika T. Compressed air blast injury with palpebral, orbital, facial, cervical, and mediastinal emphysema through an eyelid laceration: a case report and review of literature. BMC Ophthalmol. 2013;13:68.
96. Landau D, Berson D. High-pressure directed water jets as a cause of severe bilateral intraocular injuries. Am J Ophthalmol. 1995;120(4):542–3.
97. Salminen L, Ranta A. Orbital laceration caused by a blast of water: report of 2 cases. Br J Ophthalmol. 1983;67(12):840–1.
98. Duma SM, Bisplinghoff JA, Senge DM, McNally C, Alphonse VD. Evaluating the risk of eye injuries: intraocular pressure during high speed projectile impacts. Curr Eye Res. 2012;37(1):43–9.
99. Bisplinghoff JA, McNally C, Duma SM. High-rate internal pressurization of human eyes to predict globe rupture. Arch Ophthalmol. 2009;127(4):520–3.
100. Coleman DJ, Trokel S. Direct-recorded intraocular pressure variations in a human subject. Arch Ophthalmol. 1969;82(5):637–40.
101. Duma SM, Bisplinghoff JA, Senge DM, McNally C, Alphonse VD. Eye injury risk from water stream impact: biomechanically based design parameters for water toy and park design. Curr Eye Res. 2012;37(4):279–85.
102. Bullock JD, Warwar RE, Green WR. Ocular explosions from periocular anesthetic injections: a clinical, histopathologic, experimental, and biophysical study. Ophthalmology. 1999;106(12):2341–52; discussion 52–3
103. Crowley JS, Brozoski FT, Duma SM, Kennedy EA. Development of the facial and ocular countermeasures safety (FOCUS) headform. Aviat Space Environ Med. 2009;80(9):831.
104. Cormier J, Manoogian S, Bisplinghoff J, Rowson S, Santago AC, McNally C, et al. Biomechanical response of the human face and corresponding biofidelity of the FOCUS Headform. SAE Int J Passeng Cars Mech Syst. 2010;3(1):842–59.
105. Bisplinghoff JA, Duma SM. Evaluation of eye injury risk from projectile shooting toys using the focus headform–biomed 2009. Biomed Sci Instrum. 2009;45:107–12.
106. Kennedy EA, Inzana JA, McNally C, Duma SM, Depinet PJ, Sullenberger KH, et al. Development and validation of a synthetic eye and orbit for estimating the potential for globe rupture due to specific impact conditions. Stapp Car Crash J. 2007;51:381–400.

107. Allen R, Motz CT, Feola A, Chesler K, Haider R, Ramachandra Rao S, et al. Long-term functional and structural consequences of primary blast overpressure to the eye. J Neurotrauma. 2018;35(17):2104–16.
108. Shedd DF, Benko NA, Jones J, Zaugg BE, Peiffer RL, Coats B. Long term temporal changes in structure and function of rat visual system after blast exposure. Invest Ophthalmol Vis Sci. 2018;59(1):349–61.
109. Weaver AA, Stitzel SM, Stitzel JD. Injury risk prediction from computational simulations of ocular blast loading. Biomech Model Mechanobiol. 2017;16(2):463–77.
110. Notghi B, Bhardwaj R, Bailoor S, Thompson KA, Weaver AA, Stitzel JD, et al. Biomechanical evaluations of ocular injury risk for blast loading. J Biomech Eng. 2017;139(8) https://doi.org/10.1115/1.4037072.
111. Sundaramurthy A, Skotak M, Alay E, Unnikrishnan G, Mao H, Duan X, et al. Assessment of the effectiveness of combat eyewear protection against blast overpressure. J Biomech Eng. 2018;140(7):071003.
112. Hommer A, Fuchsjager-Mayrl G, Resch H, Vass C, Garhofer G, Schmetterer L. Estimation of ocular rigidity based on measurement of pulse amplitude using pneumotonometry and fundus pulse using laser interferometry in glaucoma. Invest Ophthalmol Vis Sci. 2008;49(9):4046–50.
113. Dikici AS, Mihmanli I, Kilic F, Ozkok A, Kuyumcu G, Sultan P, et al. In vivo evaluation of the biomechanical properties of optic nerve and peripapillary structures by ultrasonic shear wave elastography in glaucoma. Iran J Radiol. 2016;13(2):e36849.
114. Girard MJ, Strouthidis NG, Desjardins A, Mari JM, Ethier CR. In vivo optic nerve head biomechanics: performance testing of a three-dimensional tracking algorithm. J R Soc Interface. 2013;10(87):20130459.
115. Zeiss CJ. Translational models of ocular disease. Vet Ophthalmol. 2013;16(Suppl 1):15–33.
116. Girard MJ, Dupps WJ, Baskaran M, Scarcelli G, Yun SH, Quigley HA, et al. Translating ocular biomechanics into clinical practice: current state and future prospects. Curr Eye Res. 2015;40(1):1–18.
117. Almasieh M, Levin LA. Neuroprotection in Glaucoma: animal models and clinical trials. Annu Rev Vis Sci. 2017;3:91–120.
118. Bouhenni RA, Dunmire J, Sewell A, Edward DP. Animal models of glaucoma. J Biomed Biotechnol. 2012;2012:692609.
119. Ishikawa M, Yoshitomi T, Zorumski CF, Izumi Y. Experimentally induced mammalian models of glaucoma. Biomed Res Int. 2015;2015:281214.
120. Morrison JC. Elevated intraocular pressure and optic nerve injury models in the rat. J Glaucoma. 2005;14(4):315–7.
121. Struebing FL, Geisert EE. What animal models can tell us about glaucoma. Prog Mol Biol Transl Sci. 2015;134:365–80.
122. Toris CB, Gelfman C, Whitlock A, Sponsel WE, Rowe-Rendleman CL. Making basic science studies in glaucoma more clinically relevant: the need for a consensus. J Ocul Pharmacol Ther. 2017;33(7):501–18.
123. Weinreb RN, Lindsey JD. The importance of models in glaucoma research. J Glaucoma. 2005;14(4):302–4.
124. Agarwal R, Agarwal P. Rodent models of glaucoma and their applicability for drug discovery. Expert Opin Drug Discov. 2017;12(3):261–70.
125. Chen S, Zhang X. The rodent model of Glaucoma and its implications. Asia Pac J Ophthalmol (Phila). 2015;4(4):236–41.
126. Johnson TV, Tomarev SI. Rodent models of glaucoma. Brain Res Bull. 2010;81(2–3):349–58.
127. Morrison JC, Cepurna Ying Guo WO, Johnson EC. Pathophysiology of human glaucomatous optic nerve damage: insights from rodent models of glaucoma. Exp Eye Res. 2011;93(2):156–64.
128. Fernandes KA, Harder JM, Williams PA, Rausch RL, Kiernan AE, Nair KS, et al. Using genetic mouse models to gain insight into glaucoma: past results and future possibilities. Exp Eye Res. 2015;141:42–56.

129. Overby DR, Clark AF. Animal models of glucocorticoid-induced glaucoma. Exp Eye Res. 2015;141:15–22.
130. Rybkin I, Gerometta R, Fridman G, Candia O, Danias J. Model systems for the study of steroid-induced IOP elevation. Exp Eye Res. 2017;158:51–8.
131. Morgan JE, Tribble JR. Microbead models in glaucoma. Exp Eye Res. 2015;141:9–14.
132. Smedowski A, Pietrucha-Dutczak M, Kaarniranta K, Lewin-Kowalik J. A rat experimental model of glaucoma incorporating rapid-onset elevation of intraocular pressure. Sci Rep. 2014;4:5910.
133. Morrison JC, Cepurna WO, Johnson EC. Modeling glaucoma in rats by sclerosing aqueous outflow pathways to elevate intraocular pressure. Exp Eye Res. 2015;141:23–32.
134. Morrison JC, Moore CG, Deppmeier LM, Gold BG, Meshul CK. Johnson EC. A rat model of chronic pressure-induced optic nerve damage. Exp Eye Res. 1997;64(1):85–96.
135. Mayordomo-Febrer A, Lopez-Murcia M, Morales-Tatay JM, Monleon-Salvado D, Pinazo-Duran MD. Metabolomics of the aqueous humor in the rat glaucoma model induced by a series of intracamerular sodium hyaluronate injection. Exp Eye Res. 2015;131:84–92.
136. Pang IH, Millar JC, Clark AF. Elevation of intraocular pressure in rodents using viral vectors targeting the trabecular meshwork. Exp Eye Res. 2015;141:33–41.
137. Gross RL, Ji J, Chang P, Pennesi ME, Yang Z, Zhang J, et al. A mouse model of elevated intraocular pressure: retina and optic nerve findings. Trans Am Ophthalmol Soc. 2003;101:163–9; discussion 9–71
138. Kimball EC, Nguyen C, Steinhart MR, Nguyen TD, Pease ME, Oglesby EN, et al. Experimental scleral cross-linking increases glaucoma damage in a mouse model. Exp Eye Res. 2014;128:129–40.
139. Cao J, Yang EB, Su JJ, Li Y, Chow P. The tree shrews: adjuncts and alternatives to primates as models for biomedical research. J Med Primatol. 2003;32(3):123–30.
140. McBrien NA, Cornell LM, Gentle A. Structural and ultrastructural changes to the sclera in a mammalian model of high myopia. Invest Ophthalmol Vis Sci. 2001;42(10):2179–87.
141. Levy AM, Fazio MA, Grytz R. Experimental myopia increases and scleral crosslinking using genipin inhibits cyclic softening in the tree shrew sclera. Ophthalmic Physiol Opt. 2018;38(3):246–56.
142. Rasmussen CA, Kaufman PL. Primate glaucoma models. J Glaucoma. 2005;14(4):311–4.
143. Ho LC, Sigal IA, Jan NJ, Squires A, Tse Z, Wu EX, et al. Magic angle-enhanced MRI of fibrous microstructures in sclera and cornea with and without intraocular pressure loading. Invest Ophthalmol Vis Sci. 2014;55(9):5662–72.
144. Coudrillier B, Campbell IC, Read AT, Geraldes DM, Vo NT, Feola A, et al. Effects of peripapillary scleral stiffening on the deformation of the Lamina Cribrosa. Invest Ophthalmol Vis Sci. 2016;57(6):2666–77.
145. Clayson K, Pan X, Pavlatos E, Short R, Morris H, Hart RT, et al. Corneoscleral stiffening increases IOP spike magnitudes during rapid microvolumetric change in the eye. Exp Eye Res. 2017;165:29–34.
146. Sit AJ, Liu JH. Pathophysiology of glaucoma and continuous measurements of intraocular pressure. Mol Cell Biomech. 2009;6(1):57–69.
147. Zernii EY, Baksheeva VE, Iomdina EN, Averina OA, Permyakov SE, Philippov PP, et al. Rabbit models of ocular diseases: new relevance for classical approaches. CNS Neurol Disord Drug Targets. 2016;15(3):267–91.
148. Karl A, Makarov FN, Koch C, Korber N, Schuldt C, Kruger M, et al. The ultrastructure of rabbit sclera after scleral crosslinking with riboflavin and blue light of different intensities. Graefes Arch Clin Exp Ophthalmol. 2016;254(8):1567–77.
149. Liu TX, Wang Z. Biomechanics of sclera crosslinked using genipin in rabbit. Int J Ophthalmol. 2017;10(3):355–60.
150. Dotan A, Kremer I, Gal-Or O, Livnat T, Zigler A, Bourla D, et al. Scleral cross-linking using riboflavin and ultraviolet: a radiation for prevention of axial myopia in a rabbit model. J Vis Exp. 2016;110:e53201.

151. Palko JR, Morris HJ, Pan X, Harman CD, Koehl KL, Gelatt KN, et al. Influence of age on ocular biomechanical properties in a canine glaucoma model with ADAMTS10 mutation. PLoS One. 2016;11(6):e0156466.
152. Narfstrom K, Deckman KH, Menotti-Raymond M. Cats: a gold mine for ophthalmology. Annu Rev Anim Biosci. 2013;1:157–77.
153. Yuan Y, Li M, Chen Q, Me R, Yu Y, Gu Q, et al. Crosslinking enzyme Lysyl oxidase modulates scleral remodeling in form-deprivation myopia. Curr Eye Res. 2018;43(2):200–7.
154. Chhetri J, Jacobson G, Gueven N. Zebrafish—on the move towards ophthalmological research. Eye (Lond). 2014;28(4):367–80.
155. Yeh LK, Liu CY, Kao WW, Huang CJ, Hu FR, Chien CL, et al. Knockdown of zebrafish lumican gene (zlum) causes scleral thinning and increased size of scleral coats. J Biol Chem. 2010;285(36):28141–55.
156. Coudrillier B, Pijanka J, Jefferys J, Sorensen T, Quigley HA, Boote C, et al. Collagen structure and mechanical properties of the human sclera: analysis for the effects of age. J Biomech Eng. 2015;137(4):041006.
157. Danford FL, Yan D, Dreier RA, Cahir TM, Girkin CA, Vande Geest JP. Differences in the region- and depth-dependent microstructural organization in normal versus glaucomatous human posterior sclerae. Invest Ophthalmol Vis Sci. 2013;54(13):7922–32.
158. Lopilly Park HY, Lee NY, Choi JA, Park CK. Measurement of scleral thickness using swept-source optical coherence tomography in patients with open-angle glaucoma and myopia. Am J Ophthalmol. 2014;157(4):876–84.
159. Coudrillier B, Pijanka JK, Jefferys JL, Goel A, Quigley HA, Boote C, et al. Glaucoma-related changes in the mechanical properties and collagen micro-architecture of the human sclera. PLoS One. 2015;10(7):e0131396.
160. Rudnicka AR, Mt-Isa S, Owen CG, Cook DG, Ashby D. Variations in primary open-angle glaucoma prevalence by age, gender, and race: a Bayesian meta-analysis. Invest Ophthalmol Vis Sci. 2006;47(10):4254–61.
161. Jonas JB, Xu L. Histological changes of high axial myopia. Eye (Lond). 2014;28(2):113–7.
162. Siegwart JT, Norton TT. Regulation of the mechanical properties of tree shrew sclera by the visual environment. Vis Res. 1999;39(2):387–407.
163. Lewis JA, Garcia MB, Rani L, Wildsoet CF. Intact globe inflation testing of changes in scleral mechanics in myopia and recovery. Exp Eye Res. 2014;127:42–8.
164. McBrien NA, Jobling AI, Gentle A. Biomechanics of the sclera in myopia: extracellular and cellular factors. Optom Vis Sci. 2009;86(1):E23–30.
165. Lin X, Wang BJ, Wang YC, Chu RY, Dai JH, Zhou XT, et al. Scleral ultrastructure and biomechanical changes in rabbits after negative lens application. Int J Ophthalmol. 2018;11(3):354–62.
166. Rada JA, Nickla DL, Troilo D. Decreased proteoglycan synthesis associated with form deprivation myopia in mature primate eyes. Invest Ophthalmol Vis Sci. 2000;41(8):2050–8.
167. Liu HH, Kenning MS, Jobling AI, McBrien NA, Gentle A. Reduced scleral TIMP-2 expression is associated with myopia development: TIMP-2 supplementation stabilizes scleral biomarkers of myopia and limits myopia development. Invest Ophthalmol Vis Sci. 2017;58(4):1971–81.
168. McBrien NA, Metlapally R, Jobling AI, Gentle A. Expression of collagen-binding integrin receptors in the mammalian sclera and their regulation during the development of myopia. Invest Ophthalmol Vis Sci. 2006;47(11):4674–82.
169. Sinha Roy A, Rocha KM, Randleman JB, Stulting RD, Dupps WJ Jr. Inverse computational analysis of in vivo corneal elastic modulus change after collagen crosslinking for keratoconus. Exp Eye Res. 2013;113:92–104.
170. Liu S, Li S, Wang B, Lin X, Wu Y, Liu H, et al. Scleral cross-linking using riboflavin UVA irradiation for the prevention of myopia progression in a Guinea pig model: blocked axial extension and altered scleral microstructure. PLoS One. 2016;11(11):e0165792.

171. Wang M, Corpuz CC. Effects of scleral cross-linking using genipin on the process of form-deprivation myopia in the Guinea pig: a randomized controlled experimental study. BMC Ophthalmol. 2015;15:89.
172. Chu Y, Cheng Z, Liu J, Wang Y, Guo H, Han Q. The effects of scleral collagen cross-linking using glyceraldehyde on the progression of form-deprived myopia in Guinea pigs. J Ophthalmol. 2016;2016:3526153.
173. Dotan A, Kremer I, Livnat T, Zigler A, Weinberger D, Bourla D. Scleral cross-linking using riboflavin and ultraviolet: a radiation for prevention of progressive myopia in a rabbit model. Exp Eye Res. 2014;127:190–5.
174. Rada JA, Thoft RA, Hassell JR. Increased aggrecan (cartilage proteoglycan) production in the sclera of myopic chicks. Dev Biol. 1991;147(2):303–12.
175. Moller-Pedersen T, Ledet T, Ehlers N. The keratocyte density of human donor corneas. Curr Eye Res. 1994;13(2):163–9.
176. Siegwart JT, Norton TT. Selective regulation of MMP and TIMP mRNA levels in tree shrew sclera during minus lens compensation and recovery. Invest Ophthalmol Vis Sci. 2005;46(10):3484–92.
177. Metlapally R, Jobling AI, Gentle A, McBrien NA. Characterization of the integrin receptor subunit profile in the mammalian sclera. Mol Vis. 2006;12:725–34.
178. Qu J, Chen H, Zhu L, Ambalavanan N, Girkin CA, Murphy-Ullrich JE, et al. High-magnitude and/or high-frequency mechanical strain promotes peripapillary scleral myofibroblast differentiation. Invest Ophthalmol Vis Sci. 2015;56(13):7821–30.
179. Backhouse S, Phillips JR. Effect of induced myopia on scleral myofibroblasts and in vivo ocular biomechanical compliance in the Guinea pig. Invest Ophthalmol Vis Sci. 2010;51(12):6162–71.
180. Phillips JR, McBrien NA. Pressure-induced changes in axial eye length of chick and tree shrew: significance of myofibroblasts in the sclera. Invest Ophthalmol Vis Sci. 2004;45(3):758–63.
181. Serini G, Gabbiani G. Mechanisms of myofibroblast activity and phenotypic modulation. Exp Cell Res. 1999;250(2):273–83.
182. Qiu C, Chen M, Yao J, Sun X, Xu J, Zhang R, et al. Mechanical strain induces distinct human scleral fibroblast lineages: differential roles in cell proliferation, apoptosis, migration, and differentiation. Invest Ophthalmol Vis Sci. 2018;59(6):2401–10.

Chapter 7
Choroidal Biomechanics

Clemens A. Strohmaier and Herbert A. Reitsamer

Overview of the Structure and Function of the Choroid

The choroid is the posterior part of the uvea, located between the retina and the sclera. It forms a continuous layer starting from the pars plana of the ciliary body and extending back to the optic nerve. Most commonly, it is divided in 5 (4–6) sub-layers (from the retinal side): Bruch's membrane, the choriocapillaris, two vascular layers (Haller's and Sattler's) and the suprachoroidal space [1]. Differences in species exist and are subtle in many cases, but as far as choroidal biomechanics are concerned, for most of these differences there is no evidence of a functional significance. One exception is the possible existence of a lymphatic system within the human choroid, a subject currently being debated [2, 3].

While choroidal blood flow is amongst the highest in relation to tissue weight, the arterio-venous oxygen extraction is low [4]. The seemingly excess blood flow is necessary to deliver a sufficient oxygen gradient for diffusion to the inner retinal layers, primarily supplying oxygen to and removing metabolic waste of the photo-receptors [5, 6].

Choroidal blood flow is actively regulated in response to changes of choroidal perfusion pressure, primarily by autoregulatory mechanisms [7, 8]. Choroidal perfusion pressure can be altered by changes of either intraocular pressure (IOP), arterial pressure or venous pressure. While a broad variety of substances is known to alter choroidal blood and its ability for active regulation [9, 10], the role of the nervous system supplying the choroid is hardly known.

The innervation of the choroid is complex. While the choroidal vasculature receives sympathetic (originating in the superior cervical ganglion), as well as para-sympathetic (via the pterygopalatine ganglion) innervation, there are also neurons

C. A. Strohmaier · H. A. Reitsamer (✉)
Ophthalmology/Optometry, Paracelsus Medical University/SALK, Salzburg, Austria

© Springer Nature Switzerland AG 2021
I. Pallikaris et al. (eds.), *Ocular Rigidity, Biomechanics and Hydrodynamics of the Eye*, https://doi.org/10.1007/978-3-030-64422-2_7

within the choroid itself, the so-called intrinsic choroidal neurons [11–13]. Despite their discovery some 150 years ago, their functional role is still unknown.

Another puzzling feature of choroidal anatomy are the non-vascular smooth muscle cells [14]. Centered on the posterior pole of the eye and more numerous in species with foveae, a possible role in emmetropization has been suggested—but without functional evidence up to date.

The Choroid Has a Profound Effect on the Ocular Rigidity

Intraocular pressure arises from aqueous humor production in the ciliary body and its outflow against the resistance in the trabecular and uveoscleral pathways [15].

This outflow resistance in combination with the elasticity of the ocular coatings is the basis of the ocular pressure—volume relationship established by Friedenwald [16]:

$$E = \left[\log(IOP1) - \log(IOP2)\right]/(V1 - V2)$$

E is the ocular rigidity, $\Delta IOP = IOP1-IOP2$ is the change in intraocular pressure, $\Delta V = V1 - V2$ is the change in intraocular volume. The equation is the basis for ocular tonometry [16] and measurements of pulsatile ocular blood flow [17].

A very important assumption in these deductions is the constancy of ocular rigidity. There is, however, evidence that changes in volume and pressure within the ocular vasculature causes changes inocular rigidity. Eisenlohr et al. were the first to report a difference in the ocular rigidity between living and dead eyes [18, 19]. Arterial blood pressure influences IOP and shifts the ocular pressure volume relationship and thereby alters ocular rigidity [20]. The choroid comprises most of the ocular vascular volume and hence, has the greatest effect on ocular rigidity. The following paragraphs summarize choroidal vascular physiology as it relates to choroidal biomechanics.

Effect of Blood Pressure on Choroidal Biomechanics

As in any tissue of the body, arterial blood pressure drives blood through the choroidal vasculature and the combined resistance of all choroidal vessels cause a pressure drop to the venous side of the circulation (i.e. the vortex veins). A major difference to most circulations, however, is the compressing force exerted by intraocular pressure (IOP). This causes the choroidal veins to behave as Starling resistors, i.e. maintaining an intraluminal pressure slightly higher than IOP to prevent them from collapsing. Figure 7.1 illustrates the effect of an external compression force on the flow and transmural pressure in a vessel [21].

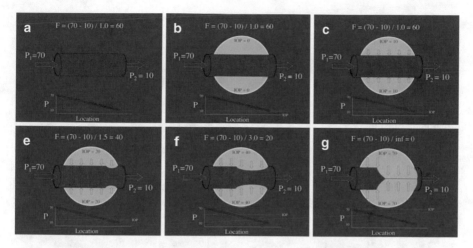

Fig. 7.1 Ocular Starling resistor. (**a**) Vessel flow (F) is a function of the pressure gradient (P1–P2) along the vessel divided by the resistance. (**b, c**) If the vessel passes through an organ (e.g., the eye) with a low tissue pressure (e.g., IOP), the pressure inside the vessel exceeds the pressure outside the vessel (i.e., the transmural pressure gradient) and so the vessel remains distended. (**d, e**) If the tissue pressure is somewhat higher and exceeds the pressure at the lowest point inside the vessel (i.e., at the "venous" end), that region of the vessel will begin to collapse. This will increase the resistance to flow in that segment thereby raising the intraluminal pressure until the transmural pressure becomes slightly positive again. (**f**) If the tissue pressure becomes greater than the arterial input pressure, the vessel will collapse completely, the resistance will be infinite, and flow through the vessel will cease. Reproduced with permission from [21]

Thus, the ocular perfusion pressure (i.e. the pressure gradient driving blood flow) can be approximated as the difference between mean arterial pressure and intraocular pressure [22]:

$$OPP = MAP - IOP$$

This equation has profound implications on choroidal biomechanics, as arterial and venous pressure in the choroid determine its elasticity. Figure 7.2 illustrates these effects during a constant-rate saline infusion (120 µl/min). The dashed line shows the IOP course as predicted by the Friedenwald equation—assuming a constant elasticity of the ocular coatings (i.e., sclera, cornea). The solid line shows the actual course of IOP in the eye of a living rabbit. The difference between both lines can be attributed to the choroidal blood volume that is expelled as IOP rises. At low volume increments—the shallow section of the curve—blood volume from the venous side is expelled and at higher IOP values the arteries are compressed. Once mean arterial pressure is reached, the choroid is devoid of blood and both curves rise at the same rate.

This behavior is dependent on the mean arterial pressure, as would be expected from Fig. 7.2. Figure 7.3 shows the effect of arterial blood pressure on ocular rigidity curves obtained by intraocular volume increments in a rabbit model [23]. The lower panel demonstrates the almost linear increase of ocular rigidity with

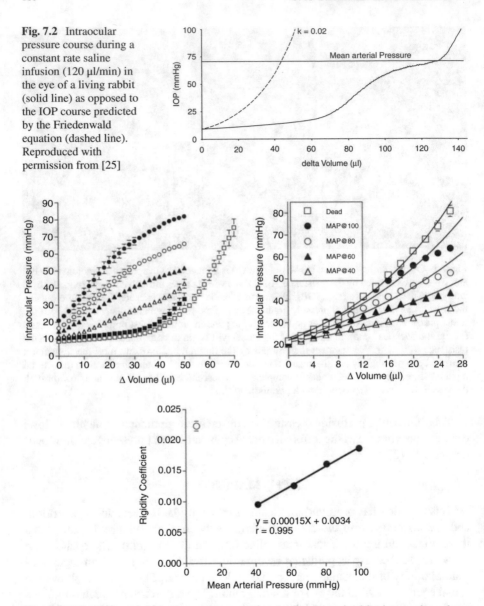

Fig. 7.2 Intraocular pressure course during a constant rate saline infusion (120 µl/min) in the eye of a living rabbit (solid line) as opposed to the IOP course predicted by the Friedenwald equation (dashed line). Reproduced with permission from [25]

Fig. 7.3 Effect of arterial blood pressure on ocular rigidity determined by intraocular volume increments [23]. The top left panel shows the data plotted with IOP uncontrolled, on the top right side the IOP was set to 20 mmHg before the start of the experiment (Reproduced with permission)

mean arterial blood pressure. While a hydraulic variation of either blood pressure or intraocular pressure over a wide range is obviously not possible in humans, the influence of blood pressure on ocular rigidity was shown in humans as well [24].

The Interaction Between Venous Pressure, Intraocular Pressure and Perfusion Pressure

In contrast to arterial pressure, the relationship between intraocular pressure and choroidal venous pressure is poorly understood. There is some evidence suggesting that the Starling resistor behavior outlined above may produce non-linear results, especially at low IOP values. Maepea was first to note that choroidal venous pressure appears to be significantly higher than IOP at low IOP values [22].

Figure 7.4 shows the author's own unpublished study on the relationship between IOP and choroidal venous pressure (measured through direct cannulation). At IOP values in a "normal" range, choroidal venous pressure clearly deviates from the assumed 1:1 relationship and thus, perfusion pressure in the choroid is less than estimated by the PP = MAP − IOP formula. From a clinical perspective, this is of high relevance in normal tension glaucoma, where low (diastolic) blood pressure might cause insufficient blood supply of the optic nerve head.

The pressures downstream the choroidal veins are poorly understood as well. They are difficult to measure in most species with the exception of rabbits, where a foramen in the scull allows direct cannulation [20]. In this model, a linear relationship between orbital venous pressure and mean arterial blood pressure was found (Fig. 7.5). Pressure in the venous system may be of high clinical relevance in ophthalmology, as the ocular veins at least partly seem to exhibit a passive behavior during pressure changes [20, 26]. This implies an effect of elevated thoracic

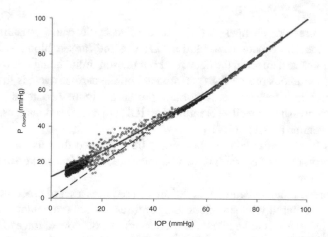

Fig. 7.4 Relationship between intraocular pressure (IOP) and choroidal venous pressure (P choroid). As expected by the Starling resistor effect, choroidal venous pressure slightly exceed intraocular pressure at medium to high IOP values. At lower IOP values, however, choroidal venous pressure deviates from this 1:1 relationship significantly, reaching 50% at values below 10 mmHg (Author's own unpublished observation)

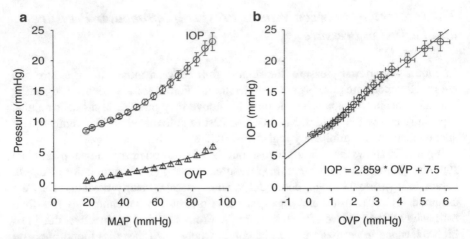

Fig. 7.5 The effect of blood pressure (MAP = mean arterial pressure) changes on intraocular pressure and orbital venous pressure (OVP) in rabbits (Reproduced with permission from [20])

pressure, as it occurs in obstructive sleep apnea syndrome but also in obesity, on the ocular circulation. A striking clinical example is the immediate choroidal thickness increase during the Valsalva maneuver [27].

Effect of Arterial Pulse on IOP and Ocular Venous Pressures

The arterial pressure changes during the cardiac cycle cause pulsatile pressure changes in the entire ocular circulation. Due to the largest blood volume, they exhibit their greatest effect in the choroidal circulation, influencing intraocular pressure as well as venous pressure. Superimposed on the cardiac cycle is the breathing rhythm, which influences the intrathoracic pressure. Figure 7.6 shows the effect of arterial pulse pressure as well as breathing on IOP, episcleral venous pressure (EVP) and orbital venous pressure (OVP).

Changes in choroidal volume can either be estimated directly (commonly via interferometry) or its effect on IOP can be measured as an indirect estimate of choroidal blood flow.

The theoretical model behind this estimation requires a set of preconditions: IOP needs to be measured with sufficient temporal resolution, the ocular pressure/volume relationship needs to be known and constant, the outflow of the eye is assumed to be constant [28]. As can be seen from the discussion in this chapter, these preconditions are not fulfilled entirely.

Clinically, the ocular pulse amplitude is most commonly measured using a dynamic contour tonometer (DCT). DCT is an IOP measurement technique that provides a continuous reading of IOP without the need for corneal applanation. Besides being less dependent on corneal thickness (as a surrogate marker for

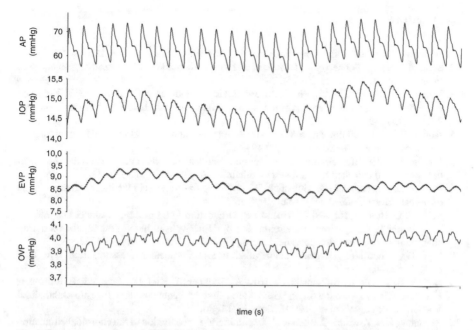

time (s)

Fig. 7.6 High speed tracing of arterial pressure (AP), intraocular pressure (IOP), episcleral venous pressure (EVP) and orbital venous pressure (OVP)—all measured through direct cannulation. Two rhythms can be seen in the tracing: a low frequency movement caused by breathing-synchronous changes in intrathoracic pressure and a high-frequency rhythm due to the cardiac cycle (Author's own unpublished observation)

corneal biomechanics), its continuous IOP measurement allows the calculation of the ocular pulse amplitude over the cardiac cycle [29, 30].

Future Directions

The present knowledge of choroidal biomechanical properties relies on measurements of surrogate parameters mainly. Future technologies based on OCT may have the potential to provide a direct measurement of choroidal volume as well as flow and, given sufficient temporal resolution, a measurement of true biomechanical properties like elasticity as well [31–33].

Another rapidly developing field is the choroidal involvement in emmetropization. The choroid reacts to retinal defocus by changing its thickness in birds and humans [34, 35] and thus, a role in emmetropization is plausible. The mechanism remains to be elucidated, but one hypothesis involves the active control of choroidal thickness by the non-vascular smooth muscle cells mentioned earlier in this chapter (reviewed in [36]). Active choroidal thickness control is of high clinical relevance, not only related to the prevention of myopia but also with regard to entities like choroidal effusion syndrome, which is poorly understood.

References

1. Wybar KC. A study of the choroidal circulation of the eye in man. J Anat. 1954;88:94–8.
2. Schrödl F, Kaser-Eichberger A, Trost A, et al. Lymphatic markers in the adult human choroid. Investig Opthalmol Vis Sci. 2015;56:7406.
3. Koina ME, Baxter L, Adamson SJ, Arfuso F, Hu P, Madigan MC, Chan-Ling T. Evidence for lymphatics in the developing and adult human choroid. Invest Ophthalmol Vis Sci. 2015;56:1310–27.
4. Alm A, Bill A. Blood flow and oxygen extraction in the cat uvea at normal and high intraocular pressures. Acta Physiol Scand. 1970;80:19–28.
5. Linsenmeier RA, Padnick-Silver L. Metabolic dependence of photoreceptors on the choroid in the normal and detached retina. Invest Ophthalmol Vis Sci. 2000;41:3117–23.
6. Braun RD, Linsenmeier RA, Goldstick TK. Oxygen consumption in the inner and outer retina of the cat. Invest Ophthalmol Vis Sci. 1995;36:542–54.
7. Schmidl D, Boltz A, Kaya S, Werkmeister R, Dragostinoff N, Lasta M, Polska E, Garhöfer G, Schmetterer L. Comparison of choroidal and optic nerve head blood flow regulation during changes in ocular perfusion pressure. Investig Opthalmol Vis Sci. 2012;53:4337.
8. Kiel JW. Choroidal myogenic autoregulation and intraocular pressure. Exp Eye Res. 1994;58:529–43.
9. Bogner B, Runge C, Strohmaier C, Trost A, Tockner B, Kiel JW, Schroedl F, Reitsamer HA. The effect of vasopressin on ciliary blood flow and aqueous flow. Investig Ophthalmol Vis Sci. 2014; https://doi.org/10.1167/iovs.13-13286.
10. Reitsamer HA, Zawinka C, Branka M. Dopaminergic vasodilation in the choroidal circulation by d1/d5 receptor activation. Invest Ophthalmol Vis Sci. 2004;45:900–5.
11. Mueller H. Ueber glatte Muskeln und Nervengeflechte der chorioidea im menschlichen Auge. Vehr Phys Ges Wurzbg. 1859;10:179–92.
12. Schroedl F. Neuropeptides in the eye. Trivandrum: Research Signpost; 2009.
13. Schroedl F, Trost A, Strohmaier C, Bogner B, Runge C, Kaser-Eichberger A, Couillard-Despres S, Aigner L, Reitsamer HA. Rat choroidal pericytes as a target of the autonomic nervous system. Cell Tissue Res. 2014; https://doi.org/10.1007/s00441-013-1769-5.
14. Poukens V, Glasgow BJ, Demer JL. Nonvascular contractile cells in sclera and choroid of humans and monkeys. Invest Ophthalmol Vis Sci. 1998;39:1765–74.
15. Goldmann H. Out-flow pressure, minute volume and resistance of the anterior chamber flow in man. Doc Ophthalmol. 1951;5–6:278–356.
16. Friedenwald JS. Contribution to the theory and practice of tonometry. Am J Ophthalmol. 1937;20:985–1024.
17. Silver DM, Farrel ME, Langham ME, O'Brien V, Schilder P. Esimation of pulsatile blood flow from intraocular pressure. Acta Ophthalmol. 1989;67:25–9.
18. Eisenlohr JE, Langham ME. The relationship between pressure and volume changes in living and dead rabbit eyes. Investig Ophthalmol. 1962;1:63–77.
19. Eisenlohr JE, Langham ME, Maumenee AE. Manometric studies of the pressure volume relationship in living and enucleated eyes of individual human subjects. Br J Ophthalmol. 1962;46:536–48.
20. Reitsamer HA, Kiel JW. A rabbit model to study orbital venous pressure, intraocular pressure, and ocular hemodynamics simultaneously. Invest Ophthalmol Vis Sci. 2002;43:3728–34.
21. Kiel JW. The ocular circulation. San Rafael: Morgan & Claypool Life Sciences; 2010.
22. Mäepea O. Pressures in the anterior ciliary arteries, choroidal veins and choriocapillaris. Exp Eye Res. 1992;54:731–6.
23. Kiel JW. The effect of arterial pressure on the ocular pressure-volume relationship in the rabbit. Exp Eye Res. 1995;60:267–78.
24. Bayerle-Eder M, Kolodjaschna J, Wolzt M, Polska E, Gasic S, Schmetterer L. Effect of a nifedipine induced reduction in blood pressure on the association between ocular pulse

amplitude and ocular fundus pulsation amplitude in systemic hypertension. Br J Ophthalmol. 2005;89:704–8.

25. Strohmaier C, Runge C, Seyeddain O, Emesz M, Nischler C, Dexl A, Grabner G, Reitsamer HA. Profiles of intraocular pressure in human donor eyes during femtosecond laser procedures: a comparative study. Investig Ophthalmol Vis Sci. 2013; https://doi.org/10.1167/iovs.12-11155.

26. Lavery WJ, Kiel JW. Effects of head down tilt on episcleral venous pressure in a rabbit model. Exp Eye Res. 2013;111:88–94.

27. Kurultay-Ersan I, Emre S. Impact of valsalva maneuver on central choroid, central macula, and disk fiber layer thickness among high myopic and hyperopic patients. Eur J Ophthalmol. 2017;27:331–5.

28. Silver DM, Farrell RA. Validity of pulsatile ocular blood flow measurements. Surv Ophthalmol. 1994;38:S72–80.

29. Kaufmann C, Bachmann LM, Robert YC, Thiel MA. Ocular pulse amplitude in healthy subjects as measured by dynamic contour tonometry. Arch Ophthalmol. 2006;124:1104.

30. Kaufmann C, Bachmann LM, Thiel MA. Comparison of dynamic contour tonometry with Goldmann Applanation tonometry. Investig Opthalmol Vis Sci. 2004;45:3118.

31. Ferrara D, Waheed NK, Duker JS. Investigating the choriocapillaris and choroidal vasculature with new optical coherence tomography technologies. Prog Retin Eye Res. 2016;52:130–55.

32. Beaton L, Mazzaferri J, Lalonde F, Hidalgo-Aguirre M, Descovich D, Lesk MR, Costantino S. Non-invasive measurement of choroidal volume change and ocular rigidity through automated segmentation of high-speed OCT imaging. Biomed Opt Express. 2015;6:1694.

33. Shin JW, Shin YU, Lee BR. Choroidal thickness and volume mapping by a six radial scan protocol on spectral-domain optical coherence tomography. Ophthalmology. 2012;119:1017–23.

34. Wallman J, Wildsoet C, Xu A, Gottlieb MD, Nickla DL, Marran L, Krebs W, Christensen AM. Moving the retina: choroidal modulation of refractive state. Vis Res. 1995;35:37–50.

35. Read SA, Collins MJ, Sander BP. Human optical axial length and defocus. Investig Opthalmol Vis Sci. 2010;51:6262.

36. Nickla DL, Wallman J. The multifunctional choroid. Prog Retin Eye Res. 2010;29:144–68.

Chapter 8
Biomechanics of the Lens and Hydrodynamics of Accommodation

Daniel B. Goldberg

Age-related changes occur in all ocular tissues [1]: "The cornea flattens and there is an attrition of endothelial cells. The shape of the trabecular meshwork changes and there is a loss of trabecular endothelium. The lens grows and becomes cataractous. The ciliary body becomes collagenized, there are choroidal vascular changes, and Bruch's membrane thickens. Retinal vessels become hyalinized and there is a loss of rods before cones in the macula. RPE morphometric changes occur with aging. The vitreous becomes liquefied and there is a loss of vitreous compartmentalization. The sclera becomes rigid and may become calcified. The optic nerve exhibits structural changes with age."

Detorakis and Pallikaris [2] have developed a useful technique to measure ocular rigidity and have shown that ocular rigidity increases with age and can be correlated with the loss of accommodative function and the progression of presbyopia in normal eyes, and also contributes to common age-related eye diseases including glaucoma and age-related macular degeneration. With age, there is an increase in ocular rigidity with resulting changes in material properties, changes in anatomic relationships, and degradation of healthy connective tissue.

Understanding the mechanism of accommodation and the changes in ocular structure which lead to presbyopia will ultimately lead to more effective treatments for presbyopia. Glasser and Campbell [3, 4] have concluded that aging changes in the lens are almost entirely responsible for the development of presbyopia, however,

Electronic Supplementary Material The online version of this chapter (https://doi.org/10.1007/978-3-030-64422-2_8) contains supplementary material, which is available to authorized users. The videos can be accessed by scanning the related images with the SN More Media App.

D. B. Goldberg (✉)
Drexel College of Medicine, Philadelphia, PA, USA

Atlantic Eye Physicians, Little Silver, NJ, USA

more recently, accommodation has been described as a complex biomechanical system, having both lenticular and extralenticular components, and we will present evidence that presbyopia occurs due to age-related changes in both lenticular and extra-lenticular structures.

Twenty-first century imaging with UBM and OCT along with new knowledge of the anatomy and movements of the accommodating structures of the eye [4–8] has enabled a computer-animated model to demonstrate all accommodating structures moving synchronously through the accommodative cycle [9, 10]. Using model-based cognitive thinking, the mechanism of accommodation can now be demonstrated and explained without relying on theory, and the factors contributing to presbyopia can be demonstrated. In this chapter, we will demonstrate the mechanism of accommodation and consider the biomechanics of the lens and extra-lenticular structures as well as the hydrodynamics of the aqueous and vitreous.

The Mechanism of Accommodation

The computer-animated model of accommodation (CAMA 2.0) [10] is shown in Fig. 8.1 in accommodation and dis-accommodation, and the animated digital file can be viewed in Video 8.1. The changes in shape and position of all anatomic elements are shown, demonstrating how the structures interconnect and function as a unit. The anatomic representation shows the configuration and movement of all zonular elements as well as the anterior hyaloid membrane and Weiger ligament.

Accommodation results in a dioptric change in the optical power of the lens due to an increase in the lens thickness, and steepening of the curvature of the anterior and posterior capsule of the lens. As many investigators have noted, the architecture of the zonular fibers determines the way the forces of ciliary muscle contraction are distributed. There are 6 zonular pathways (see Fig. 8.2) which can be divided into 3 groups based on structure and function. During accommodation, the anterior zonule

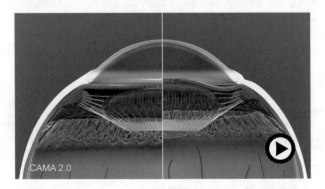

Fig. 8.1 Computer-animated model of accommodation showing structures in accommodation (right side) and dis-accommodation (left side). (Video 8.1 Animated digital file). https://doi.org/10.1007/000-2a8

Fig. 8.2 Six zonular
pathways, Weiger ligament,
and anterior vitreous
membrane. Anterior zonule
(blue), Anterior vitreous
zonule (yellow), Intermediate
vitreous zonule (red),
Posterior vitreous zonule
(gray), Pars plana zonule
(green), Posterior insertion
zone to lens equator zonule
(purple), Weiger
ligament (white)

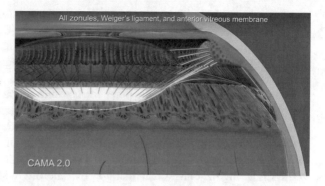

(Zinn) loses tension due to the anterior and centripetal movement of the ciliary
body, allowing the lens to 'round-up' due to the intrinsic elasticity of the lens and
lens capsule. In disaccommodation, the ciliary body relaxation and return to resting
position results in tension on the anterior zonular fibers, with flattening of the lens
and loss of accommodative effect. The anterior zonule (composed of anterior and
posterior tines, plus equatorial fibers) are the first zonular group and their function
is tension and release on the lens. The second division of the zonule are the crossing
zonules including the anterior vitreous zonule (shown in yellow in Fig. 8.2), and the
recently discovered PIZ-LE zonule (posterior insertion zone to lens equator zonule-
shown in purple in Fig. 8.2). Along with the Weiger ligament, the crossing zonular
fibers cradle, shape and stabilize the lens and vitreous—maintaining the lens in it's
position in the central fossa formed by the anterior vitreous membrane. The crossing zonules prevent outside forces from displacing the lens while at the same time
the anterior and posterior zonules work reciprocally to keep focused vision. The
primary function of the crossing zonule is to support the lens. In addition, from the
model (Fig. 8.1 and Video 8.1) it appears that the ciliary muscle contraction causes
angular rotation of the anterior vitreous zonule which likely helps to shape the lens
as it rounds up during accommodation. The third functional group of zonular fibers
are the posterior zonular fibers, which include the intermediate vitreous zonule
(shown in red), the posterior vitreous zonule (shown in gray), and the pars plana
zonule (shown in green). The posterior zonule anchors the ciliary body and extends
posteriorly at the posterior insertion zone to attach to the elastic foundation in
Bruch's membrane and peripheral choroid. When the ciliary muscle contracts, the
posterior zonular fibers, attached to the elastic elements of the choroid, stretch and
store energy for disaccommodation. When the ciliary muscle relaxes, the elastic
fibers of the choroid pull the posterior zonular fibers and the ciliary body posteriorly. As the ciliary body moves posteriorly, the anterior zonules stretch and flatten
the lens. The posterior vitreous zonule is a sponge-like structure at the vitreous base
with obliquely crossing fibers forming a network capable of dampening the forces
of accommodation and preventing trauma to the peripheral retina, as suggested by
Lutjen-Drecoll et al. [5] As a group, the posterior zonular fibers, in concert with the
anterior zonular fibers, create the reciprocal zonular action that occurs during the

accommodative cycle. The posterior zonular fibers transfer tension and release from the ciliary muscle to the elastic foundation in the choroid.

Perhaps the major reason that the mechanics of accommodation was not understood until recently is recognizing that disaccommodation occurs due to stored energy in Bruch's elastic foundation in the choroid. This elastic structure surrounds the vitreous and conforms to the inner form of the sclera in the shape of a circumferential girdle posterior to the ora serrata. Muscle movements throughout the body involve sets of agonist and antagonist muscles to achieve back and forth movements. In the case of accommodation, there is only one muscle moving—the ciliary muscle, and the muscle acts by releasing tension on the lens during accommodation while stretching the elastic foundation in the choroid to store energy for disaccommodation. Thus, the accommodative system functions with one muscle providing tension and release to 2 opposing elastic structures. During disaccommodation, the elastic tension in the choroid pulls the posterior zonule and ciliary muscle back to the resting position. Since this physiology is unique, the mystery of accommodation was elusive.

In 2013, Croft [6, 7] showed the dynamic movement of the choroid and retina, and demonstrated that the stretch and movement of the tissues extends at least to 4.0–7.0 mm posterior to the ora serrata. Further studies [11] using optical coherence reflectometry showed that the choroidal stretch and thinning extends to the fovea at the back of the eye and that axial elongation occurs during accommodation [12]. Thus, accommodation causes changes in all elements of the uveal tract from the iris/pupil to the sub-foveal choroid.

Croft et al. [7] demonstrated scleral deformation of the outer limbus in the nasal quadrant during accommodation. In addition, inward bowing of the sclera in this region occurs with age. These changes indicate traction in the area of the limbus overlying the scleral spur where the ciliary muscle and uveal tract are anchored to the sclera. In 2013, Ni et al. [13] demonstrated changes in corneal volume, curvature, and corneal high order aberrations with accommodation. Thus, the movements of accommodation also cause changes in the sclera and cornea, the outer tunic of the globe.

Biomechanics of the Lens

Accommodative changes in the lens account almost entirely for the increased dioptric power of the eye during accommodation. The lens thickness increases, and the anterior and posterior capsule curvature increases. Fincham [14] demonstrated that the elasticity of the lens and lens capsule enables the lens to round up during accommodation when ciliary muscle contraction results in relaxation of tension in the anterior zonular fibers. During disaccommodation, the increasing tension of the anterior zonular fibers pull outward on the capsule to flatten the lens. The lens diameter does not increase with accommodation or age [15, 16]. This finding refutes the Schachar theory.

Fincham [14] demonstrated that the lens capsule is comprised of variable thickness with the capsule thickest at the mid-peripheral anterior surface and thinner towards the lens equatorial region with a posterior peripheral thickening but thinnest at the posterior pole of the lens. The lens capsule is a thin, transparent, elastic membrane. During accommodation the tension of the anterior zonule is reduced, which then enables the lens to 'round up' due to the intrinsic elasticity of the lens capsule. The variable thickness of the capsule when zonular tension is released determines the accommodative shape of the lens. Experimentally, when the lens is isolated from the zonule, the lens shape changes to the accommodative shape due to the effect of the elastic lens capsule and its varying regional thickness. When the lens capsule is removed, the lens substance takes on an unaccommodative shape, indicating that the elasticity and shape of the lens capsule is the driving force for accommodative lens shape change when zonular stretch is released. With age, the lens capsule thickens, and loses elasticity.

The lens substance consists of lens fiber cells composing the lens nucleus and cortex. Beneath the capsule is a layer of lens epithelial cells, and the deeper layers of lens epithelial cells differentiate to become lens fiber cells. This process continues throughout life, and results in lens thickness increasing with age, along with an increase in the anterior surface and posterior surface curvatures, but without increase in the lens diameter with age [17]. Since the aging lens increases in thickness and capsule curvatures, the lens power might be expected to increase and result in myopic progression with age; however, there is a gradual age-related decrease in the refractive index of the lens which accounts for this 'lens paradox' [18].

In addition to shape changes with age, the human lens loses elasticity, and lenticular rigidity and stiffness increases until ultimately the lens is unable to undergo optical change even when the ciliary muscle is still capable of contraction.

Hydrodynamics of Accommodation

By modeling the aqueous and vitreous spaces, we can add to our understanding of the hydrodynamics of accommodation. Figure 8.3 and Video 8.2 demonstrates the accommodative movements.

The aqueous space includes both anterior and posterior chambers. During accommodation, the anterior chamber shallows centrally as the lens moves anteriorly, and deepens peripherally as the peripheral iris bends posteriorly. This iris configuration has been clearly demonstrated with video ultrasound biomicroscopy [10]. At the onset of accommodation, the lens moves anteriorly and contacts the posterior iris centrally which may obstruct aqueous flow from posterior to anterior chamber during the accommodative phase. During the later phase of accommodation, the anterior chamber deepens peripherally, and increases the force pressing the iris against the anterior lens capsule. At the same time, the ciliary muscle contraction stretches the scleral spur and facilitates the outflow of aqueous thru the trabecular meshwork. Aqueous is continuously produced in the posterior chamber by the ciliary processes

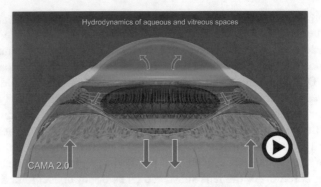

Fig. 8.3 Hydrodynamics of aqueous and vitreous space—early phase of accommodation. (Video 8.2 Accommodative movements). https://doi.org/10.1007/000-2a7

at a rate of approximately 2.5 µL/min. "During disaccommodation, the lens moves posteriorly and the iris returns to the resting position, and during this phase of the accommodative cycle the aqueous inflow can replenish the anterior chamber volume". During ciliary muscle contraction, the insertion of the ciliary muscle into the scleral spur and adjacent trabecular meshwork results in stretching the trabecular meshwork and enhancing aqueous outflow. This supports the pumping model for trabecular outflow [19] in contrast to static resistance. Other sources of pulsatile flow include the systole of the cardiac cycle, as well as blinking and extraocular muscle movement. Further, the reduction of accommodative movement with age may contribute to a reduced outflow of aqueous with age thereby contributing to the occurrence of glaucoma with age. Through the accommodative cycle, aqueous production and drainage are in equilibrium; however, there may be a relative pupillary block during the accommodative phase resulting in net outflow in the anterior chamber during the accommodative phase and net inflow in the posterior chamber during the accommodative phase. During disaccommodation, the flow from posterior to anterior chamber is able to replenish the anterior chamber volume. Also, there is a convection flow of aqueous in the anterior chamber—downward close to the cornea where the temperature is cooler, and upward near the lens where the temperature is warmer [20].

The movement of aqueous in the posterior chamber has been beautifully demonstrated by Croft et al [6, 7] with endoscopy using triamcinolone particles. At the same time that aqueous is moving posteriorly through the circumlental space into the anterior hyaloid cleft, the anterior hyaloid in the region between the Weiger ligament, and the peripheral shoulder of the vitreous bows backwards (Video 8.2). This is evidence that the hydraulic pressure in the posterior aqueous space overcomes the hydraulic pressure in the vitreous space. This is contrary to the Coleman theory of accommodation which posits that vitreous pressure presses the lens and anterior hyaloid forward. Croft and Kaufman [7] also showed that the portion of the hyaloid membrane that was adjacent to, and interconnected with, the intermediate vitreous zonule up to the anterior hyaloid cleft also was pulled forward. The accommodative forward movement of this portion of the vitreous membrane pulls forward much of the neighboring inner vitreous near and posterior to the region of the ora serrata. Axially, the posterior lens capsule moves posteriorly during accommodation, resulting in posterior movement of the vitreous in this area behind Berger's space. There may be an additional effect of the aqueous movement in the posterior chamber during ciliary muscle contraction since the movement of aqueous into the hyaloid cleft may facilitate the rounding up of the lens in addition to the effect of the elastic lens capsule, and the angular rotation of the anterior vitreous zonule which occur at the same time.

The documented movements within the vitreous space include the posterior movement of the axial vitreous due to the posterior displacement of the lens during accommodation, and the anterior movement of the peripheral anterior vitreous adjacent to the posterior zonule. This peripheral anterior movement of the vitreous membrane is due to attachments of the intermediate vitreous zonule to the peripheral hyaloid. Worst [21] has demonstrated a cisternal anatomy of the vitreous body. It is possible that the cisternal anatomy of the vitreous body directs the flow; however, further study of vitreous movements during accommodation is needed, especially to document the movement of posterior vitreous. Croft et al. [22] have suggested that the posterior fluid movement in the vitreous may extend to the optic nerve head and may be implicated in the pathogenesis of glaucoma.

The catenary/hydraulic theory of Coleman [23, 24] and Coleman and Fish [25] is based on measurement of vitreous pressure spikes in sequence with ciliary muscle contraction. However, the posterior movement of the anterior hyaloid membrane during accommodation, and the posterior movement of the capsule following ECCE [26] demonstrate that the aqueous pressure during accommodation is higher than the vitreous pressure, and that the findings of vitreous pressure spike by Coleman have been misleading. It seems possible that the experimental model of vitreous pressure measurement utilizing a needle penetrating the sclera and choroid with the tip in the vitreous may represent detection of pressure in the elastic Bruch's membrane rather than in the vitreous. Regardless, the vitreous consists of a transparent gel without contractile elements, and is contained within the hyaloid membrane. The movements within the vitreous are secondary to movement of surrounding structures e.g. the lens, ciliary body, and aqueous (higher hydraulic pressure in aqueous causes anterior hyaloid to bow backwards). The vitreous is a visco-elastic structure which contains 99% water, and which contains properties of both fluids and elastic tissues. Viscoelastic tissues can deform under stress and return to their original form. With stress, viscoelastic materials can rearrange to accommodate the stress (this is called creep), and following stress, the viscoelastic returns to its original shape. Certainly, the vitreous provides support for the lens, and the hydraulic interactions of the lens and vitreous are subject to physical properties of viscoelastic tissue contained in elastic membranes, similar to the Coleman model of 2 fluid filled balloons one on top of the other as occurs in the eye with the lens located directly anterior to and attached by the Weiger ligament to the central fossa of the anterior hyaloid.

Further, the elastic foundation in Bruch's membrane stretches in the anterior-posterior direction due to the traction of the posterior zonule which pulls the choroid and retina anteriorly with ciliary muscle contraction. The forward movement at the ora serrata is approximately 1 mm, and is proportional to the anterior movement of the ciliary apex, and the accommodative change in the lens [8]. Since the vitreous posterior to the anterior hyaloid membrane is surrounded by and shaped by the sclera, there could be a fractional vector of force acting on the vitreous anterior to the equator consisting of anterior and centripetal vectors. This may facilitate the accommodative movement of the vitreous.

Presbyopia

The presbyopic eye demonstrates thickening and stiffening of lens and capsule with steepening of the anterior capsule curvature; also, the lens equator moves forward with age and the insertion of the anterior zonules moves anteriorly with on the lens capsule. The presbyopic lens fails to flatten in disaccommodation and, compared to that of the normal 25-year-old, the presbyopic lens is almost frozen in a thicker state. It should also be noted that the anterior movement of the ora serrata is markedly reduced in presbyopia, which is related to the loss of elasticity in the ciliary body and choroid. Lenticular sclerosis and lens stiffness increase with age, ultimately causing complete loss of the ability of the lens to undergo accommodative change in optical power. As per Croft et al. [6] and Richdale et al. [7] there are proportionate reductions in lenticular accommodation, ciliary apex movement, and movement of the ora serrata. The ciliary muscle retains the ability to contract and to undergo accommodative movement in the presbyopic eye, whereas presbyopia results ultimately in the complete loss in accommodative ability in the lens. There is an increase in ocular rigidity and loss of elasticity with age that effects all ocular tissues. The model does not demonstrate that the changes in the lens and lens capsule determine the stage of presbyopia, exclusively. It is evident that the aging of the extralenticular structures, including the ciliary body and elastic foundation in the choroid is also a major factor causing presbyopia. The ciliary muscle undergoes degenerative changes, but maintains its ability to contract long after the lens stops accommodating. A model of a 75 year-old presbyope would show residual ciliary muscle movements while the accommodative movements of the lens and ora serrata has stopped. This is evidence that age-related changes in the lens, and in the elastic foundation in the choroid, are both contributing to the restriction of accommodative movement with age.

In regard to the etiology of presbyopia, there are strong arguments that aging of the lens, including thickening of lens capsule with loss of capsular elasticity, and growth and hardening of the lens nucleus are paramount. However, the proportional loss of movement of the ora serrata and elastic foundation in the choroid are evidence that both lenticular and extra-lenticular elements develop ocular rigidity and loss of elasticity, and deterioration of function. Further research is needed to determine the relative contributions of each restrictive element (lens, choroid, zonules and ciliary muscle). This knowledge will help guide the development of future therapeutic treatments for presbyopia. For example, there may be separate benefits from treatments to reverse lenticular sclerosis, such as femtosecond laser lens softening, and from treatments to compensate for loss of choroidal elasticity, such as scleral laser or scleral implants. Or, possibly, there will be a pharmacologic agent to reverse the loss of elasticity in both the lens and the choroidal foundation for accommodation. Most promising would be development of better accommodating IOLs based on our improved understanding of the biomechanics of accommodation.

References

1. Grossniklaus HE, Nickerson JM, Edelhauser HF, et al. Anatomic alterations in aging and age-related diseases of the eye. Invest Ophth Vis Sci. 2013;54(14):ORSF 23–7.
2. Detorakis ET, Pallikaris IG. Ocular rigidity: biomechanical role, in vivo measurements and clinical significance. Clin Exp Ophthalmol. 2013;41(1):73–81.
3. Glasser A, Campbell MC. Presbyopia and the optical changes in the human crystalline lens with age. Vis Res. 1998;38(2):209–29.
4. Glasser A, Campbell MC. On the potential causes of presbyopia. Vis Res. 1999;39(7):1267–72.
5. Lutjen-Drecoll E, Kaufman PL, Wasielewski R, et al. Morphology and accommodative function of the vitreous zonule in human and monkey eyes. Invest Ophthalmol Vis Sci. 2010;51(3):1554–64.
6. Croft MA, McDonald JP, Katz A, et al. Extralenticular and lenticular aspects of accommodation and presbyopia in human versus monkey eyes. Invest Ophthalmol Vis Sci. 2013;54(7):5035–48.
7. Croft MA, Nork TM, McDonald JP, et al. Accommodative movements of the vitreous membrane, choroid and sclera in young and presbyopic human and non-human primate eyes. Invest Ophthalmol Vis Sci. 2013;54(7):5049–58.
8. Richdale K, Sinnott MA, Bullimore MA, et al. Quantification of age-related and per diopter accommodative changes of the lens and ciliary muscle in the emmetropic human eye with age and accommodation. Invest Ophthalmol Vis Sci. 2013;54(2):1095–105.
9. Goldberg DB. Computer-animated model of accommodation and theory of reciprocal zonular action. Clin Ophthalmol. 2011;5:1559–66.
10. Goldberg DB. Computer-animated model of accommodation and presbyopia. J Cataract Refract Surg. 2015;41(2):437–45.
11. Woodman EC, Read SA, Collins MJ. Axial length and choroidal thickness changes accompanying prolonged accommodation in myopes and emmetropes. Vis Res. 2012;72:34–41.
12. Zhong J, Tao A, Xu Z, et al. Whole eye axial biometry during accommodation using ultra-long scan depth optical coherence tomography. Am J Ophthalmol. 2014;157:1064–9.
13. Ni Y, Liu X, Lin Y, et al. Evaluation of corneal changes with accommodation in young and presbyopic populations using Pentacam high resolution Scheimpflug system. Clin Exp Ophth. 2013;41:244–50.
14. Fincham EF. The mechanism of accommodation. Br J Ophthalmol. 1937;21:5.
15. Wendt M, Croft MA, McDonald PL, et al. Lens diameter and thickness as a function of age and pharmacologically stimulated accommodation in rhesus monkeys. Exp Eye Res. 2008;86:746–52.
16. Strenck SA, Semmlow JL, Strenck LM, et al. Age-related changes in human ciliary muscle and lens: a magnetic resonance imaging study. Invest Ophthalmol Vis Sci. 1999;40:1162–9.
17. Glasser A. Accommodation. In: Kaufman PL, Alm A, editors. Adler's physiology of the eye. 11th ed; 2011. p. 40–70.

18. Atchison DA, Markwell EL, Kasthurirangan S, et al. Age-related changes in optical and biometric characteristics of emmetropic eyes. J Vis. 2008;8:29.
19. Johnstone MA. The aqueous outflow system as a mechanical pump. Evidence from examination of tissue and aqueous movement in human and non-human primates. J Glauc. 2004;13:421.
20. Kaufman PL, True Gabelt BA. Production and flow of aqueous humor. In: Kaufman PL, Alm A, editors. Adler's physiology of the eye. 11th ed; 2011. p. 285–6.
21. Worst JGF. Cisternal systems of the fully developed vitreous in young adults. Trans Ophthalmol Soc UK. 1977;97:550.
22. Croft MA, Lutjen-Drecoll E, Kaufman PL. Age related posterior ciliary muscle restriction—a link between trabecular meshwork and optic nerve head physiology. Exp Eye Res. 2016;2016:1–3.
23. Coleman DJ. Unified model for accommodative mechanism. Am J Ophthalmol. 1970;69:1063–79.
24. Coleman DJ. On the hydraulic suspension theory of accommodation. Trans Am Ophthalmol Soc. 1986;84:846–68.
25. Coleman DJ, Fish SK. Presbyopia, accommodation and the mature catenary. Ophthalmology. 2001;108:1544–51.
26. Croft MA, Heatley G, McDonald JP, et al. Accommodative movements of the lens/capsule and the strand that extends between the posterior vitreous zonule insertion zone and the lens equator, in relation to the vitreous face and aging. Ophthalmic Physiol Opt. 2016;36:21–32.

Chapter 9
Influence of Ocular Rigidity and Ocular Biomechanics on the Pathogenesis of Age-Related Presbyopia

Ann Marie Hipsley and Brad Hall

Biomechanics is the study of the relationship between the mechanical laws relating to the movement and structure of living systems. The application of biomechanics principles play a critical role in understanding the forces and function of mechanisms inside of the living body. Over the past decade there has been a growing body of literature in ocular biomechanics regarding the importance of characterizing ocular tissue properties for clinical applications. Ocular biomechanics is an emerging field of study and there have been significant advances in translational biomechanical strategies in ophthalmology to establish more effective treatment and management solutions for ophthalmic diseases and conditions of the eye such as glaucoma, myopia, and keratoconus [1]. Models for the anterior globe are emerging but published literature in this area are scant. Most of these efforts have focused on the characterization of the posterior scleral globe [2–6]. More recently, however, the biomechanical behavior of the sclera as it relates to the correlation between the progressive increase in biomechanical stiffness and concomitant loss of visual accommodation has been investigated. In one study, relationships between ocular stiffness and accommodative ability were explored in the anterior globe through age-matched crosslinking porcine eyes ex vivo [7]. Scleral crosslinking was performed chemically using 2% glutaraldehyde and ocular rigidity was measured individually for each eye with a custom measurement system. Chemically crosslinking the porcine sclera significantly increased ocular rigidity compared to non-crosslinked controls, and both crosslinked and non-crosslinked eyes correlated well with the ocular rigidities observed in 30- and 60-year old human eyes. Using a novel laser scleral therapy, the authors were able to reduce the ocular rigidity by changing the

A. M. Hipsley (✉)
Ace Vision Group, Newark, CA, USA
e-mail: ahipsley@acevisiongroup.com

B. Hall
Sengi, Penniac, NB, Canada
e-mail: bhall@sengiclinical.com

© Springer Nature Switzerland AG 2021
I. Pallikaris et al. (eds.), *Ocular Rigidity, Biomechanics and Hydrodynamics of the Eye*, https://doi.org/10.1007/978-3-030-64422-2_9

viscoelastic modulus of the scleral tissue in both the crosslinked and non-crosslinked eyes, demonstrating that ocular rigidity and age-related biomechanical dysfunction can be reversed.

There are complex biomechanics involved in the accommodation mechanism in order to achieve an "on demand" change of the shape of the lens to see at various distances [8]. When viewing a far object the ciliary muscle is relaxed and the anterior zonules, which are under tension, stretch the lens into a flatter shape [9]. Conversely, to view a near object, the ciliary muscle contracts, releasing tension on the anterior zonules, releasing tension on the lens and allowing the material properties of the lens to return its more natural convex shape [9, 10]. Goldberg described this biomechanical relationship of the zonular tension on the lens as reciprocal zonular function [11]. Accommodation has traditionally been described as the ability of the crystalline lens of the eye to change dioptric power dynamically to see objects clearly when changing focus from far to near [12]. However, the accommodative mechanism is much more complex, and involves both lenticular and extralenticular components [11, 13–19]. The lens, lens capsule, zonules, ciliary muscle, sclera, and the choroid all have significant biomechanical roles in the accommodative mechanism [11, 13–22]. There are numerous lenticular and extralenticular changes that decrease accommodative ability and lead to presbyopia with age [14, 15, 20, 23–28].

An understanding of biomechanics is particularly useful to understand the complexity of accommodative function as well as the biomechanical dysfunction that occurs with age-related eye diseases (glaucoma, AMD) and myopia [29, 30]. Age-related changes in the crystalline lens have long been understood and reported [31–34]. Recent endeavors, however, have demonstrated how stiffening of all ocular tissues manifest in presbyopia [16, 29]. This research has gleaned more evidence that age-related changes in the biomechanical properties of extralenticular structures are correlated with a clinically significant loss of accommodation such as ocular rigidity, geometric changes in the zonular apparatus, and loss of elasticity in the choroid [16, 29]. These new findings have changed our understanding of how the accommodation mechanism works together with optical demands and has opened up new ideas to restore this function in the eye rather than the previous monolithic paradigms of refractive corrections either in the cornea or the lens.

Biomechanics of the Lens

The crystalline lens is the part of the eye which acts as a zooming lens to change focus at various distances. The average crystalline lens has an optical power of 20 D [35]. The outermost part of the ocular lens is known as the lens capsule. It is a membrane comprised of mostly type IV collagen by weight and surrounds the lens like a transparent envelope [36]. Inside this envelope (lens capsule) are the lens cortex and the lens nucleus (most internal). The lens cortex and lens nucleus are made up of fiber cells arranged in annular layers, which contains mostly alpha, beta, and gamma crystalline proteins and provide unique biomechanical properties to the lens [37]. Fischer observed that the modulus of elasticity of a young human lens is 750 N/m^2 anterior to posterior and 850 N/m^2 equatorially, making the crystalline lens a suitable material capable of being molded into shape by the forces of the ciliary muscles [38]. The forces of the ciliary muscle are transmitted to the lens via the anterior zonules and the lens capsule. The lens capsule can more easily mold an elastic substance, such as a rubber ball (1.5×10^6 N/m^2), versus a stiffer substance, such as a ball made of cast iron (1.65×10^{11} N/m^2) [39]. Thus the lens capsule is a crucial part of the accommodative mechanism since the shape of the lens directly affects the power of the lens. Equation 9.1 demonstrates the calculation for central optical power (COP), where n_1 and n_a are the refractive indices for the lens and the aqueous and vitreous respectively, r_a and r_p are the radii of curvature for the anterior and posterior lens surfaces respectively, and t is the central lens thickness [40].

$$COP = \frac{n_1 - n_a}{r_a} - \frac{n_1 - n_a}{r_p} + \frac{t(n_1 - n_a)^2}{r_a r_p n_1} \tag{9.1}$$

The zonular apparatus maintains a "pre-stretch" tension on the crystalline lens when it is in the state of disaccommodation for viewing distant objects. The forces of the ciliary muscle relieve this zonular tension to allow the lens to change shape in order to focus on near objects at various distances [9]. During accommodation as the lens adapts its more natural convex shape, the lens thickness increases by approximately 0.043–0.085 mm per diopter of accommodation (Fig. 9.1) [13, 41–47]. The forces produced by the ciliary muscles (circular, longitudinal, radial) increase lens thickness during accommodation which directly increases the COP of the lens (Eq. 9.1). There is also a corresponding decrease in the radii of curvature of the anterior and posterior surfaces, which further increases the COP of the lens (Eq. 9.1) [27, 28]. The equatorial diameter of the lens decreases by 0.07–1.12 mm per diopter during accommodation, corresponding with the increase in lens thickness [13, 24, 48]. This has been quantified by measurements taken with ocular coherence tomography (OCT) and magnetic resonance imaging (MRI). Moreover, some studies have also shown that the anterior lens surface moves anteriorly and the posterior surface moves slightly posteriorly during accommodation [27, 49–51], corresponding with concomitant changes in lens thickness and anterior and posterior radii of curvature during accommodation. This leads to a further increase in the optical power of the lens. All of the biomechanical mechanisms involved in

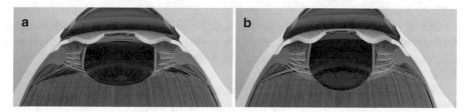

Fig. 9.1 Computer-animated model of the accommodative mechanism when viewing an object at **a** far and **b** near

accommodation are precisely designed in order to allow the crystalline lens to be very specifically modulated for clear vision at all distances allowing perfect 'on demand' vision at every possible focal point from an average of 10 cm to infinity [52].

Age-Related Changes in the Biomechanics of the Lens

The crystalline lens is not static and undergoes numerous biomechanical changes with age that affect both the disaccommodated and the accommodated lens. The crystalline lens yellows with increasing age [53]. The lens capsular elasticity increases with increasing age [54]. However, the lens stiffens with age, having an elastic modules 3 times that of a young lens at 3000 N/m² anterior to posterior and equatorially [10]. The change in stiffness is more pronounced in the lens nucleus compared to the lens cortex [55]. A stiffer lens is more resistant to the forces generated by the ciliary muscle and less deformable by the lens capsule [56]. These age-related changes create biomechanical dysfunctions which lead to decreased efficiency of the accommodation mechanism and therefore decreased resultant COP of the lens during accommodation. The overall weight of the lens has also been shown to increase by 150% with age [57], which can impact the accommodative system from a force exertion standpoint as the larger lens weight is more difficult to move. Furthermore, the lens cortex continues to grow with age [33], which can affect lens thickness. There is compelling evidence that supports the claim that the age-related increase in both anterior/posterior (AP) thickness and lens equatorial diameter during the disaccommodated state affect the capabilities of the ciliary muscles to impose forces on the accommodation apparatus to impact the COP power of the lens [13, 14, 24, 31, 58–60]. Continuous growth of the lens cortex reduces circumlental space and causes the anterior zonules to be positioned in a more slackened state thereby disallowing the lens to return to its fully disaccommodated state wherein the anterior zonules would be in a more ideal biomechanical "pre-stretch" tensile state [14]. This reduces not only the available range of motion for the lens to move upon demand of the ciliary muscles, but it effectively reduces the potential energy of the neuromuscular system involved in the accommodative reflex and therefore reduces the resultant dynamic accommodation potential [14, 24, 34]. Additionally, growth of the lens cortex can diverge the insertions of the anterior zonules on the lens, which may reduce their disaccommodated tension, further affecting accommodative potential [61–63]. There is also an additional increase in the radii of curvature during accommodation for the anterior and posterior lens surfaces with age, which decreases the potential COP of the lens [13, 31, 58, 64, 65].

It is interesting to note that the lens equatorial diameter and anterior/posterior lens thickness which occur during accommodation are unaffected by increasing age [13, 41, 44]. Therefore, this should be an indication that despite the numerous biomechanical changes in the lens with age the lens could still have enough capability to change COP to see clearly at near if there were no age-related dysfunctions in extralenticular components of accommodation. Therefore, *both* lenticular and extralenticular components must be considered together in order to fully understand the impact that biomechanical functions have on the ability of the accommodative mechanism to change COP in conjunction with the optical and visuals functions involved in achieving clear quality binocular vision at various distances.

Ocular Rigidity and Presbyopia

Presbyopia literally means 'old eye' [12] and it has traditionally been used interchangeably with accommodation loss. However, it should be emphasized that accommodation loss is just one clinical manifestation of the consequences of an aging (or presbyopic) eye. There are numerous changes to the lens and surrounding tissues with increasing age, which may contribute to accommodation loss (Fig. 9.2). Age-related changes in the vitreous membrane, peripheral choroid, sclera, ciliary muscle, and zonules have been reported and could influence the loss of accommodative ability with age [13–15, 19]. Indeed, the amount of accommodation lost with age, which is related to extralenticular factors (primarily the zonules, choroid, and sclera) have only been relatively recently investigated [66, 67]. The ciliary muscle is responsible not only for the efficiency of the visual accommodative system but plays a critical role in aqueous hydrodynamics (outflow/inflow, pH regulation, and IOP) [68–70]. The ciliary muscle is comprised of smooth muscle which is oriented in a complex architecture and involves three different fiber directions, circular, radial, and longitudinal [71]. The innermost region is Müller's muscle (circular muscle), which has fibers oriented in a circular direction who's contraction lowers tension on the anterior zonules [71]. The outermost region is Brücke's muscle (longitudinal muscle), which has fibers oriented in a longitudinal direction and who's contraction pulls forward the choroid [71]. In between the circular and longitudinal fibres is the radial muscle, which has fibres oriented in a radial direction and who's contraction pulls forward the ciliary muscle [71]. With age, the longitudinal and radial muscles decrease in size while the circular muscle increase in size, but these changes do not appear to affect the contractile force generated by the ciliary muscle [24, 72–74].

One of the phenomena that can be measured to evaluate accommodative capability is the change in the distance between the scleral spur and the ora serrata. During accommodation, the ciliary muscle movement pulls the ora serrata upward and inward toward the scleral spur demonstrating the muscle contraction and the ability of the ciliary muscles to impose fine-tuned resultant forces on the lens to allow accommodation. There is a notable decrease in this distance with age by approximately 85% [14]. Another important biomechanical role in the extralenticular anatomy is the function of the posterior insertion zone-to-lens equator zonules (PIZ-INS-LE) [15]. Croft et al. identified an attachment zone (posterior insertion zone) of the PIZ-INS-LE, intermediate and posterior vitreous zonules, and the pars

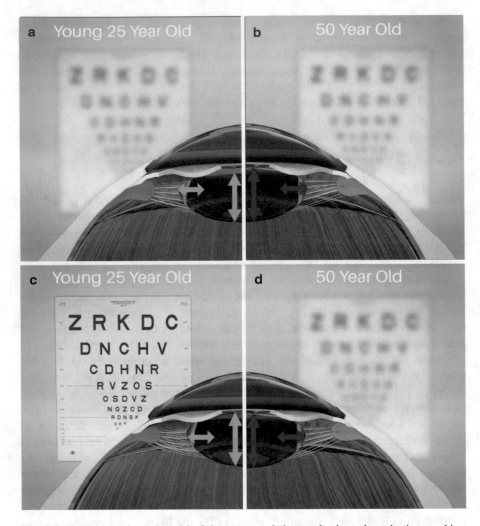

Fig. 9.2 Computer-animated model of the accommodative mechanism when viewing an object with (**a**) normal eye at far and (**b**) presbyopic eye at far (**c**) normal eye at near and (**d**) presbyopic eye at near

plana zonules adjacent to the ora serrata by utilizing UBM of the anterior segment. As the choroid stiffens with age, the forces from the longitudinal muscle, which support the upward inward thrust on the lens, become dampened. This is thought to be the etiology of the decrease in the excursion of the ciliary muscle from the ora serrata to the scleral spur which occurs in young healthy eye accommodation [16]. Croft et al. measured the changes in the distance between two landmarks (sclera spur & ora serrata), correlated to COP, and found that 0.1 mm of movement has been is equated to 1 D of COP [14].

There is also a complex action and biomechanical relationship of the zonules which is suspected to be reciprocal, as described by Goldberg [11]. For example, while the anterior zonules are relaxed, they reduce their tension on the lens such that the lens changes shape anteriorly. Accordingly, the posterior zonules are tensioned, moving the posterior capsule backward [16]. In addition the vitreal-zonular complex stiffens with age, losing its elasticity or ability to efficiently manage the force translation from the ciliary muscles to the lens [29, 66, 67, 75]. Moreover, the choroid and ciliary muscle could be considered to have an agonist/synergist relationship during accommodation and disaccommodation in the young eye. The ciliary muscle forces are supported by the elastic choroid mechanism during accommodation which stores energy to recoil the system back to disaccommodation. However, in the ageing eye the choroid stiffens which now dampens the ciliary muscle forces for accommodation and disaccommodation becomes an antagonist to this movement in an older eye [76]. It is also now known that the sclera becomes less deformable during accommodation in the nasal area with age due to ocular rigidity. This creates an additional antagonistic force to accommodation which further impacts the ciliary muscle biomechanical efficiency to translate forces to the lens therefore resulting in decreased COP capability.

Influence of Ocular Rigidity on Loss of Accommodative Ability

Increases in ocular rigidity or "stiffness" of the sclera and the cornea have been correlated with increasing age, lending support to the idea that presbyopia and ocular rigidity share a common biomechanical factor [29, 67]. Ocular rigidity may lead to accommodation loss in presbyopia by impacting the biomechanical relationships and functions of the accommodation complex [75, 77, 78]. Ocular rigidity may also decrease the ability of the structures of the eye to return from an accommodated to a disaccommodated state by affecting the elastic recoil of the choroid [11, 67, 79]. This creates an important biomechanical dysfunction since the lens posture is never able to fully accommodate therefore losing capability for "pre-stretch" zonular tension and lens shape change.

The sclera is made up of dense irregular connective tissue including collagen (50–75%), elastin (2–5%), and proteoglycans [80], and has an elastic modulus of approximately 1.61×10^6 N/m^2 [79, 81]. Age has a distinct effect on all connective tissues including those in the sclera. With age, the connective tissue in the sclera begins to crosslink and form bonds between the protein chains. These crosslinks decrease the elasticity of the connective tissues and stiffen the sclera, increasing the elastic modulus to approximately 2.85×10^6 N/m^2 [79, 81]. This 'sclerosclerosis' [82], as well as a concomitant increase in metabolic physiological stress, creates the cycle of pathophysiology related to the aging sclera which becomes less compliant when subjected to forces, such as contraction of the ciliary muscle. The biomechanical dysfunction becomes a vicious cycle resulting in less accommodative efficiency as well as the potential of disruption of other physiological functions of the eye organ which lie beneath the scleral coat.

Chronic stress that exceeds the healing ability of tissues can lead to chronic inflammation and eventual cell death, which technically describes the pathophysiology of aging [83]. The underlying factors of the change in the scleral material properties which leads to the loss of scleral compliance may include age-related and race-related increases in collagen crosslinks, along with loss of elastin-driven recoil, and/or collagen microarchitectural changed [84]. As this pathophysiology progresses, the sclera may exert compression and loading stresses on underlying structures, creating further biomechanical dysfunction, specifically those related to accommodation which affects not only visual accommodation but other physiological functions of the eye organ [85].

Age-related material property and architectural changes within the sclera also affect the mobility of connective tissues of the scleral fibers, directly leading to the loss of compliance. This causes a decrease in the normal maintenance and turnover of proteoglycans (PG) in the sclera, leading to the loss of PG and eventual tissue atrophy [86]. However, if the compliance and mobility of scleral connective tissues are restored, this PG loss could be reversed and flexibility restored [87]. The potential to improve property characteristics of the aging sclera could allow for restoration of biomechanical efficiency for the ciliary muscles to work more effectively in molding the lens.

Presbyopia: Theory and Treatment

Helmholtz theory of accommodation, wherein as the lens stiffens with age accommodative ability decreases [9], is the traditional definition of presbyopia. Following from this traditional definition, presbyopia treatments primarily modify optics along the visual axis to allow the clear focusing of objects at near. Non-invasive spectacles and contact lens use are most common treatments, however surgically treating the lens or cornea is also widespread [88, 89]. These surgical treatments aim to induce multifocality or create changes in asphericity and facilitate a large depth of focus for clear vision [88]. These procedures do not attempt to restore true physiological accommodation to the presbyopic eye, and may sacrifice distance visual acuity, binocularity, and stereopsis for clear vision at near [90–92].

Schachar and colleagues argued that presbyopia is caused by a decrease in circumlental space with age which crowds the lens [93–95]. Following from this theory, several iterations of scleral implants have been used in an attempt to lift the sclera to increase the area between the lens and the ciliary muscle, uncrowd the lens, tighten the anterior zonules, and restore accommodative ability. There is some evidence to suggest that these procedures were effective at restoring near visual acuity, however most versions of scleral implants were abandoned due to poor patient satisfaction and mixed results [96]. The only remaining scleral implant with the CE mark is the VisAbility Micro-Insert scleral implant (Refocus Group, Dallas, TX,

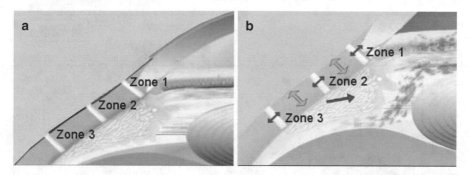

Fig. 9.3 LaserACE surgical procedure. (**a**) the three critical zones of significance as measured from the anatomical limbus; (**b**) restored mechanical efficiency and improved biomechanical mobility (procedure objectives). Reprinted with permission from [99]

USA), which is currently is FDA clinical trials [97]. Visual acuity and patient satisfaction results are encouraging, despite risks of anterior segment ischemia, implant infection, implant displacement, and subconjunctival erosion [98].

Following from the theory that ocular rigidity has a large influence on the pathogenesis of age-related loss in accommodative ability, laser scleral therapies were developed. Laser anterior ciliary excision (LaserACE) is the first iteration of the new laser scleral therapies. LaserACE is an eye laser therapy designed to create an 'uncrosslinking' effect in the sclera by uncoupling the fibrils and microfibrils in the scleral layers. The biomechanical properties are manipulated by using a laser with a spot size of 600 μm to create a 5 mm by 5 mm matrix of microablations (microexcisions) in the sclera in 3 critical zones overlaying key anatomy of the accommodative mechanism (Fig. 9.3). This results in improving the compliance in the scleral tissue upon stress of the ciliary muscle forces. The 3 critical zones are as follows [11, 14, 16, 82, 100]:

- Zone 1: The scleral spur at the origin of the ciliary muscle (0.5–1.1 mm from AL).
- Zone 2: The mid ciliary muscle body (1.1–4.9 mm from AL).
- Zone 3: Insertion of the longitudinal muscle fibers of the ciliary muscle, just anterior to the ora serrata at the insertion zone of the posterior vitreous zonules (4.9–5.5 mm from AL).

LaserACE uses an erbium: yttrium–aluminum–garnet (Er:YAG) laser (VisioLite®) to create the microablations in the sclera, with the aim to increase scleral compliance. This would alleviate any compression and loading stresses that a rigid sclera could exert onto underlying accommodative structures. There is evidence demonstrating that LaserACE can reduce the ocular rigidity of scleral tissue by uncrosslinking. In a study presented at the American Society of Cataract and Refractive Surgery (ASCRS) annual meeting in 2013 [7], enucleated porcine sclera was chemically crosslinked to mimic the ocular rigidity observed in presbyopic 60-year-old human patients. The LaserACE procedure was then performed on the crosslinked porcine sclera and reduced its ocular rigidity by 30%, which was

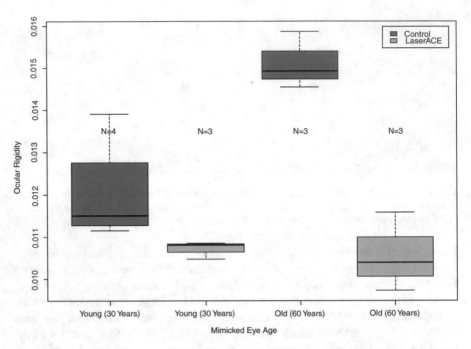

Fig. 9.4 Box-and-whiskers plot of the ocular rigidity for control (blue) and Laser Anterior Ciliary Excision treated (green) porcine eyes. The upper and lower extremities of the box represent the 75th and 25th percentiles, the bar within the box represents the median, and the whiskers represent the full extent of the data ranges

statistically significant (Fig. 9.4; p = 0.0009). After LaserACE treatment, the rigidity in the porcine sclera returned to the ocular rigidity levels observed in pre-presbyopic 30-year-old human patients.

Previous studies have also shown that LaserACE can improve accommodative ability. A multicenter pilot study of 80 eyes in 40 patients measured objective accommodation preoperatively and up to 18 months after the LaserACE procedure [100]. Accommodation was measured with either wavefront aberrometry with the iTrace dynamic aberrometer (Tracey Technologies, Houston, TX) or the COAS Shack-Hartmann aberrometer with dynamic stimulation aberrometry (AMO Wavefront Sciences, Albuquerque, NM) [101]. The results are shown in Fig. 9.5. Patients received an average improvement in accommodative amplitude of 1.25–1.5 D following the LaserACE procedure, which was sustained for 18 months postoperatively. No patient lost accommodative amplitude. In another study, effective range of focus (EROF), true physiological accommodation, and pseudoaccommodation were measured in 6 eyes of 3 patients (average age 59.3 years) for up to 13 years postoperatively after LaserACE treatment [102]. Measurements were done using wavefront aberrometry with the iTrace dynamic aberrometer (Tracey Technologies, Houston, TX). The EROF is the range of focus with acceptable blur and is the sum of the true physiological accommodation and the

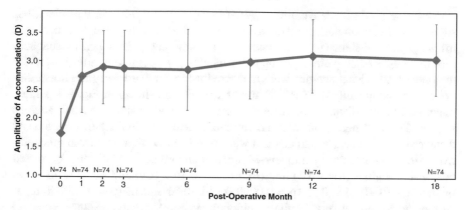

Fig. 9.5 Objectively-measured patient accommodative amplitude. Error bars represent mean ± SD. Reprinted with permission from SLACK Incorporated [101]

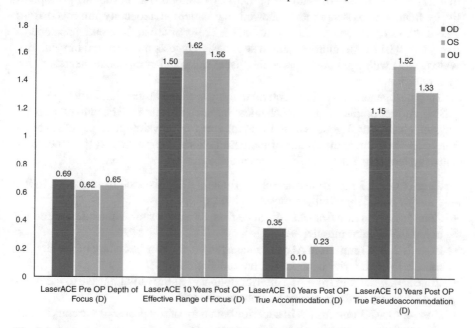

Fig. 9.6 Patient averages of depth of focus, effective range of focus, true accommodation, pseudoaccomodation: OD (dark blue), OS (green), OU (light blue). Adapted with permission from [102]

pseudoaccommodation. The results are summarized in Fig. 9.6. Clinical accommodation for these patients averaged 0.92 ± 0.61 D preoperatively. The average EROF for all patient eyes (n = 6) was higher than preoperative accommodation at 1.56 ± 0.36 D postoperatively. The EROF included 0.23 ± 0.24 D and 1.33 ± 0.38 D of true and pseudoaccommodation respectively. This was significant, as these presbyopic patients would likely have no true physiological accommodation if they had not received LaserACE treatment.

Restoring accommodative ability by targeting ocular rigidity in the sclera, has significant effects on patient visual acuity. An IRB approved phase 3 clinical trial investigated the distance (4 m), intermediate (60 cm), and near (40 cm) visual acuities of 52 eyes of 26 patients for up to 24 months postoperatively after LaserACE treatment [99]. Visual acuities were measured using standard early treatment diabetic retinopathy study (ETDRS) charts and results are shown in Fig. 9.7. Patient uncorrected and distance corrected intermediate and distance visual acuities improved or remained stable after the LaserACE treatment. Patient uncorrected and distance corrected near visual acuities were significantly improved from preoperative up to 24 months postoperatively. Monocular uncorrected and distance corrected near visual acuities (logMAR) improved from +0.36 ± 0.20 and +0.34 ± 0.18 preoperatively, to +0.25 ± 0.18 (p = 0.00005) and +0.21 ± 0.18 (p = 0.00000002) at 24 months postoperatively. Similarly, binocular uncorrected and distance corrected visual acuities at near improved from +0.20 ± 0.16 and +0.21 ± 0.17 preoperatively, to +0.12 ± 0.14 (p = 0.001) and +0.11 ± 0.12 (p = 0.0003) at 24 months postoperatively. Randot stereoscopic tests showed that patient stereoacuity improved from 74.8 ± 30.3 s of arc preoperatively, to 58.8 ± 22.9 s of arc at 24 months postoperatively (p = 0.012). An improvement in stereopsis suggests that restored binocularity which is lost with age may improve the visual skills and components necessary for quality vision.

The latest generation of laser scleral therapy is called laser scleral microporation (LSM). Animal studies and biomechanical research unveiled the need to expand the physiological critical zones from 3 critical zones of physiological significance to 5 in order to optimize the effects of increased scleral compliance on the accommodative system (Fig. 9.8). The five zones are:

- Zone 0: 0.0–1.3 mm from anatomical limbus (AL); distance from the AL to the superior boundary of ciliary muscle/scleral spur;
- Zone 1: 1.3–2.8 mm from AL; distance from the sclera spur to the inferior boundary of the circular muscle;
- Zone 2: 2.8–4.7 mm from AL; distance from the inferior boundary of the circular muscle to the inferior boundary of the radial muscle;
- Zone 3: 4.7–6.6 mm from AL; inferior boundary of the radial muscle to the superior boundary of the posterior vitreous zonule zone; and
- Zone 4: 6.6–7.3 mm from AL; superior boundary of the posterior vitreous zonule zone to the superior boundary of the ora serrata.

The LSM procedure utilizes an Er:YAG laser in the wavelength of 2.94 μm (VisioLite®) to create a matrix of microporations in the sclera arranged in an array, with the aim to uncrosslink scleral tissue overlying the ciliary muscles in the eye. Early results of the LSM procedure show significant improvements for distance (4 m), intermediate (60 cm), and near (40 cm) visual acuities (Fig. 9.9) [103]. Thirty-two eyes of 16 patients aged >40 years who showed loss of accommodative ability and near visual acuity of 20/50 or worse were treated with LSM. Visual outcomes were assessed using the Early Diabetic Retinopathy Study (EDTRS) logMAR charts up to 1 month postoperatively. Binocular uncorrected visual acuities

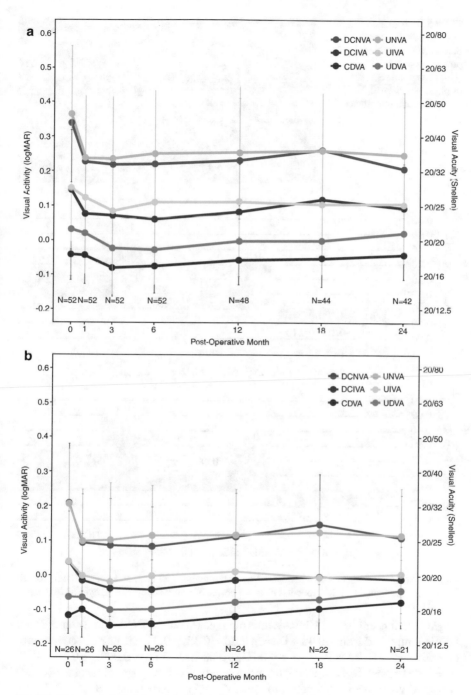

Fig. 9.7 Uncorrected (lightly colored) and distance-corrected (darkly colored) visual acuity at a distance 4 m, intermediate (60 cm), and near (40 cm) for (**a**) Monocular and (**b**) Binocular patient eyes. Error bars represent mean ± SD. Reprinted with permission from [99]

Fig. 9.8 Schematic representation of the Laser Scleral Microporation procedure over the five critical anatomical zones of physiological and biomechanical importance

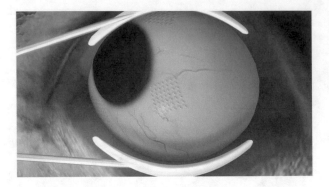

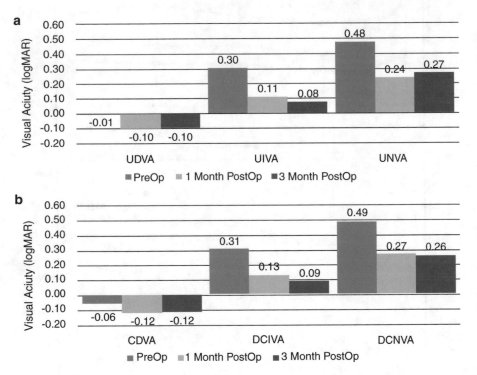

Fig. 9.9 Mean visual acuity at a distance 4 m, intermediate (60 cm), and near (40 cm) for (**a**) Binocular uncorrected and (**b**) Binocular distance corrected patient eyes. N = 32 eyes of 16 patients

(logMAR) at near (40 cm; UNVA), intermediate (60 cm; UIVA), and distance (4 m; UDVA) improved from +0.48 ± 0.16, +0.30 ± 0.15, −0.01 ± 0.12 respectively pre-operatively, to +0.27 ± 0.17 (p < 0.001), +0.08 ± 0.13 (p = 0.008), −0.10 ± 0.10 (p = 0.05) respectively at 3 months postoperatively. Similarly, binocular distance corrected visual acuities at near (40 cm; DCNVA), intermediate (60 cm; DCIVA), and distance (4 m; CDVA) improved from +0.49 ± 0.15 (logMAR), +0.31 ± 0.15 (logMAR), −0.06 ± 0.10 (logMAR) respectively preoperatively, to +0.26 ± 0.19

(logMAR) (p = 0.003), +0.09 ± 0.14 (logMAR) (p = 0.001), −0.12 ± 0.09 (log-MAR) (p > 0.05) respectively at 3 months postoperatively. These early experimental results are very encouraging and also corroborate previous findings.

Summary

In summary, recent literature has illuminated that the lens together with the extral-enticular structures including the lens capsule, zonules, choroid, vitreous, sclera, ciliary muscles, all play a critical role in accommodation. These structures like all other connective tissues in the body are all affected by increasing age. Increasing ocular rigidity with age produces stress and strain on all of the ocular structures and can affect accommodative ability and biomechanical efficiency.

Scleral therapies may have an important role in treating age-related biomechanical deficiencies in presbyopes, by providing at least one means to address the true etiology of the clinical manifestation of the loss of accommodation seen with age. LaserACE and LSM treatments, utilizing laser microporation of the sclera to restore more pliable biomechanical properties, appear to be safe procedures, and can improve visual outcomes in aging adults. These technologies continue to be further explored and optimized. The field of ocular biomechanics is in its infancy, however with the advent of improved biometry, imaging, and research focus, information about how the accommodation complex works and how it impacts the entire eye organ is not far from reach. This is a severely understudied field, however, the relevance of the biomechanics of accommodation is more overarching than simply the loss of near vision, and of worthwhile relevance to pursue further. Further investigation could lead to the unveiling of even greater significance than the focus we currently have. There are quintessential questions that remain to be pursued, therefore more research is needed in this area to further identify and understand all the relevant biomechanical factors contributing to ocular rigidity and presbyopia. It is notable to admit that we still do not fully understand the biomechanics of accommodation and that there currently exists no whole eye accommodation model that can fully encapsulate the biomechanical interactions of the optical, physiological, and neuromuscular functions of accommodation. Moreover, we are lacking a model of the complex biomechanics of the ciliary muscle forces on the lens during accommodation and disaccommodation with regard to age-related ocular rigidity. More biomechanical studies that account for all the physiological implications of the loss of accommodation as mentioned in this paper need to be done to further illuminate the relationships between presbyopia dysfunction and age-related tissue changes. Fundamental studies about the complex biomechanics of accommodation are still needed to understand the comprehensive mechanisms underlying presbyopia. Improved modelling along with a better understanding of the precepts and dynamics of the biomechanics of accommodation could lead to prevention or even delay of the onset of age-related eye dysfunction and disease.

References

1. Girard MJ, Dupps WJ, Baskaran M, et al. Translating ocular biomechanics into clinical practice: current state and future prospects. Curr Eye Res. 2015;40:1–18.
2. Pavlatos E, Perez BC, Morris HJ, et al. Three-dimensional strains in human posterior sclera using ultrasound speckle tracking. J Biomech Eng. 2016;138:021015.
3. MJA G, Downs JC, Burgoyne CF, JKF S. Peripapillary and posterior scleral mechanics—part I: development of an anisotropic hyperelastic constitutive model. J Biomech Eng. 2009;131:051011.
4. Girard MJ, Suh JK, Bottlang M, Burgoyne CF, Downs JC. Scleral biomechanics in the aging monkey eye. Invest Ophthalmol Vis Sci. 2009;50:5226–37.
5. Downs JC. Viscoelastic characterization of peripapillary sclera: material properties by quadrant in rabbit and monkey eyes. J Biomech Eng. 2003;125:124–31.
6. Jia X, Yu J, Liao SH, Duan XC. Biomechanics of the sclera and effects on intraocular pressure. Int J Ophthalmol. 2016;9:1824–31.
7. Hipsley A, Waring GO, Wang J-L, Hsiao E. Novel method using collagen cxl to evaluate ability of laser anterior ciliary excision procedure to decrease ocular rigidity for restoring accommodation. In: American Society of Cataract and Refractive Surgery. San Francisco, CA: ASCRS; 2013.
8. Ethier CR, Johnson M, Ruberti J. Ocular biomechanics and biotransport. Annu Rev Biomed Eng. 2004;6:249–73.
9. von Helmholtz H. Mechanism of accommodation. Helmholtz's treatise on physiological optics, Vol 1, Trans from the 3rd German ed. 1924;143–172.
10. Fisher RF. The elastic constants of the human lens. J Physiol. 1971;212:147–80.
11. Goldberg DB. Computer-animated model of accommodation and presbyopia. J Cataract Refract Surg. 2015;41:437–45.
12. Millodot M. Dictionary of optometry and visual science. 7th ed. Oxford, UK: Elsevier Health Sciences; 2014. p. xix–8.
13. Richdale K, Sinnott LT, Bullimore MA, et al. Quantification of age-related and per diopter accommodative changes of the lens and ciliary muscle in the emmetropic human eyelens and ciliary muscle with age and accommodation. Invest Ophthalmol Vis Sci. 2013;54:1095–105.
14. Croft MA, McDonald JP, Katz A, et al. Extralenticular and lenticular aspects of accommodation and presbyopia in human versus monkey eyes. Invest Ophthalmol Vis Sci. 2013;54:5035–48.
15. Croft MA, Nork TM, McDonald JP, et al. Accommodative movements of the vitreous membrane, choroid, and sclera in young and presbyopic human and nonhuman primate eyes. Invest Ophthalmol Vis Sci. 2013;54:5049–58.
16. Lütjen-Drecoll E, Kaufman PL, Wasielewski R, Ting-Li L, Croft MA. Morphology and accommodative function of the vitreous zonule in human and monkey eyes. Investig Ophthalmol Vis Sci. 2010;51:1554–64.
17. Nankivil D, Manns F, Arrieta-Quintero E, et al. Effect of anterior zonule transection on the change in lens diameter and power in cynomolgus monkeys during simulated accommodation. Invest Ophthalmol Vis Sci. 2009;50:4017–21.
18. Croft MA, Glasser A, Heatley G, et al. Accommodative ciliary body and lens function in rhesus monkeys, I: Normal lens, zonule and ciliary process configuration in the iridectomized eye. Invest Ophthalmol Vis Sci. 2006;47:1076–86.
19. Strenk SA, Strenk LM, Guo S. Magnetic resonance imaging of the anteroposterior position and thickness of the aging, accommodating, phakic, and pseudophakic ciliary muscle. J Cataract Refract Surg. 2010;36:235–41.
20. Croft MA, Heatley G, McDonald JP, Katz A, Kaufman PL. Accommodative movements of the lens/capsule and the strand that extends between the posterior vitreous zonule insertion zone & the lens equator, in relation to the vitreous face and aging. Ophthalmic Physiol Opt. 2016;36:21–32.

21. Croft MA, Lutjen-Drecoll E, Kaufman PL. Age-related posterior ciliary muscle restriction–a link between trabecular meshwork and optic nerve head pathophysiology. Exp Eye Res. 2017;158:187–9.
22. Flugel-Koch CM, Croft MA, Kaufman PL, Lutjen-Drecoll E. Anteriorly located zonular fibres as a tool for fine regulation in accommodation. Ophthalmic Physiol Opt. 2016;36:13–20.
23. Tamm S, Tamm E, Rohen JW. Age-related changes of the human ciliary muscle. A quantitative morphometric study. Mech Ageing Dev. 1992;62:209–21.
24. Strenk SA, Semmlow JL, Strenk LM, et al. Age-related changes in human ciliary muscle and lens: a magnetic resonance imaging study. Invest Ophthalmol Vis Sci. 1999;40:1162–9.
25. Pardue MT, Sivak JG. Age-related changes in human ciliary muscle. Optom Vis Sci. 2000;77:204–10.
26. Bito LZ, Miranda OC. Accommodation and presbyopia. Ophthalmol Annual. 1989;1989:103–28.
27. Dubbelman M, Van der Heijde GL, Weeber HA. Change in shape of the aging human crystalline lens with accommodation. Vis Res. 2005;45:117–32.
28. Brown N. The change in shape and internal form of the lens of the eye on accommodation. Exp Eye Res. 1973;15:441–59.
29. Detorakis ET, Pallikaris IG. Ocular rigidity: biomechanical role, in vivo measurements and clinical significance. Clin Exp Ophthalmol. 2013;41:73–81.
30. Pallikaris IG, Kymionis GD, Ginis HS, et al. Ocular rigidity in patients with age-related macular degeneration. Am J Ophthalmol. 2006;141:611–5.
31. Glasser A, Campbell MC. Presbyopia and the optical changes in the human crystalline lens with age. Vis Res. 1998;38:209–29.
32. Glasser A, Campbell MC. On the potential causes of presbyopia. Vis Res. 1999;39:1267–72.
33. Fisher R. Presbyopia and the changes with age in the human crystalline lens. J Physiol Lond. 1973;228:765–79.
34. Koretz JF, Cook CA, Kaufman PL. Aging of the human lens: changes in lens shape at zero-diopter accommodation. J Opt Soc Am A. 2001;18:265–72.
35. Smith G. The optical properties of the crystalline lens and their significance. Clin Exp Ophthalmol. 2003;86:3–18.
36. Barnard K, Burgess SA, Carter DA, Woolley DM. Three-dimensional structure of type iv collagen in the mammalian lens capsule. J Struct Biol. 1992;108:6–13.
37. Truscott RJ. Presbyopia. Emerging from a blur towards an understanding of the molecular basis for this most common eye condition. Exp Eye Res. 2009;88:241–7.
38. Atchison DA. Accommodation and presbyopia. Ophthalmic Physiol Opt. 1995;15:255–72.
39. Cambridge University Engineering Department. Materials data book. 2003;13.
40. Schachar RA. The mechanism of accommodation and presbyopia. Amsterdam: Kugler Publications; 2012.
41. Laughton DS, Sheppard AL. Davies LN. A longitudinal study of accommodative changes in biometry during incipient presbyopia. Ophthalmic Physiol Opt. 2016;36:33–42.
42. Sheppard AL, Evans CJ, Singh KD, et al. Three-dimensional magnetic resonance imaging of the phakic crystalline lens during accommodation. Invest Ophthalmol Vis Sci. 2011;52:3689–97.
43. Richdale K, Bullimore MA, Zadnik K. Lens thickness with age and accommodation by optical coherence tomography. Ophthalmic Physiol Opt. 2008;28:441–7.
44. Koretz JF, Cook CA, Kaufman PL. Accommodation and presbyopia in the human eye. Changes in the anterior segment and crystalline lens with focus. Invest Ophthalmol Vis Sci. 1997;38:569–78.
45. Ostrin L, Kasthurirangan S, Win-Hall D, Glasser A. Simultaneous measurements of refraction and a-scan biometry during accommodation in humans. Optom Vis Sci. 2006;83:657–65.
46. Bolz M, Prinz A, Drexler W, Findl O. Linear relationship of refractive and biometric lenticular changes during accommodation in emmetropic and myopic eyes. Br J Ophthalmol. 2007;91:360–5.

47. Garner LF, Yap MK. Changes in ocular dimensions and refraction with accommodation. Ophthalmic Physiol Opt. 1997;17:12–7.
48. Richdale K, Bullimore MA, Sinnott LT, Zadnik K. The effect of age, accommodation, and refractive error on the adult human eye. Optom Vis Sci. 2016;93:3–11.
49. Beauchamp R, Mitchell B. Ultrasound measures of vitreous chamber depth during ocular accommodation. Am J Optom Physiol Opt. 1985;62:523–32.
50. Coleman DJ. Unified model for accommodative mechanism. Am J Ophthalmol. 1970;69:1063–79.
51. Raphael J. Accommodational variations in Israel, 1949-1960. Br J Physiol Opt. 1961;18:181–5.
52. Mordi JA, Ciuffreda KJ. Static aspects of accommodation: age and presbyopia. Vis Res. 1998;38:1643–53.
53. Artigas Verde J, Felipe Marcet A, Navea A, et al. Age-induced change in the color of the human crystalline lens. Acta Ophthalmol. 2011;89 https://doi.org/10.1111/j.1755-3768.2011.256.x.
54. Fisher RF. Elastic constants of the human lens capsule. J Physiol. 1969;201:1–19.
55. Heys KR, Cram SL, Truscott RJ. Massive increase in the stiffness of the human lens nucleus with age: the basis for presbyopia? Mol Vis. 2004;10:956–63.
56. Weeber HA, van der Heijde RG. On the relationship between lens stiffness and accommodative amplitude. Exp Eye Res. 2007;85:602–7.
57. Glasser A, Campbell MC. Biometric, optical and physical changes in the isolated human crystalline lens with age in relation to presbyopia. Vis Res. 1999;39:1991–2015.
58. Rosen AM, Denham DB, Fernandez V, et al. In vitro dimensions and curvatures of human lenses. Vis Res. 2006;46:1002–9.
59. Cook CA, Koretz JF, Pfahnl A, Hyun J, Kaufman PL. Aging of the human crystalline lens and anterior segment. Vis Res. 1994;34:2945–54.
60. Dubbelman M, van der Heijde GL, Weeber HA. The thickness of the aging human lens obtained from corrected scheimpflug images. Optom Vis Sci. 2001;78:411–6.
61. Farnsworth PN, Shyne SE. Anterior zonular shifts with age. Exp Eye Res. 1979;28:291–7.
62. Sakabe I, Oshika T, Lim SJ, Apple DJ. Anterior shift of zonular insertion onto the anterior surface of human crystalline lens with age. Ophthalmology. 1998;105:295–9.
63. Brown N. The shape of the lens equator. Exp Eye Res. 1974;19:571–6.
64. Brown N. The change in lens curvature with age. Exp Eye Res. 1974;19:175–83.
65. Dubbelman M, Van der Heijde GL. The shape of the aging human lens: curvature, equivalent refractive index and the lens paradox. Vis Res. 2001;41:1867–77.
66. Wilde GS. Measurement of human lens stiffness for modelling presbyopia treatments. (Doctoral dissertation, Oxford University) 2011.
67. Pallikaris IG, Kymionis GD, Ginis HS, Kounis GA, Tsilimbaris MK. Ocular rigidity in living human eyes. Invest Ophthalmol Vis Sci. 2005;46:409–14.
68. Read SA, Collins MJ, Becker H, et al. Changes in intraocular pressure and ocular pulse amplitude with accommodation. Br J Ophthalmol. 2010;94:332–5.
69. Crawford K, Kaufman PL. Pilocarpine antagonizes prostaglandin f2α-induced ocular hypotension in monkeys: evidence for enhancement of uveoscleral outflow by prostaglandin f2α. Arch Ophthalmol. 1987;105:1112–6.
70. Croft MA, Kaufman PL. Accommodation and presbyopia: the ciliary neuromuscular view. Ophthalmol Clin. 2006;19:13–24.
71. Tamm ER, Lutjen-Drecoll E. Ciliary body. Microsc Res Tech. 1996;33:390–439.
72. Fisher RF. The mechanics of accommodation in relation to presbyopia. Eye (Lond). 1988;2(Pt 6):646–9.
73. Fisher R. The force of contraction of the human ciliary muscle during accommodation. J Physiol Lond. 1977;270:51–74.
74. Koretz JF, Kaufman PL, Neider MW, Goeckner PA. Accommodation and presbyopia in the human eye–aging of the anterior segment. Vis Res. 1989;29:1685–92.

75. Dastiridou AI, Tsironi EE, Tsilimbaris MK, et al. Ocular rigidity, outflow facility, ocular pulse amplitude, and pulsatile ocular blood flow in open-angle glaucoma: a manometric study. Invest Ophthalmol Vis Sci. 2013;54:4571–7.

76. Schor CM. Bharadwaj SR. a pulse-step model of accommodation dynamics in the aging eye. Vis Res. 2005;45:1237–54.

77. Dastiridou AI, Ginis HS, De Brouwere D, Tsilimbaris MK, Pallikaris IG. Ocular rigidity, ocular pulse amplitude, and pulsatile ocular blood flow: the effect of intraocular pressure. Invest Ophthalmol Vis Sci. 2009;50:5718–22.

78. Ravalico G, Toffoli G, Pastori G, Croce M, Calderini S. Age-related ocular blood flow changes. Invest Ophthalmol Vis Sci. 1996;37:2645–50.

79. Friberg TR, Lace JW. A comparison of the elastic properties of human choroid and sclera. Exp Eye Res. 1988;47:429–36.

80. Watson PG, Young RD. Scleral structure, organisation and disease. Exp Eye Res. 2004;78:609–23.

81. Eilaghi A, Flanagan JG, Tertinegg I, et al. Biaxial mechanical testing of human sclera. J Biomech. 2010;43:1696–701.

82. Hipsley A, Dementiev D. Visiodynamics theory: a biomechanical application for the aging eye and LaserAceTM natural vision restoration. In: Ashok G, K MC EHJ, Roberto P, editors. Mastering the techniques of corneal refractive surgery. New Delhi: Jaypee Brothers Pvt Ltd; 2006. p. 490–506.

83. Diamant J, Keller A, Baer E, Litt M, Arridge R. Collagen; ultrastructure and its relation to mechanical properties as a function of ageing. Proc R Soc Lond B Biol Sci. 1972;180:293–315.

84. Grytz R, Fazio MA, Libertiaux V, et al. Age- and race-related differences in human scleral material properties. Invest Ophthalmol Vis Sci. 2014;55:8163–72.

85. Swartz TS, Rocha KM, Jackson M, et al. Restoration of accommodation: new perspectives. Arq Bras Oftalmol. 2014;77:V–VII.

86. Shephard RJ, Wetzler HP. Physiology and biochemistry of exercise. J Occup Environ Med. 1982;24:440.

87. Buckwalter J. Maintaining and restoring mobility in middle and old age: the importance of the soft tissues. Instr Course Lect. 1996;46:459–69.

88. Charman WN. Developments in the correction of presbyopia II: surgical approaches. Ophthal Physiol Optics. 2014;34:397–426.

89. Charman WN. Developments in the correction of presbyopia I. spectacle and contact lenses. Ophthal Physiolog Opt. 2014;34:8–29.

90. O'Keefe M, O'Keeffe N. Corneal surgical approach in the treatment of presbyopia. J Clin Exp Ophthalmol. 2016;7:1–4.

91. Evans BJW. Monovision: a review. Ophthalmic Physiol Opt. 2007;27:417–39.

92. Gil-Cazorla R, Shah S, Naroo SA. A review of the surgical options for the correction of presbyopia. Br J Ophthalmol. 2015;100:62–70.

93. Schachar RA. Zonular function: a new hypothesis with clinical implications. Ann Ophthalmol. 1993;26:36–8.

94. Schachar RA. Pathophysiology of accommodation and presbyopia. Understanding the clinical implications. J Fla Med Assoc. 1994;81:268.

95. Schachar RA. Cause and treatment of presbyopia with a method for increasing the amplitude of accommodation. Ann Ophthalmol. 1992;24:445.

96. Malecaze FJ, Gazagne CS, Tarroux MC, Gorrand J-M. Scleral expansion bands for presbyopia. Ophthalmology. 2001;108:2165–71.

97. Trials USNIoHC. A clinical trial of the visability micro insert system for presbyopic patients.

98. Charters L. Refocus scleral implants for presbyopia. Ophthalmol Times. 2013;

99. Hipsley A, Ma DH-K, Sun C-C, et al. Visual outcomes 24 months after LaserACE. Eye Vis. 2017;4:15.

100. Hipsley A, McDonald M. Laser scleral matrix microexcisions (laserace/erbium yag laser). In: Pallikaris IG, Plainis S, Charman WN, editors. Presbyopia: origins, effects, and treatment. Thorofare, NJ: Slack Incorporated; 2012. p. 219–25.
101. Hipsley A, Ma DH, Rocha KM, Hall B. Laser scleral microporation procedure. In: Wang M, editor. Surgical correction of presbyopia: the fifth wave. Thorofare, NJ: Slack Incorporated; 2019.
102. Hipsley A, Hall B, Rocha KM. Long-term visual outcomes of laser anterior ciliary excision. Am J Ophthalmol Case Rep. 2018;10:38–47.
103. Jackson MA, Hipsley A, Ma DH, et al. Multi-center clinical trial results of laser scleral microporation in presbyopic eyes. In: American Society of Cataract and Refractive Surgery. Virtual annual meeting; 2020.

Chapter 10
Biomechanical Properties of the Trabecular Meshwork in Aqueous Humor Outflow Resistance

VijayKrishna Raghunathan

Introduction

Primary open angle glaucoma (POAG), age associated macular degeneration (AMD), and cataract are the three most common age associated ocular disorders worldwide, leading to vision loss. Among these vision loss in POAG and AMD are irreversible. The etiology and progression of these diseases are multifactorial [1, 2] although fibrosis, oxidative and senescence have been thought to be significant contributing factors. A key facet of fibrosis is a dynamic change in the extracellular matrix leading the tissue to become stiffer. The context in which this 'stiffness' is measured is dependent on the type of tissue, sample preparation, or the method by which it was measured. Regardless, a change in the biomechanical property of a tissue has profound implications on how cells respond to changes in their microenvironment. This is indeed true of the trabecular meshwork as well. Responsible for drainage of approximately 80% of the aqueous humor of the eye, dysfunction in the TM is thought to be the primary site of resistance, and lowering the intraocular pressure is the only modifiable risk factor in glaucoma, a major cause of irreversible blindness in the aging population [3–9]. The increased resistance to aqueous humor in POAG is thought to be due to dependent on a number of factors—senescence, matrix composition/morphology/mechanics, loss of intra- and inter-cellular pores, deposition of plaque like material, changes in segmental regions, loss of cells, and/or collapsing of the beams. With age, accumulation of extracellular matrix,

V. Raghunathan (✉)
The Ocular Surface Institute, University of Houston, Houston, TX, USA

Department of Basic Sciences, College of Optometry, University of Houston, Houston, TX, USA

Department of Biomedical Engineering, Cullen College of Engineering, University of Houston, Houston, TX, USA
e-mail: vraghunathan@uh.edu

© Springer Nature Switzerland AG 2021
I. Pallikaris et al. (eds.), *Ocular Rigidity, Biomechanics and Hydrodynamics of the Eye*, https://doi.org/10.1007/978-3-030-64422-2_10

thickening of the beams, and loss of TM cells have all been documented [10–14]. Lutjen-Drecoll et al. [15] demonstrated that with age the elastic fibers of the TM thicken with minimal changes to the elastin containing central core. Classical studies by Tripathi [16, 17] have shown elevated amounts of matrix proteins in the TM that were postulated to contribute to increased resistance to outflow. Data emanating from studies over the past 4 decades are yet to identify the molecular mechanisms or the implications of mechanical changes in the TM contributing to the etiology and progression of glaucoma. Such increase in thickness may contribute to the changing biomechanics in glaucoma or age, and this is yet to be demonstrated.

The Importance of Studying Biomechanics of the Outflow Pathway

The anterior segment of the eye is complex and includes the cornea, lens, iris, ciliary body, trabecular meshwork (TM) and Schlemm's canal (SC). The TM and SC are located at the iridocorneal angle and primarily regulate and drive the drainage of aqueous humor. The TM is an incredibly complex structure (Fig. 10.1) comprised primarily of three regions which differ in both structure and function [18–22]. Anterior to posterior, first is the <20 μm thin juxtracanalicular (JCT) or cribiform region (primary site of resistance to outflow) that is separated from the endothelial cells of inner wall of the Schlemm's canal via a discontinuous basement membrane. The JCT is a made of 2–5 layers of cells embedded in a wide variety of macromolecules and residing over loose fibrillar ECM. This is followed by the corneo-scleral trabecular meshwork (CTM) comprised of thick 8–15 trabecular beams/lamellae made of Col I/III, and elastic fibers. Each layer is covered by cells on a basal lamina rich in laminin and Col IV. Posteriorly, this is followed by 1–3 layers of uveal trabecular meshwork (UTM) whose lamellae are thinner than those observed in the CTM. These together form a sponge-like filter whose porosity varies between and within the three layers.

Approximately 75% of all aqueous humor flows through the TM and SC [23, 24]. The inner wall cells are currently thought to contribute only about 10% of the total resistance [25]. Since the cells in the JCT of the meshwork are not continuous, the bulk of outflow resistance would lie with the extracellular matrix (ECM) of the meshwork at the JCT. ECM components include fibrillar scaffolding proteins (e.g. fibronectin, laminin, collagen etc), non-structural matricellular proteins (e.g. SPARC, matrix gla protein, periostin, CCN family of proteins, thrombospondin, tenascin etc), and glycosylated proteoglycans. Common proteoglycans observed in the TM are glycosaminoglycans [(chondroitin sulfate, heparan sulfate, hyaluronan etc), and versican, perlecan, decorin, biglycan etc]. These together provide structural and mechanical properties to the tissue and adequate surface for the attachment of cells and by acting as load bearing structures. Further, through the presentation of various ligands, ECM components can bind, sequester, and stabilize signaling molecules to modulate essential cellular processes such as migration, proliferation, differentiation, and cell fate determination.

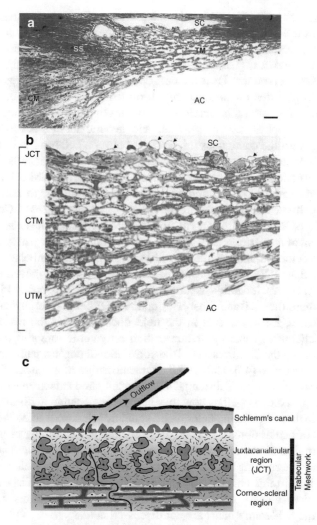

Fig. 10.1 The trabecular meshwork: (**a**) Shows a view of the trabecular meshwork that separates the aqueous humor in the anterior chamber from the canal of Schlemm. *TM* trabecular meshwork; *SC* Schlemm's canal; *AC* anterior chamber; *SS* scleral spur; *CM* ciliary muscle. Magnification bar is 20 μm. (**b**) A magnification of the trabecular meshwork demonstrating the 3 regions: *UTM* uveal trabecular meshwork; *CTM* corneoscleral trabecular meshwork; *JCT* Juxtacanalicular tissue. Magnification bar is 5 μm. (**c**) Schematic illustrates the direction of outflow across the trabecular meshwork. (**a, b**) are reproduced with permission from Tamm [18]

For any tissue, the intimate interaction between cells and their matrix contribute to the mechanical properties. The contribution of either component in defining these properties are quite difficult to isolate. Biomechanical stimuli—such as mechanical stretch, pulsatile motion, compression, shear, pressure, static cell guidance cues etc. are all integral components of the cellular microenvironment in the tissue. That cells are sensitive to dynamic mechanical forces such as shear stress, pressure, and stretch are well recognized [26, 27]. Nevertheless, a plethora of passive biophysical tissue attributes of tissue exists such as stiffness or nanotopography alter cellular proliferation, migration, expression, and differentiation [28–32]. Whilst these cues may appear to be passive at a given instant, they are capable of changing with time, stimulus, and/or intervention. Over the past decade a number of groups have demonstrated the impact that biophysical stimuli on tissue homeostasis, development, differentiation and disease. It is therefore paramount to place these in the context of tissue function. Biophysical, biochemical, and genetic factors act in concert to dynamically govern the continuous interactions between cells and their extracellular microenvironment. Using other cell systems it was shown that cells cultured on stiffer substrates adopt a more contractile tone [33–36]. Truly, TM cells have been reported to be contractile [37, 38], and this is thought to contribute to matrix changes observed in the tissue in POAG leading to outflow resistance [39–41]. Congruently, the importance of Rho signaling and its effect on lowering IOP has been the target for development of novel drugs targeting the conventional outflow pathway [42–44].

Despite the demonstrated importance of biophysics on cellular behaviors, and its potential to mediate IOP, the complexity of the outflow tract has prevented its complete mechanical characterization. Nearly a decade ago, Overby et al. [45] proposed a paradigm where the JCT and inner wall endothelial cells synergistically control outflow resistance. Emerging data in the field document that the resistance goes beyond the Schlemm's canal by demonstrating a dynamic range in resistance to aqueous outflow by the distal vessels of the conventional outflow pathway when the TM was excised ex vivo [46]. Thus, a full characterization of mechanical properties is essential to account for the substantial heterogeneity and anisotropic organization of the tissues involved, as well as how these properties change in disease. It would be wise to note that there are no determined standards that exist to define mechanical properties of ocular tissues. Despite these challenges, a number of laboratories have made significant inroads in characterizing the material properties using various techniques and determining how these properties may influence cell behavior and outflow function. In this chapter we shall explore further the published data, and relevance of biomechanics to TM mechanobiology and outflow resistance. Data pertaining to the Schlemm's canal are not discussed here.

Parameters Defining the Mechanical Properties of Biological Materials

Biological materials such as tissues are difficult to define due to the complex nature of their compositions: ECM, cells, soluble factors, and interstitial fluid. The trabecular meshwork is unique in the sense that it potentially has both *isotropic* (direction independent) and *anisotropic* (direction dependent) characteristics. The way the collagen lamellae are organized around the circumference is highly aligned while the loosely packed matrix of the JCT is stochastic in organization. Further, judging by the anatomical organization of the TM, it is *inhomogeneous in toto* although there may be certain localized regions where the material may be considered *homogeneous*. For example, flow across the TM has been recognized to be segmental i.e. there are regions of high, low, and medium flow with marked differences in the expression of select matrix/matricellular proteins [47–53]. However, whether there are intrinsic structural changes between these segments, and if these vary with time, stimulus, disease are unknown. As such, cells aligned with the collagen fibers may experience 'contact guidance' and experience *static* stretch. It is been postulated that the aqueous system behaves like a mechanical pump [54, 55] to produce *cyclical* strain that is capable of transferring cyclical stretch and compression to the tissue/cells/ECM. Thus the forces experienced by cells are both tangential and perpendicular to their alignment on matrix fibers/bundles. Combined with a possible pulsatile motion, the tissue (cells & matrix) potentially thus experience localized and bulk tensile and compressive loading. Such a property that defines the negative of the ratio of transverse strain to corresponding axial strain is defined as Poisson's ratio (ν) and is essentially constant for any given material. Isotropic materials have a Poisson's ratio between -1.0 and 0.5. The Poisson's ratio of most engineering materials is typically $0.2 < \nu < 0.5$, incompressible materials with elastic deformations will have $\nu = 0.5$, while $\nu = 0$ demonstrates that there is no change in transverse strain.

Combining all these attributes, the most commonly used term to define the mechanical property of a biological tissue in the ocular field is elastic modulus often referred to simply as 'stiffness'. It is a measure of the tendency of a material to resist deformation under stress (force applied per unit area). The ratio of stress to strain (change in deformation per original length) when load is applied in plane is defined as the Young's modulus. The term Young's modulus is true when a material's property is such that the relationship between stress and strain is linear. This is often not the case for biological materials where the modulus varies with the amount and rate of strain, and direction of loading. As such, tissue 'stiffness' is simply referred to as elastic modulus/apparent elastic modulus/tensile modulus etc. depending on the method used. That being said, measures of TM tissue stiffness cannot be taken as absolute unless the methods by which samples are prepared, instrumentation/techniques used, parameters applied for determination are all taken into consideration. Nonetheless values reported in literature provide information on the differences observed between homeostasis and disease to a reasonable extent.

Box 1 Definition of Basic Parameters

Elastic modulus: The modulus of elasticity or elastic modulus is the property of a material that defines how deformable it is under various loads applied. Elastic materials do not have a permanent irreversible change in structure and behavior when a load is applied. The factors that describe the relation between deformation and applied force are termed as 'elastic constants' and the modulus is just one such constant. In biological science research, stiffness and elastic modulus are often used interchangeable, and this has not been without controversy. However, in engineering context, stiffness refers to the force-deformation relationship of the whole system, rather than an intrinsic property of the material. The most commonly used parameter to define the mechanical property of the trabecular meshwork is the elastic modulus, which is defined as Young's modulus. It must be noted that the Young's modulus usually refers to the modulus determined by tensile testing and is defined as follows: For an isotropic material, when a uniaxial tensile stress is applied, the initial slope, where a linear relationship exists between axial stress and axial strain, is defined as the tensile modulus of elasticity or Young's modulus (E) i.e. $E = \sigma/\varepsilon$ in units of N/m^2 or Pa. This linear relationship is also termed Hooke's law (Fig. 10.2).

Viscoelasticity: A number of materials have an elastic component and a viscous component whose stress-strain relationship depends on 'time'. It must be noted that viscoelastic materials will return to their original shape when the applied force is removed (elastic response) although with prolonged time (viscous response) this will not occur. (Figure 10.2 shows difference between elastic loading and viscoelastic loading also termed hysteresis). Cells and tissues have viscoelastic properties with small perturbations at a cell membrane eliciting an elastic response while larger forces eliminate this elastic response.

Reported Mechanical Characterization of the Trabecular Meshwork

Very few studies have actually evaluated the mechanical properties of trabecular meshwork either _in vitro_ or _ex vivo_. The most common parameter reported is the elastic modulus; very little is known about the viscoelastic properties of the TM. These measurements have been made directly and indirectly using a number of techniques. To our knowledge, there are no studies that have reported any mechanical characterization of the TM tissue in vivo. Further, the effects of drugs used to lower IOP on TM biomechanics is largely lacking. However, recent studies combing imaging and computational methodologies hold great promise in accurately characterizing the TM.

Human

The trabecular meshwork, while under constant circumferential stress, is also subjected to compressive loading by dynamic remodeling of the extracellular matrix in addition to modulation in cellular cytoskeletal dynamics. Atomic force microscopy is an indentation technique used to determine the mechanical properties in a localized environment and is thus suitable method for TM. Less than a decade ago, the

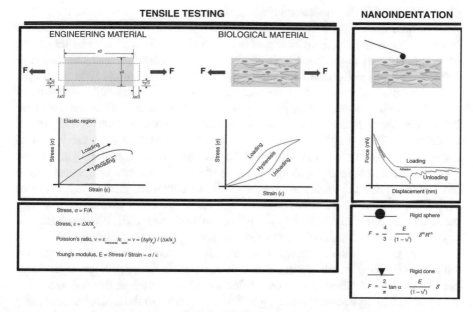

Fig. 10.2 Tensile testing vs nanoindentation. A comparison of uniaxial tensile behavior of engineering vs biological materials is illustrated. Biological materials are viscoelastic and exhibit hysteresis. Nanoindentation methods enable the determination of mechanical properties at a localized area rather than the bulk of the material. General equations governing the definition of elastic modulus are provided. F force; E elastic modulus; δ indentation; R radius of spherical indenter; α half angle of cone; A area; ν Poisson's ratio of material; ε strain; σ stress

elastic modulus of the human TM, at the JCT side, was quantified using AFM [56]. This study was particular important as it the first to report that the apparent elastic moduli of human TM isolated from glaucomatous donors was significantly greater (~20 fold at ~80 kPa) than from normal donors (~4 kPa). There has been skepticism with the manner in which the tissue was prepared and speculation that the cyanoacrylate glue used to adhere the sample may have resulted in an artifactually high value. However, in the same study the authors demonstrate a large range of values for the elastic modulus along the TM suggesting there may have some regional variations. More recently, Vranka et al. [53], using AFM, demonstrated that the elastic moduli of TM (JCT side) varied between the segmental flow regions with mean values for low flow (LF) regions at ~7 kPa vs ~3 kPa for high flow (HF) regions in normal TM obtained from 24 h ex vivo anterior segment perfusion cultures at 1x pressure. Further, they demonstrated that with elevated pressure (2×) for 24 h in normal tissues, HF regions became softer (~1.3 kPa) while LF regions appeared to become stiffer (~9.7 kPa). In a further recent follow up, Raghunathan et al. [57] demonstrate that glaucomatous LF tissues have a mean elastic modulus of ~75 kPa while glaucomatous HF tissues were ~2 kPa. These two recent studies did not use any glue as a mounting agent to adhere the TM tissue [58] and measured the JCT side. These values are in agreement with those reported by Last et al. [56] for glaucomatous TM. In another study [59], using AFM, the elastic modulus of TM from normal eyes was ~1.37 kPa while that of glaucomatous eyes was ~2.75 kPa and observed no significant differences between HF or LF regions in either group; here, the TM was not excised from the corneo-scleral wedge, thus the measurements were likely performed away from the JCT and on the uveo/corneo-scleral side.

Using uni-axial tensile testing, the most commonly and traditionally used method to determine tissue mechanical property, the tensile modulus of human TM from both normal and glaucomatous donors has been reported. Camras et al. [60–62] reported that the Young's modulus of glaucomatous TM 51.5 MPa while that of non-glaucomatous tissues was 12.5 MPa. Additionally, Camras et al. [60] also noted substantial inhomogeneity, with variations in modulus in different segments within the TM, implying the meshwork may exhibit segmental mechanics suggestive of segmental outflow [49, 51, 63–66] although these were not investigated. Whilst these values appear to contradict the findings of Last et al. [56], it is imperative to understand that the methods used in the two studies are vastly different. Also, the organization of fibrillar structural components in tissues can exhibit substantial anisotropy, making tensile testing highly dependent on the orientation of the sample. All of these challenges are exemplified in the TM. Further, the elastic moduli values reported depends on (i) the applied stress/strain, (ii) the hydration state, (iii) time between tissue excision and measurement, (iv) alignment with the tissue grips, (v) temperature, (vi) storage and bathing medium, and (vii) precise location/anatomy of tissue tested [67–70]. Any method used to determine the mechanical property of soft tissues will have to simulate the native environment during testing. It is likely that the contribution of the corneo-scleral portion of the meshwork is greater with the tensile testing than that of JCT. Although, why the values reported for the TM are significantly larger than values reported for scleral biomechanics are unclear. A major factor with tensile measurements is the clamping force applied to hold the tissue. In the case of the TM measurements, it is unclear what these were or how they affect the moduli values reported. Also, tensile testing informs us of the bulk properties of tissue and do not account for the individual contribution of cells versus matrix components or the contribution from segmental regions.

Other methods have also been used to estimate the modulus of the TM, notably by combining optical coherence tomography (OCT) images and engineering models. Johnson et al. [71] estimated the elastic modulus of the TM to be 128 kPa using an analytical model of beam-bending under uniform load for a linearly elastic material with simplified geometry and based on changes in TM and SC thickness. Subsequently, using a nearly incompressible neo-Hookean solid model, Pant et al. [72] estimate the elastic modulus for TM as 5.75 kPa by inverse finite element modeling (FEM). In these above methods, the influence of TM compressibility was not taken into account, although the values estimated by Pant et al. [72] are closer to those reported using AFM by Last [56], Vranka [53], Raghunathan [57] and Wang et al. [59]. Values obtained from FEM and AFM must be compared only with caution since the methods in which the load is applied are quite different (tension in OCT imaging, vs compression in AFM). Interestingly, using inverse FEM, Wang et al. [59] estimated normal TM modulus at 70 ± 20 kPa and glaucomatous TM modulus at 97 ± 19 kPa which is approximately 10–15 times greater than that estimated by Pant et al. [72]. A major difference between these two studies are in how the images were collected, analyzed, and thus used to create the mesh required for FEM. Further, a major factor contributing to the discrepancy in the values in these two studies is how the areas and thickness of Schlemm's canal were factored.

Non-human Primate

The structure of the eye's aqueous humor outflow system and its influence on IOP have been studied in humans and animals for many years and continue to be investigated. Of the available animal models, experimental glaucoma (ExGl) in the non-human primate (NHP), induced by subtotal laser photocoagulation of the trabecular meshwork (TM), is considered the most predictive for drug efficacy in the human [73]. Morphological and hydrodynamic data in this model suggest that fibrosis of the TM and adjacent inner wall of Schlemm's canal (SC) reduces the area for conventional aqueous outflow, leading to decreased outflow facility, and elevated IOP [74–78]. Furthermore, the classic arcuate mid-peripheral visual field losses observed in human patients with primary open angle glaucoma (POAG) and elevated IOP have also been observed in visual field testing of NHPs with ExGl [79]. Additional evidence suggests that aqueous humor flow in eyes with ExGl is largely diverted to the small unlasered area of TM, suggesting a capacity for this tissue to dynamically compensate both structurally and functionally, accommodating the increased flow [76]. However, very little is known about the mechanical properties of the NHP TM and if there is any relevance to glaucoma. To the best of our knowledge, there is only one study [80] that reports the elastic modulus in NHPs; mean elastic modulus as determined by AFM was 3.3 ± 0.32 kPa for control animals, while the unlasered regions of TM in ExGl NHPs were approximately 300 Pa (0.30 kPa). This data suggested dynamic compensation for chronic IOP elevation in ExGl and that a softer TM promotes increased outflow, provided by the capacity for unlasered primate TM cells in normal primate eyes to compensate for increased IOP and reduced overall outflow from the eye by altering the composition and subsequent mechanical properties of the matrix in the JCT region. However, a principal limitation of that investigation is the lack of knowledge as to the mechanism of action or class of the topical agents previously administered to these NHPs, as well as the need for sporadic to frequent treatment to manage excessively high IOP in eyes with ExGl.

Mice

Mice are extensively used to study pathophysiology of the TM due to their ease of genetic manipulation, ability to administer treatments, and similarity of the conventional outflow pathway with humans. However mechanical characterization of rodent TM, although much sought after, has been quite challenging to perform, and as such only a couple of studies have reported the elastic modulus of the mouse TM using various methods. The first report was by Li et al. [81] combining spectral domain OCT images and mathematical modeling. They made the following assumptions for these measurements: that a decrease in Schlemm's canal lumen was by TM deformation, that there was change in the width of SC, that pressure inside SC lumen was independent of IOP, and that TM was linearly elastic. The elastic modulus was reported as 2.16 kPa in control eyes and 3.46 or 5.01 kPa in BMP2 overexpressing eyes (as a model for ocular hypertension) after 7 or 10 days respectively. It is important to note that the parameters used for mathematical modeling were identical for all mice across the groups, and thus differences in anatomical and pressure parameters between animals or regional variations were not considered.

More recently, Wang et al. [82] measured TM modulus in 10–20 μm thick sagittal cryosections after whole globe perfusions. They compared two freezing techniques one with a cryoprotectant (15% glycerol) and one without. In this initial study, the authors found no correlation between outflow facility and TM modulus in 5 eyes (C57BL/6J) whose TM were frozen with a cryoprotectant or in 11 eyes (CBA/J) whose TM were frozen without cryoprotectant. The elastic modulus of the TM in cryosections obtained with cryoprotectant was 3.22 ± 1.84 kPa while those without cryoprotectant was 3.84 ± 3.37 kPa. Segmental flow observations were not taken into account in this study. In a follow up study, Wang et al. [83] report that TM modulus from 18 C57BL/6J mice was 2.20 ± 1.12 kPa vs 3.08 ± 3.55 kPa in 10 CBA/J mice. Further, they demonstrated that TM modulus was 2.38 ± 1.31 kPa in mice treated with dexamethasone for 14 days vs 1.99 ± 0.91 kPa in vehicle control mice. For the first time, this study report a small but significant correlation between TM modulus and outflow resistance but not IOP with dexamethasone treatment using two strains (C57BL/6J and CBA/J) of mice. This is especially important considering mechanical properties were first suggested to impact the resistance to aqueous outflow. Although rehydrated frozen sections have been used for AFM but non-ocular investigators, this is not without limitation. Whether such freeze-thaw cycles alters GAG content that contribute to tissue compression resistance were not reported or discussed.

Rabbit

Using AFM, we reported that the elastic modulus of the TM (JCT side) in adult New Zealand white rabbits as 1.03 ± 0.55 kPa and that its modulus was elevated threefold to 3.89 ± 2.55 kPa with 3 weeks of 0.1% (w/v) topical dexamethasone treatment in vivo. In our study irrespective of any measured change in IOP, a change in the mechanical property of the TM was observed. Long-term consequences of steroid administration on IOP changes or TM biomechanics in rabbits were not determined, although steroid induced IOP elevation in humans and mice have been reported [84, 85].

Rat

Huang et al. [86] report a method of estimating the elastic modulus of the TM in rat eyes. This involved perfusion of the eyes with Evans blue (a non-specific tracer to the TM), flat mounting the anterior segments, subsequently measuring indentation on the uveal side of the TM by AFM to estimate elastic modulus, and finally using the indentation values with a mathematical model for non-Hookean materials to verify the moduli measurements. The geometric mean elastic modulus of the TM was reported as 162 ± 1.2 Pa.

Porcine

Elastic modulus of the porcine TM has been evaluated both by AFM and tensile testing. Camras et al. [60, 62] reported the tensile elastic modulus of porcine TM as 2.49 MPa, while Yuan et al. [87] reported the indentation modulus by AFM as 1.38 kPa.

Considerations While Interpreting AFM Moduli Measurements

Sample preparation: Preparation of biological samples is crucial in biomechanical characterization. One of the major advantages of using AFM is that the tissue needn't be fixed or dehydrated and can be characterized in a biomimetic environment without the need for fixation or dehydration. The most common method to immobilize biological samples is by using cyanoacrylate or fibrin based glues that can potentially introduce artifacts [88, 89]. For very small samples, Cell-Tak or poly-L-lysine may be used. While minimizing the amount glue to minimize errors or discarding artifactual data are feasible, it is preferred that sample preparation is objective and controlled. This problem is increasingly being recognized and glue-free methods are being developed [58, 90]. Similarly, avoiding freeze-thaw of tissues to prevent alterations in tissue composition should be preferred.

Anatomical location: This is undoubtedly an important consideration while performing AFM on TM. The TM is defined by 3 major regions: uveo-scleral meshwork, corneo-scleral meshwork, JCT and cribiform plexus. Thus whether measurements are performed on the JCT side or the uveal-/corneo-scleral side is critical. Further, how the cells differ in each region and what their contribution to mechanics is poorly defined. Depending on the region of the TM, cells may either form sheets covering ECM structures or they may be scattered throughout the ECM forming occasional gap and adherens junctions. Elastic fibers in the TM have a circumferential alignment, yet the JCT is loosely organized with large open spaces.

Segmental flow regions of the TM also ought to be considered while performing experiments.

Hydration medium: Tissues are hydrated in vivo and thus have to be adequately and appropriately hydrated while performing AFM. Physiological buffer like phosphate buffered saline or Hank's balanced salt solution with divalent salts (Ca^{2+}/ Mg^{2+}) will minimize electrostatic interactions and osmotic pressure, and prevent potential swelling artifacts.

Cantilever considerations: Since AFM is dependent on deflection of a cantilever; the choice of appropriate cantilever stiffness (spring constant) should be matched with the sample stiffness. i.e. if a stiff cantilever is used to measure a sample softer by orders of magnitude, large deformations would not lead to detectable cantilever deflection. At the same time, the spring constant cannot be too small such that drag force due to motion through the buffer generates appreciable deflection. Further, the osmolarity and viscosity of the medium being used to perform the measurements are important to consider as they can influence cantilever deflection. In addition, prior to every experiment, it is important to calibrate the spring constant and optical sensitivity of the cantilever. For all samples, optimal parameters for approach velocity and indentation depth have to be kept consistent. When using elastic approximations for viscoelastic tissues, approach velocity of the cantilever must be carefully controlled.

Indenter shape and depth: This is a critical factor while obtaining force versus indentation curves for AFM analysis. The models used to fit force versus indentation curves are geometry specific: rigid cone, sphere, or flat cylinder [91, 92]. If cantilevers are modified with a sphere, the diameter of the sphere factors heavily in indentation depth and subsequent analysis of elastic modulus [93–96]. For thin samples such as tissues or cell derived matrices, it is essential to consider the influence of the underlying substrate, which is typically far stiffer. To mitigate substrate effects the general rule is to limit the indentation depth to approximately 10% of the total sample thickness [97, 98]. Further, due to the viscoelastic nature of biological tissues, the velocity of indentation is critical while performing measurements.

A Brief Glimpse on the Cellular Consequences or Mechanobiology of the Trabecular Meshwork

Besides using genetic or ocular hypertension models by steroid administration, most of our understanding of TM biology including the study of cell signaling pathways come from traditional cell culture of primary human TM cells isolated from whole eye globes or corneo-scleral rims on rigid non-physiological polystyrene/ tissue culture plastic (TCP) or glass bottom dishes. These surfaces have elastic moduli of the order of >1 GPa which is several orders of magnitude greater than what TM cells sense in the native environment, are generally topographically flat compared to a topographic rich ECM in vivo, chemically devoid of functional heterogeneity unlike the TM tissue. An overwhelmingly large body of literature document the biology of cells are vastly different when presented with relevant substratum biophysical properties (stiffness, topography, chemical and physical heterogeneity, porosity) in vitro [99, 100]. It is thus evident that TCP dishes do not provide the necessary cues that may be essential to dictate cell fate.

Considering just one factor, substrate rigidity, a number of studies have demonstrated that TM cells respond differentially in the presence or absence of a number of soluble factors when cultured on hydrogels of biomimetic elastic modulus. For example, Schlunck et al. [101] demonstrated that cell spreading and focal adhesion size, FAK activation, serum-induced ERK phosphorylation, expression and recruitment of αSMA to stress fibers and all increased with substrate rigidity. They further demonstrated that the morphology of fibronectin deposits differed on the various matrices. Interestingly, elevated amounts of myociling and αB-crystallin were observed on softer gels. Subsequently, Han et al. [102] further showed that with increasing substratum rigidity and TGFβstimulus, protein expression (collagen VI, αSMA, fibronectin etc) similar to that reported in primary open-angle glaucoma was observed and partially mediated via non-Smad signaling (ERK, AKT, or PI3K). We previously showed that an increase in substrate stiffness increases secreted frizzled related protein 1 (SFRP1, a potent antagonist of the Wnt pathway [103]) expression level in HTM cells [104]. SFRP increases with senescence, with steroid treatment in HTM cells, and can actually increase senescence in these cells [105]. Using glass/plastic surfaces increases in TM cell stiffness have been observed with dexamethasone treatment, Wnt inhibition (both canonical and non-canonical), or with replicative senescence [106–108]. The modulatory effects of Wnt signaling in cells cultured on substrates of varying rigidity are yet to be evaluated.

In other studies, Wood et al. [109], Thomasy et al. [110, 111] demonstrate that substratum rigidity modulates TM cell response to actin disruption (by Latrunculin-B) partially via mechanotransducers YAP and YAZ. Cells on softer substrates demonstrated lower cell proliferation and attachment. Further data from these studies demonstrated that TM cells cultured on hydrogels of normal or glaucomatous tissue stiffness responded differently to Latrunculin-B treatment in comparison with when cultured on TCP; notably decreases in ECM protein expression, and lower cellular responses to mechanotransducers when treated with Lat-B were observed on softer gels. McKee et al. [112] demonstrated that primary HTM cells adhered to stiffer substrates were significantly more responsive to Lat-B suggesting that the effects of Lat-B treatment would be most pronounced in glaucomatous eyes with a stiffer HTM. They also show a rebound effect on HTM cell stiffness as the actin cytoskeleton was reforming after the Lat-B treatment. Considering a number of cytoskeletal modulators are in clinical trial for IOP reduction, there is a possibility that a number of drugs may be inadvertently considered ineffective because pre-clinical tests were performed on irrelevant substrates.

Other biomechanical stimuli such as stretch (due to anisotropy of the ECM, or dynamic strain due to pulsatile motion) also have profound effects on TM cell behaviors. Static stretch, due to anisotropy of or underlying substrates, was sufficient to increase myocilin and versican expression in TM cells in a size dependent manner [113]. Non-topographic static stretch was shown to elevate aquaporin-1 levels and inversely correlated with lactate dehydrogenase release suggesting a possible role in cytoprotection [114]. From non-ocular systems it is evident that both cyclic and static strain modulate mechanosensors (integrins and focal adhesion complexes) differentially to effect a plethora a signaling cascades downstream. Similarly, in the context of TM cell culture in vitro, dynamic stretch elicited by cyclic strain has been shown to affect a myriad of cellular function and gene/protein expression. Again, not all genes/proteins are modulated in a similar or expected manner. Cyclic stain, on the other hand, has been shown to alter the actin cytoskeleton, transiently decrease αB-crystallin, significantly increase both secretion and transcription of IL-6, elevated production of metalloproteinase-2 (MMP-2), MMP-14 and tissue inhibitor of metalloproteinase-1 (TIMP-1) but not MMP9 or TIMP-2, increased extracellular secretion of ATP and adenosine, increased phosphorylation of protein kinase B, elevated expression of vertebrate lonesome kinase, secretion of autotaxin, and modulate mTOR signaling/autophagy to name a few [115–126]. Such phenomena are not unique to the TM and are prevalent in almost every tissue/disease model. Whether substratum stiffness plays a role in stretch mediated cellular outcomes remains to be seen. Despite all these, studies are continued to be performed on 2D surfaces with artificial chemistry. In an attempt to move towards a biomimetic approach, our lab and others have begun to move towards the use of 3D scaffolds or cell derived matrices to evaluate TM behavior [57, 108, 127–129]. Such models have been used to both evaluate the effects of drugs [129] or to simply demonstrate that pathologic matrices are capable to driving healthy cells towards a glaucomatous phenotype [57].

Summary

The overview presented here is by no means exhaustive, but is meant to demonstrate the complexities and differences in quantifying TM mechanics and how it influences their biology. Changes in mechanics by themselves are insufficient to understand the fundamental question: what drives outflow resistance and how this regulates subsequent elevated intraocular pressure? It would appear from the existing knowledge that a better means to integrate the biomechanics with the cell biology concurrent with sophisticated tools to dissect the signal transduction pathways as it pertains to cytoskeleton/ECM/tissue remodeling would be ideal. Recent advances in multi-photon microscopy and second harmonic imaging capabilities are capable of providing high resolution spatial distribution of cellular and extracellular structures and proteins. Particularly, they are useful to resolve the associations between tissue architecture, cells and ECM proteins [130–132]. In addition to static imaging, dynamic motion of the TM has recently been imaged by phase-sensitive optical coherence tomography [55] allowing for live visualization of TM in vivo. When all the data from various techniques are integrated, they can then be used for predictive mathematical modeling in silico. Computational modeling of TM behavior will provide valuable information to predict the effects of drugs that alter aqueous humor drainage and regulation of IOP restricting the number of animal studies that may be required for drug development.

References

1. Seddon JM. Genetic and environmental underpinnings to age-related ocular diseases. Invest Ophthalmol Vis Sci. 2013;54:ORSF28–30. https://doi.org/10.1167/iovs.13-13234.
2. Chew EY. Nutrition effects on ocular diseases in the aging eye. Invest Ophthalmol Vis Sci. 2013;54:ORSF42–7. https://doi.org/10.1167/iovs13-12914.
3. Quigley HA. Open-angle glaucoma. N Engl J Med. 1993;328:1097–106. https://doi.org/10.1056/NEJM199304153281507.
4. Johnson M. What controls aqueous humour outflow resistance? Exp Eye Res. 2006;82:545–57. https://doi.org/10.1016/j.exer.2005.10.011.
5. Gottanka J, Johnson DH, Martus P, Lutjen-Drecoll E. Severity of optic nerve damage in eyes with POAG is correlated with changes in the trabecular meshwork. J Glaucoma. 1997;6:123–32.
6. Lutjen-Drecoll E. Morphological changes in glaucomatous eyes and the role of TGFbeta2 for the pathogenesis of the disease. Exp Eye Res. 2005;81:1–4. https://doi.org/10.1016/j.exer.2005.02.008.
7. Rohen JW, Lutjen-Drecoll E, Flugel C, Meyer M, Grierson I. Ultrastructure of the trabecular meshwork in untreated cases of primary open-angle glaucoma (POAG). Exp Eye Res. 1993;56:683–92.
8. Quigley HA, Broman AT. The number of people with glaucoma worldwide in 2010 and 2020. Br J Ophthalmol. 2006;90:262–7. https://doi.org/10.1136/bjo.2005.081224.
9. Klein R, Klein BE. The prevalence of age-related eye diseases and visual impairment in aging: current estimates. Invest Ophthalmol Vis Sci. 2013;54:ORSF5–ORSF13. https://doi.org/10.1167/iovs.13-12789.
10. Alvarado J, Murphy C, Polansky J, Juster R. Age-related changes in trabecular meshwork cellularity. Invest Ophthalmol Vis Sci. 1981;21:714–27.
11. Alvarado J. Presence of matrix vesicles in the trabecular meshwork of glaucomatous eyes. Graefes Arch Clin Exp Ophthalmol. 1982;218:171–6.
12. Alvarado J, Murphy C, Juster R. Trabecular meshwork cellularity in primary open-angle glaucoma and nonglaucomatous normals. Ophthalmology. 1984;91:564–79. https://doi.org/10.1016/S0161-6420(84)34248-8.
13. Miyazaki M, Segawa K, Urakawa Y. Age-related changes in the trabecular meshwork of the normal human eye. Jpn J Ophthalmol. 1987;31:558–69.
14. McMenamin PG, Lee WR, Aitken DA. Age-related changes in the human outflow apparatus. Ophthalmology. 1986;93:194–209.
15. Lütjen-Drecoll E, Rohen JW. Morphology of aqueous outflow pathways in normal and glaucomatous eyes. In: Ritch R, Shields MB, Krupin T, editors. The glaucomas. St. Louis: Mosby; 1996. p. 89–123.
16. Tripathi RC. Pathologic anatomy of the outflow pathway of aqueous humour in chronic simple glaucoma. Exp Eye Res. 1977;25:403–7. https://doi.org/10.1016/S0014-4835(77)80035-3.
17. Tripathi RC, Tripathi BJ. Contractile protein alteration in trabecular endothelium in primary open-angle glaucoma. Exp Eye Res. 1980;31:721–4. https://doi.org/10.1016/S0014-4835(80)80056-X.
18. Tamm ER. The trabecular meshwork outflow pathways: structural and functional aspects. Exp Eye Res. 2009;88:648–55. https://doi.org/10.1016/j.exer.2009.02.007.
19. Lütjen-Drecoll E. Functional morphology of the trabecular meshwork in primate eyes. Prog Retina Eye Res. 1999;18:91–119. https://doi.org/10.1016/S1350-9462(98)00011-1.

20. Lütjen-Drecoll E, Schenholm M, Tamm E, Tengblad A. Visualization of hyaluronic acid in the anterior segment of rabbit and monkey eyes. Exp Eye Res. 1990;51:55–63. https://doi.org/10.1016/0014-4835(90)90170-Y.
21. Lütjen-Drecoll E, Tektas OY. In: Dartt DA, editor. Encyclopedia of the eye. New York: Academic Press; 2010. p. 224–8.
22. Tektas O-Y, Lütjen-Drecoll E. Structural changes of the trabecular meshwork in different kinds of glaucoma. Exp Eye Res. 2009;88:769–75. https://doi.org/10.1016/j.exer.2008.11.025.
23. Toris CB, Yablonski ME, Wang Y-L, Camras CB. Aqueous humor dynamics in the aging human eye. Am J Ophthalmol. 1999;127:407–12.
24. Toris CB, Koepsell SA, Yablonski ME, Camras CB. Aqueous humor dynamics in ocular hypertensive patients. J Glaucoma. 2002;11:253–8.
25. Johnson M, Shapiro A, Ethier CR, Kamm RD. Modulation of outflow resistance by the pores of the inner wall endothelium. Invest Ophthalmol Vis Sci. 1992;33:1670–5.
26. Janmey PA, McCulloch CA. Cell mechanics: integrating cell responses to mechanical stimuli. Annu Rev Biomed Eng. 2007;9:1–34. https://doi.org/10.1146/annurev.bioeng.9.060906.151927.
27. Mendez MG, Janmey PA. Transcription factor regulation by mechanical stress. Int J Biochem Cell Biol. 2012;44:728–32. https://doi.org/10.1016/j.biocel.2012.02.003.
28. Discher DE, Janmey P, Wang YL. Tissue cells feel and respond to the stiffness of their substrate. Science. 2005;310:1139–43. https://doi.org/10.1126/science.1116995.
29. Janmey PA, Wells RG, Assoian RK, McCulloch CA. From tissue mechanics to transcription factors. Differentiation. 2013;86:112–20. https://doi.org/10.1016/j.diff.2013.07.004.
30. Engler A, et al. Substrate compliance versus ligand density in cell on gel responses. Biophys J. 2004;86:617–28. https://doi.org/10.1016/S0006-3495(04)74140-5.
31. Engler AJ, Rehfeldt F, Sen S, Discher DE. In: Yu-Li W, Dennis ED, editors. Methods in cell biology, vol. 83. New York: Academic Press; 2007. p. 521–45.
32. Engler AJ, Sen S, Sweeney HL, Discher DE. Matrix elasticity directs stem cell lineage specification. Cell. 2006;126:677–89. https://doi.org/10.1016/j.cell.2006.06.044.
33. Califano JP, Reinhart-King CA. The effects of substrate elasticity on endothelial cell network formation and traction force generation. Conf Proc IEEE Eng Med Biol Soc. 2009;2009:3343–5. https://doi.org/10.1109/iembs.2009.5333194.
34. Califano JP, Reinhart-King CA. Substrate stiffness and cell area predict cellular traction stresses in single cells and cells in contact. Cell Mol Bioeng. 2010;3:68–75. https://doi.org/10.1007/s12195-010-0102-6.
35. Casey MK-R, Shawn PC, Joseph PC, Brooke NS, Cynthia AR-K. The role of the cytoskeleton in cellular force generation in 2D and 3D environments. Phys Biol. 2011;8:015009.
36. Kraning-Rush CM, Carey SP, Califano JP, Reinhart-King CA. Quantifying traction stresses in adherent cells. Methods Cell Biol. 2012;110:139–78. https://doi.org/10.1016/b978-0-12-388403-9.00006-0.
37. Lepple-Wienhues A, Stahl F, Wiederholt M. Differential smooth muscle-like contractile properties of trabecular meshwork and ciliary muscle. Exp Eye Res. 1991;53:33–8. https://doi.org/10.1016/0014-4835(91)90141-Z.
38. Wiederholt M, Lepple-Wienhues A, Stahl E. Electrical properties and contractility of the trabecular meshwork. Exp Eye Res. 1992;55(Suppl 1):41. https://doi.org/10.1016/0014-4835(92)90345-S.
39. Fuchshofer R, Tamm ER. In: Dartt DA, editor. Encyclopedia of the eye. New York: Academic Press; 2010. p. 28–36.
40. Tamm ER, Braunger BM, Fuchshofer R. In: Hejtmancik JF, John MN, editors. Progress in molecular biology and translational science, vol. 134. New York: Academic Press; 2015. p. 301–14.
41. Braunger BM, Fuchshofer R, Tamm ER. The aqueous humor outflow pathways in glaucoma: a unifying concept of disease mechanisms and causative treatment. Eur J Pharm Biopharm. 2015;95:173–81. https://doi.org/10.1016/j.ejpb.2015.04.029.

42. Rao PV, Deng P, Sasaki Y, Epstein DL. Regulation of myosin light chain phosphorylation in the trabecular meshwork: role in aqueous humour outflow facility. Exp Eye Res. 2005;80:197–206. https://doi.org/10.1016/j.exer.2004.08.029.
43. Pattabiraman PP, Rao PV. Mechanistic basis of Rho GTPase-induced extracellular matrix synthesis in trabecular meshwork cells. Am J Physiol Cell Physiol. 2010;298:C749–63. https://doi.org/10.1152/ajpcell.00317.2009.
44. Ren R, et al. Netarsudil increases outflow facility in human eyes through multiple mechanisms. Invest Ophthalmol Vis Sci. 2016;57:6197–209. https://doi.org/10.1167/iovs.16-20189.
45. Overby DR, Stamer WD, Johnson M. The changing paradigm of outflow resistance generation: towards synergistic models of the JCT and inner wall endothelium. Exp Eye Res. 2009;88:656–70. https://doi.org/10.1016/j.exer.2008.11.033.
46. McDonnell F, Dismuke WM, Overby DR, Stamer WD. Pharmacological regulation of outflow resistance distal to Schlemm's Canal. Am J Physiol Cell Physiol. 2018; https://doi.org/10.1152/ajpcell.00024.2018.
47. Carreon TA, Edwards G, Wang H, Bhattacharya SK. Segmental outflow of aqueous humor in mouse and human. Exp Eye Res. 2017;158:59–66. https://doi.org/10.1016/j.exer.2016.08.001.
48. Cha EDK, Xu J, Gong L, Gong H. Variations in active outflow along the trabecular outflow pathway. Exp Eye Res. 2016;146:354–60. https://doi.org/10.1016/j.exer.2016.01.008.
49. de Kater AW, Melamed S, Epstein DL. Patterns of aqueous humor outflow in glaucomatous and nonglaucomatous human eyes. A tracer study using cationized ferritin. Arch Ophthalmol. 1989;107:572–6.
50. Hann CR, Bahler CK, Johnson DH. Cationic ferritin and segmental flow through the trabecular meshwork. Invest Ophthalmol Vis Sci. 2005;46:1–7. https://doi.org/10.1167/iovs.04-0800.
51. Swaminathan SS, Oh D-J, Kang MH, Rhee DJ. Aqueous outflow: segmental and distal flow. J Cataract Refract Surg. 2014;40:1263–72. https://doi.org/10.1016/j.jcrs.2014.06.020.
52. Vranka JA, Acott TS. Pressure-induced expression changes in segmental flow regions of the human trabecular meshwork. Exp Eye Res. 2016; https://doi.org/10.1016/j.exer.2016.06.009.
53. Vranka JA, et al. Biomechanical rigidity and quantitative proteomics analysis of segmental regions of the trabecular meshwork at physiologic and elevated pressures. Invest Ophthalmol Vis Sci. 2018;59:246–59. https://doi.org/10.1167/iovs.17-22759.
54. Johnstone MA. The aqueous outflow system as a mechanical pump - evidence from examination of tissue and aqueous movement in human and non-human primates. J Glaucoma. 2004;13:421–38. https://doi.org/10.1097/01.ijg.0000131757.63542.24.
55. Li P, Shen TT, Johnstone M, Wang RK. Pulsatile motion of the trabecular meshwork in healthy human subjects quantified by phase-sensitive optical coherence tomography. Biomed Opt Express. 2013;4:2051–65. https://doi.org/10.1364/boe.4.002051.
56. Last JA, et al. Elastic modulus determination of normal and glaucomatous human trabecular meshwork. Invest Ophthalmol Vis Sci. 2011;52:2147–52. https://doi.org/10.1167/iovs.10-6342.
57. Raghunathan VK, et al. Glaucomatous cell derived matrices differentially modulate nonglaucomatous trabecular meshwork cellular behavior. Acta Biomater. 2018;71:444–59. https://doi.org/10.1016/j.actbio.2018.02.037.
58. Morgan JT, Raghunathan VK, Thomasy SM, Murphy CJ, Russell P. Robust and artifact-free mounting of tissue samples for atomic force microscopy. BioTechniques. 2014;56:40–2. https://doi.org/10.2144/000114126.
59. Wang K, et al. Estimating human trabecular meshwork stiffness by numerical modeling and advanced OCT imaging. Invest Ophthalmol Vis Sci. 2017;58:4809–17. https://doi.org/10.1167/iovs.17-22175.
60. Camras LJ, Stamer WD, Epstein D, Gonzalez P, Yuan F. Differential effects of trabecular meshwork stiffness on outflow facility in normal human and porcine eyes. Invest Ophthalmol Vis Sci. 2012;53:5242–50. https://doi.org/10.1167/iovs.12-9825.
61. Camras LJ, Stamer WD, Epstein D, Gonzalez P, Yuan F. Circumferential tensile stiffness of glaucomatous trabecular meshwork. Invest Ophthalmol Vis Sci. 2014;55:814–23. https://doi.org/10.1167/iovs.13-13091.

62. Camras LJ, Stamer WD, Epstein D, Gonzalez P, Yuan F. Erratum. Invest Ophthalmol Vis Sci. 2014;55:2316. https://doi.org/10.1167/iovs.12-9825a.
63. Chang JY, Folz SJ, Laryea SN, Overby DR. Multi-scale analysis of segmental outflow patterns in human trabecular meshwork with changing intraocular pressure. J Ocul Pharmacol Ther. 2014;30:213–23. https://doi.org/10.1089/jop.2013.0182.
64. Keller KE, Bradley JM, Vranka JA, Acott TS. Segmental versican expression in the trabecular meshwork and involvement in outflow facility. Invest Ophthalmol Vis Sci. 2011;52:5049–57. https://doi.org/10.1167/iovs.10-6948.
65. Overby DR. The role of segmental outflow in the trabecular meshwork. ARVO SIG, e-SIG # 1221, 2010.
66. Stamer WD, Acott TS. Current understanding of conventional outflow dysfunction in glaucoma. Curr Opin Ophthalmol. 2012;23:135–43. https://doi.org/10.1097/ICU. 0b013e32834ff23e.
67. Hatami-Marbini H, Etebu E. Hydration dependent biomechanical properties of the corneal stroma. Exp Eye Res. 2013;116:47–54. https://doi.org/10.1016/j.exer.2013.07.016.
68. Hatami-Marbini H, Rahimi A. Effects of bathing solution on tensile properties of the cornea. Exp Eye Res. 2014; https://doi.org/10.1016/j.exer.2013.11.017.
69. Hatami-Marbini H, Rahimi A. Evaluation of hydration effects on tensile properties of bovine corneas. J Cataract Refract Surg. 2015;41:644–51. https://doi.org/10.1016/j.jcrs.2014.07.029.
70. Hatami-Marbini H, Rahimi A. The relation between hydration and mechanical behavior of bovine cornea in tension. J Mech Behav Biomed Mater. 2014;36:90–7. https://doi.org/10.1016/j.jmbbm.2014.03.011.
71. Johnson M, Schuman JS, Kagemann L. Trabecular meshwork stiffness in the living human eye. Invest Ophthalmol Vis Sci. 2015;56:3541.
72. Pant AD, Kagemann L, Schuman JS, Sigal IA, Amini R. An imaged-based inverse finite element method to determine in-vivo mechanical properties of the human trabecular meshwork. J Model Ophthalmol. 2017;1:100–11.
73. Stewart WC, Magrath GN, Demos CM, Nelson LA, Stewart JA. Predictive value of the efficacy of glaucoma medications in animal models: preclinical to regulatory studies. Br J Ophthalmol. 2011;95:1355–60. https://doi.org/10.1136/bjo.2010.188508.
74. Johnstone MA, Grant WM. Pressure-dependent changes in structures of the aqueous outflow system of human and monkey eyes. Am J Ophthalmol. 1973;75:365–83.
75. Zhang Y, Toris CB, Liu Y, Ye W, Gong H. Morphological and hydrodynamic correlates in monkey eyes with laser induced glaucoma. Exp Eye Res. 2009;89:748–56. https://doi.org/10.1016/j.exer.2009.06.015.
76. Melamed S, Epstein DL. Alterations of aqueous humour outflow following argon laser trabeculoplasty in monkeys. Br J Ophthalmol. 1987;71:776–81.
77. Melamed S, Pei J, Epstein DL. Delayed response to argon laser trabeculoplasty in monkeys. Morphological and morphometric analysis. Arch Ophthalmol. 1986;104:1078–83.
78. Koss MC, March WF, Nordquist RE, Gherezghiher T. Acute intraocular pressure elevation produced by argon laser trabeculoplasty in the cynomolgus monkey. Arch Ophthalmol. 1984;102:1699–703.
79. Harwerth RS, et al. Visual field defects and neural losses from experimental glaucoma. Prog Retin Eye Res. 2002;21:91–125.
80. Raghunathan V, et al. Biomechanical, ultrastructural, and electrophysiological characterization of the non-human primate experimental glaucoma model. Sci Rep. 2017;7:14329. https://doi.org/10.1038/s41598-017-14720-2.
81. Li G, et al. Disease progression in iridocorneal angle tissues of BMP2-induced ocular hypertensive mice with optical coherence tomography. Mol Vis. 2014;20:1695–709.
82. Wang K, Read AT, Sulchek T, Ethier CR. Trabecular meshwork stiffness in glaucoma. Exp Eye Res. 2017;158:3–12. https://doi.org/10.1016/j.exer.2016.07.011.
83. Wang K, et al. The relationship between outflow resistance and trabecular meshwork stiffness in mice. Sci Rep. 2018;8:5848. https://doi.org/10.1038/s41598-018-24165-w.

84. Whitlock NA, McKnight B, Corcoran KN, Rodriguez LA, Rice DS. Increased intraocular pressure in mice treated with dexamethasone. Invest Ophthalmol Vis Sci. 2010;51:6496–503. https://doi.org/10.1167/iovs.10-5430.
85. Weinreb RN, Polansky JR, Kramer SG, Baxter JD. Acute effects of dexamethasone on intraocular pressure in glaucoma. Invest Ophthalmol Vis Sci. 1985;26:170–5.
86. Huang J, Camras LJ, Yuan F. Mechanical analysis of rat trabecular meshwork. Soft Matter. 2015; https://doi.org/10.1039/c4sm01949k.
87. Yuan F, Camras LJ, Gonzalez P. Trabecular meshwork stiffness in ex vivo perfused porcine eyes. Invest Ophthalmol Vis Sci. 2011;52:6693.
88. Ebenstein DM, Pruitt LA. Nanoindentation of biological materials. Nano Tod. 2006;1:26–33. https://doi.org/10.1016/S1748-0132(06)70077-9.
89. Oyen ML. Nanoindentation of biological and biomimetic materials. Exp Tech. 2013;37:73–87. https://doi.org/10.1111/j.1747-1567.2011.00716.x.
90. Dias JM, Ziebarth NM. Anterior and posterior corneal stroma elasticity assessed using nanoindentation. Exp Eye Res. 2013;115:41–6. https://doi.org/10.1016/j.exer.2013.06.004.
91. Harding J, Sneddon I. The elastic stresses produced by the indentation of the plane surface of a semi-infinite elastic solid by a rigid punch. Cambridge: Cambridge University Press; 2008. p. 16–26.
92. Love AEH. Boussingesq's problem for a rigid cone. Q J Math. 1939;10:161–75.
93. Cheng L, Xia X, Scriven LE, Gerberich WW. Spherical-tip indentation of viscoelastic material. Mech Mater. 2005;37:213–26. https://doi.org/10.1016/j.mechmat.2004.03.002.
94. Cheng Y-T, Cheng C-M. Relationships between initial unloading slope, contact depth, and mechanical properties for spherical indentation in linear viscoelastic solids. Mater Sci Eng A. 2005;409:93–9. https://doi.org/10.1016/j.msea.2005.05.118.
95. Rodriguez ML, McGarry PJ, Sniadecki NJ. Review on cell mechanics: experimental and modeling approaches. Appl Mech Rev. 2013;65:060801. https://doi.org/10.1115/1.4025355.
96. Rodríguez R, Gutierrez I. Correlation between nanoindentation and tensile properties: influence of the indentation size effect. Mater Sci Eng A. 2003;361:377–84. https://doi.org/10.1016/S0921-5093(03)00563-X.
97. Oliver WC, Pharr GM. Improved technique for determining hardness and elastic modulus using load and displacement sensing indentation experiments. J Mater Res. 1992;7:1564–83.
98. Pharr G, Oliver W, Brotzen F. On the generality of the relationship among contact stiffness, contact area, and elastic modulus during indentation. J Mater Res. 1992;7:613–7.
99. Gasiorowski JZ, Murphy CJ, Nealey PF. Biophysical cues and cell behavior: the big impact of little things. Annu Rev Biomed Eng. 2013;15:155–76. https://doi.org/10.1146/annurev-bioeng-071811-150021.
100. Gasiorowski JZ, Russell P. Biological properties of trabecular meshwork cells. Exp Eye Res. 2009;88:671–5. https://doi.org/10.1016/j.exer.2008.08.006.
101. Schlunck G, et al. Substrate rigidity modulates cell–matrix interactions and protein expression in human trabecular meshwork cells. Invest Ophthalmol Vis Sci. 2008;49:262–9. https://doi.org/10.1167/iovs.07-0956.
102. Han H, Wecker T, Grehn F, Schlunck G. Elasticity-dependent modulation of TGF-β responses in human trabecular meshwork cells. Invest Ophthalmol Vis Sci. 2011;52:2889–96.
103. Morgan JT, Murphy CJ, Russell P. What do mechanotransduction, Hippo, Wnt, and TGFbeta have in common? YAP and TAZ as key orchestrating molecules in ocular health and disease. Exp Eye Res. 2013;115:1–12. https://doi.org/10.1016/j.exer.2013.06.012.
104. Raghunathan VK, et al. Role of substratum stiffness in modulating genes associated with extracellular matrix and mechanotransducers YAP and TAZ. Invest Ophthalmol Vis Sci. 2012;54:378–86.
105. Babizhayev MA, Yegorov YE. Senescent phenotype of trabecular meshwork cells displays biomarkers in primary open-angle glaucoma. Curr Mol Med. 2011;11:528–52.

106. Morgan JT, Raghunathan VK, Chang Y-R, Murphy CJ, Russell P. Wnt inhibition induces persistent increases in intrinsic stiffness of human trabecular meshwork cells. Exp Eye Res. 2015;132:174–8.
107. Morgan JT, Raghunathan VK, Chang Y-R, Murphy CJ, Russell P. The intrinsic stiffness of human trabecular meshwork cells increases with senescence. Oncotarget. 2015; https://doi.org/10.18632/oncotarget.3798.
108. Raghunathan VK, et al. Dexamethasone stiffens trabecular meshwork, trabecular meshwork cells, and matrix. Invest Ophthalmol Vis Sci. 2015;56:4447–59. https://doi.org/10.1167/iovs.15-16739.
109. Wood JA, et al. Substratum compliance regulates human trabecular meshwork cell behaviors and response to latrunculin B. Invest Ophthalmol Vis Sci. 2011;52:9298–303. https://doi.org/10.1167/iovs.11-7857.
110. Thomasy SM, Wood JA, Kass PH, Murphy CJ, Russell P. Substratum stiffness and latrunculin B regulate matrix gene and protein expression in human trabecular meshwork cells. Invest Ophthalmol Vis Sci. 2012;53:952–8. https://doi.org/10.1167/iovs.11-8526.
111. Thomasy SM, Morgan JT, Wood JA, Murphy CJ, Russell P. Substratum stiffness and latrunculin B modulate the gene expression of the mechanotransducers YAP and TAZ in human trabecular meshwork cells. Exp Eye Res. 2013;113:66–73. https://doi.org/10.1016/j.exer.2013.05.014.
112. McKee CT, et al. The effect of biophysical attributes of the ocular trabecular meshwork associated with glaucoma on the cell response to therapeutic agents. Biomaterials. 2011;32:2417–23. https://doi.org/10.1016/j.biomaterials.2010.11.071.
113. Russell P, Gasiorowski JZ, Nealy PF, Murphy CJ. Response of human trabecular meshwork cells to topographic cues on the nanoscale level. Invest Ophthalmol Vis Sci. 2008;49:629–35. https://doi.org/10.1167/iovs.07-1192.
114. Baetz NW, Hoffman EA, Yool AJ, Stamer WD. Role of aquaporin-1 in trabecular meshwork cell homeostasis during mechanical strain. Exp Eye Res. 2009;89:95–100. https://doi.org/10.1016/j.exer.2009.02.018.
115. Liton PB, et al. Induction of IL-6 expression by mechanical stress in the trabecular meshwork. Biochem Biophys Res Commun. 2005;337:1229–36. https://doi.org/10.1016/j.bbrc.2005.09.182.
116. Porter KM, Jeyabalan N, Liton PB. MTOR-independent induction of autophagy in trabecular meshwork cells subjected to biaxial stretch. Biochim Biophys Acta. 2014;1843:1054–62. https://doi.org/10.1016/j.bbamcr.2014.02.010.
117. Okada Y, Matsuo T, Ohtsuki H. Bovine trabecular cells produce TIMP-1 and MMP-2 in response to mechanical stretching. Jpn J Ophthalmol. 1998;42:90–4. https://doi.org/10.1016/S0021-5155(97)00129-9.
118. Wu J, et al. Endogenous production of extracellular adenosine by trabecular meshwork cells: potential role in outflow regulation. Invest Ophthalmol Vis Sci. 2012;53:7142–8. https://doi.org/10.1167/iovs.12-9968.
119. Luna C, et al. Extracellular release of ATP mediated by cyclic mechanical stress leads to mobilization of AA in trabecular meshwork cells. Invest Ophthalmol Vis Sci. 2009;50:5805–10. https://doi.org/10.1167/iovs.09-3796.
120. Maddala R, Skiba NP, Rao PV. Vertebrate lonesome kinase regulated extracellular matrix protein phosphorylation, cell shape, and adhesion in trabecular meshwork cells. J Cell Physiol. 2017;232:2447–60. https://doi.org/10.1002/jcp.25582.
121. Iyer P, et al. Autotaxin-lysophosphatidic acid axis is a novel molecular target for lowering intraocular pressure. PLoS One. 2012;7:e42627. https://doi.org/10.1371/journal.pone.0042627.
122. Mitton KP, et al. Transient Loss of αB-crystallin: an early cellular response to mechanical stretch. Biochem Biophys Res Commun. 1997;235:69–73. https://doi.org/10.1006/bbrc.1997.6737.

123. Tumminia SJ, et al. Mechanical stretch alters the actin cytoskeletal network and signal transduction in human trabecular meshwork cells. Invest Ophthalmol Vis Sci. 1998;39:1361–71.
124. WuDunn D. The effect of mechanical strain on matrix metalloproteinase production by bovine trabecular meshwork cells. Curr Eye Res. 2001;22:394–7.
125. Bradley JM, et al. Effects of mechanical stretching on trabecular matrix metalloproteinases. Invest Ophthalmol Vis Sci. 2001;42:1505–13.
126. Bradley JM, Kelley MJ, Rose A, Acott TS. Signaling pathways used in trabecular matrix metalloproteinase response to mechanical stretch. Invest Ophthalmol Vis Sci. 2003;44:5174–81.
127. Raghunathan VK, et al. Transforming growth factor Beta 3 modifies mechanics and composition of extracellular matrix deposited by human trabecular meshwork cells. ACS Biomater Sci Eng. 2015;1:110–8. https://doi.org/10.1021/ab500060r.
128. Torrejon KY, et al. Recreating a human trabecular meshwork outflow system on microfabricated porous structures. Biotechnol Bioeng. 2013;110:3205–18. https://doi.org/10.1002/bit.24977.
129. Torrejon KY, et al. TGFβ2-induced outflow alterations in a bioengineered trabecular meshwork are offset by a rho-associated kinase inhibitor. Sci Rep. 2016;6:38319. https://doi.org/10.1038/srep38319.
130. Chu ER, Gonzalez JM, Tan JCH. Tissue-based imaging model of human trabecular meshwork. J Ocul Pharmacol Ther. 2014;30:191–201. https://doi.org/10.1089/jop.2013.0190.
131. Gonzalez JM, Hamm-Alvarez S, Tan JCH. Analyzing live cellularity in the human trabecular meshwork. Invest Ophthalmol Vis Sci. 2013;54:1039–47. https://doi.org/10.1167/iovs.12-10479.
132. Gonzalez JM, Heur M, Tan JCH. Two-photon immunofluorescence characterization of the trabecular meshwork in situ. Invest Ophthalmol Vis Sci. 2012;53:3395–404. https://doi.org/10.1167/iovs.11-8570.

Chapter 11
Aqueous Humor Outflow

Goichi Akiyama, Thania Bogarin, Sindhu Saraswathy, and Alex S. Huang

The Purpose of Aqueous Humor, Outflow, and Intraocular Pressure

Stable vision demands, among many variables, a semi-rigid eye for predictable optics and a clear visual axis. Aqueous humor and its intraocular flow (aqueous humor outflow [AHO]) supports this by performing several functions. Aqueous humor provides nourishment in the form of oxygen and micro-/macro-molecules such as glucose to avascular tissues like the crystalline lens and cornea. AHO creates an intraocular pressure (IOP) which reliably firms the globe and cornea for stable optics. As a fluid, aqueous humor can wash out intraocular particulate matter (such as inflammation) that otherwise, if replaced by an optically clear but solid media (like cornea), would cause scarring and block light. As a clear fluid, aqueous humor allows uninterrupted passage of light that would be prevented if blood were the substituted medium. Therefore, like any physiological process, AHO is critical to organ function, and AHO can be associated with disease such as elevated IOP and glaucoma when AHO is impeded.

G. Akiyama · T. Bogarin
Department of Ophthalmology, David Geffen School of Medicine at UCLA, Los Angeles, CA, USA
e-mail: gakiyama@doheny.org; tbogarin@doheny.org

S. Saraswathy
Doheny Eye Institute, Los Angeles, CA, USA
e-mail: ssaraswathy@doheny.org

A. S. Huang (✉)
Department of Ophthalmology, David Geffen School of Medicine at UCLA, Los Angeles, CA, USA

Doheny Eye Institute, Los Angeles, CA, USA
e-mail: ahuang@Doheny.org

© Springer Nature Switzerland AG 2021
I. Pallikaris et al. (eds.), *Ocular Rigidity, Biomechanics and Hydrodynamics of the Eye*, https://doi.org/10.1007/978-3-030-64422-2_11

169

Anatomy of Intraocular Pressure and Aqueous Humor Outflow

IOP has many determinants and is a product of the balance between production of fluid and outflow of fluid (regulated at the level of the eye or as a backup of fluid from more distal sources). This relationship is modeled in the Goldman equation where IOP = (F)(R) + EVP (IOP = intraocular pressure [mm Hg]; F = aqueous production [μl/min]; R = outflow resistance [mmHg*min/μl], and EVP = episcleral venous pressure [mm Hg]) [1].

Anatomically, aqueous humor production ("F" in the Goldman equation) occurs at the epithelial layers of the ciliary body via three mechanisms: ultrafiltration, passive diffusion, and active secretion [2, 3]. Aqueous production is centrally regulated [2, 4] and a major target of therapeutic IOP reduction. However, its role in disease pathophysiology is not firmly established.

After production, aqueous then moves between the iris and lens, into the anterior chamber, and toward the angle where two outflow pathways (trabecular and uveoscleral) reside. In trabecular outflow, aqueous humor passes through the trabecular meshwork (TM and primary source of "R" in the Goldman equation) into Schlemm's Canal (SC), then collector channels (CCs), into an intrascleral venous plexus, and eventually to aqueous and episcleral veins [2]. EVP arises in episcleral veins and can be altered by pathological distal venous congestion (such as in a carotid-cavernous fistula [5]) to impact the Goldman equation.

Since a second outflow pathway (unconventional/uveoscleral) also exists [6], the Goldman equation can be expanded into IOP = (Fin − Fout)(R) + EVP where "Fin" represents aqueous production and "Fout" represents uveoscleral outflow [7]. In the uveoscleral outflow pathway, aqueous humor passes through the ciliary body of the angle, into ciliary body clefts, draining either into the supraciliary space, through the sclera, or into lymphatics [7, 8].

Since trabecular outflow represents the majority of aqueous humor outflow (~50%–85%) [9, 10], occurs on a faster time scale compared to uveoscleral outflow [11], is more superficial relative to the ocular surface compared to uveoscleral outflow, and whose diminished capacity has been implicated in high pressure glaucoma [12], it will be the focus of this chapter and heretofore designated as trabecular, conventional or simply aqueous humor outflow (AHO).

Resistance to AHO in Normal and Diseased Eyes

Seminal work by Morton Grant, using post-mortem human eyes, demonstrated that the primary resistor (50–75%) to AHO was the TM [12] (Fig. 11.1). The TM is a multi-layered biological filter [13] and one-way valve that teleologically acts to prevent blood reflux into the eye that can result in blocked vision. Specifically, AHO resistance has been pin-pointed to the border between the juxtacanalicular TM and contiguous inner-wall of SC [13]. In glaucoma, Morton Grant noted that there was

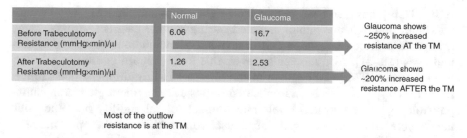

	Normal	Glaucoma
Before Trabeculotomy Resistance (mmHg×min)/µl	6.06	16.7
After Trabeculotomy Resistance (mmHg×min)/µl	1.26	2.53

Glaucoma shows ~250% increased resistance AT the TM

Glaucoma shows ~200% increased resistance AFTER the TM

Most of the outflow resistance is at the TM

Fig. 11.1 Glaucoma as a Resistance Problem, Both at the TM and Past the TM. Outflow facility values were taken from Grant, WM (1963) [12]. Normal values (n = 15) were obtained from Table 5 [12]. Open angle glaucoma values (n = 6) were taken from Table 8 [12]. Outflow facility values were averaged and the reciprocal calculated to determine the resistance. This table organizes measured resistance in normal and glaucoma eyes before and after trabeculotomy. Vertical Arrow: a drop in resistance in both normal and glaucoma eyes after trabeculotomy demonstrated that the primary resistor to outflow in the eye was the trabecular meshwork (TM). However, residual resistance (after trabeculotomy) was still present, denoting the amount of distal (post-TM) outflow resistance. Top Horizontal Arrow: comparing normal to glaucoma eyes, there was increased outflow resistance in glaucoma eyes implicating increased overall resistance as the cause of increased intraocular pressure in glaucoma. Bottom Horizontal Arrow: after trabeculotomy there was increased distal (post-TM) resistance in glaucoma compared to normal eyes at approximately the same magnitude as was seen for overall resistance (Top Horizontal Arrow). This suggested that the underlying pathology in glaucoma impacted the whole eye, TM and post-TM. Glaucoma = Open Angle Glaucoma

elevated TM AHO resistance to explain elevated IOP [12] (Fig. 11.1). At a cellular level it has been hypothesized that increased extracellular matrix (ECM) deposition [13], theories of funneling [13], alterations in TM biomechanics/rigidity [14], or defective cellular pore formation [15] may cause this increased resistance. In addition to the TM, Morton Grant also identified additional resistance and potential impact of disease past the TM. After trabeculotomy (TM removal) in normal eyes there was residual resistance meaning that resistance was still present in regions past the TM in the distal outflow pathways (SC to episcleral veins) [12, 16] (Fig. 11.1). Then in glaucoma eyes, while trabeculotomy dropped outflow resistance, the residual distal outflow resistance was not only present but still elevated compared to the distal outflow resistance of normal eyes (Fig. 11.1) [12, 16]. In fact, the magnitude of increased distal outflow resistance in diseased compared to normal eyes (~2-fold) was about the same as the increased overall resistance comparing the same diseased to normal eyes (~ 2.5-fold) [12, 16] (Fig. 11.1). This implied that glaucoma is not only a TM outflow resistance disease but potentially a whole-eye outflow resistance problem requiring a molecular mechanism to explain both TM and post-TM changes.

Influence of TGF-β

Among many actions, TGF-β is a master regulator of fibrosis in the body. In the eye, TGF-β's multiple pathways have been implicated in ocular functions including maintaining corneal integrity and regulating wound healing [17]. For

AHO, TGF-β has also been implicated in glaucoma and the TM. As an example, analyzing aqueous humor sampled during routine cataract surgery, many groups have detected elevated TGF-β levels in glaucomatous compared to normal eyes [18–21]. At a molecular level, this TGF-β could cause the cellular-level increased TM ECM deposition and elevated TM rigidity described above. In fact, TGF-β has even been implicated in posterior segment glaucoma pathophysiology where elevated levels may impact scleral rigidity near the optic nerve, potentially increasing the structural vulnerability of the optic nerve to high IOP [22].

For understanding TGF-β impact on distal aqueous humor outflow, it is important to recall that while outflow resistance (and hence IOP) is increased, total AHO should be the same in normal and glaucomatous eyes. This is the case because (a) aqueous humor production is believed to be relatively stable in most eyes, and (b) outflow has to equal inflow. At any time, if outflow is more than inflow, the anterior chamber eventually becomes lost over time. Therefore, intact eyes act as constant-flow systems. It's just that in glaucoma (because of increased AHO resistance), aqueous humor has to be pushed much harder (elevated IOP) to achieve the same rate of flow.

Therefore, any pathological agent in the aqueous humor that is implicated in glaucomatous TM alterations, in reality, just flows past the TM to potentially alter the distal outflow pathways as well. Similar to TGF-β mediated scleral changes near the optic nerve, TGF-β mediated changes have also been seen in the sclera surrounding the distal outflow pathways with increased levels of alpha-smooth muscle actin and fibro nectin EDA [23]. This might explain the pathological distal outflow resistance seen by Morton Grant above [12].

Thus, to better study AHO, and in particular distal AHO, better tools are necessary to visualize where and how the fluid is flowing. To image trabecular/conventional AHO, tools can be divided into two categories: structural vs. functional imaging with each category sub-divided into static vs. real-time methods.

Structural AHO Assessment

Structural AHO assessment focuses on the evaluation of the physical outflow pathways themselves. In static methods (including histological techniques), the presence of outflow pathways can only be observed after tissue processing and sectioning. Real-time methods, like optical coherence tomography (OCT), are available for live subjects and amenable to longitudinal study, such as before and after manipulations.

Static Structural AHO Assessment

Static structural AHO pathway assessments have been very important for unveiling the basic outflow pathway anatomy and for studying disease. This is particularly true for the TM where a robust literature exists [13]. The same holds for the distal outflow pathways as well. Decades ago, histological evaluation suggested sclerosis of distal AHO pathways in ocular hypertensive glaucomatous eyes [24]. More recently, tissue herniation into CCs has been shown at high pressures [25]. Using electron microscopy, outflow pathways have been shown to be more complicated than straightforward pathways and openings. For example, CCs can have different configurations such as standard circular (direct oval openings off the posterior wall of SC) or atypical complex (composed of tethered flaps or bridges) [26]. So, while unveiling fundamental pathology, the disadvantage of these approaches has been the reliance on sampling sectioned tissue so that more global approaches visualizing AHO 360° around the eye have been needed.

To better visualize AHO as one unit in an intact eye, early work on the structural anatomy of AHO pathways also used casting agents which were injected into the eye, allowed to polymerize, and then after removal or digestion of ocular tissue isolated as three-dimensional (3D) casts [27, 28]. The advantage was that the entire circumferential outflow pathways around the limbus could be identified from SC to episcleral veins. The disadvantage was the need for firm (supraphysiologic) pressure to deliver the agent and the high likelihood that artifactual anatomy was introduced. More recently, 3D micro-CT has been performed on eyes that were perfusion fixed at physiologic pressures [29]. Identifying AHO pathways as radiolucent signal, SC and CC were re-constructed into a 3D representation [29]. In these cases, while demonstrating global AHO in an eye, the disadvantage of such methods were their incompatibility with live subjects.

Real-Time Structural AHO Assessment

To better study structural AHO pathways in live subjects and to conduct studies in a more longitudinal fashion, variations of anterior-segment OCT have been crucial. Here, visualization of TM, SC, and CCs have been reported by structural OCT. TM measurements have been made in live patients across different races [30] and over time at different ages [31]. Phase-based OCT (ph-OCT) has shown pulsatile TM motion in both enucleated non-human primate [32] and live human eyes [33]. Simultaneously imaged with digital pulse-oximetry, pulsatile TM motion synchronized with the digital pulse (despite a temporal offset), implying a cardiac origin.

SC and CC have been studied by OCT as well. Like 3D-micro-CT, fluid-filled SC and CCs provide a clear OCT hypo-reflective signal that can be identified. However, OCT has the advantage of being applicable to post-mortem human eyes

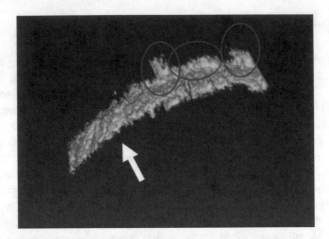

Fig. 11.2 Optical Coherence Tomography (OCT) structural aqueous humor outflow assessment. Anterior-segment OCT was performed on the right eye of a 35-year old male circumferentially around the limbus. Automated segmentation identified outflow lumens (Schlemm's canal [SC] and collector channels [CC]) that were reconstructed to show small a small 3D segment containing SC (white arrow) and CCs (blue circles)

and intact eyes of living normal [34] and glaucomatous [35] individuals. Automated segmentation methods for SC and CCs using OCT images have been developed [36]. Extrapolation of SC 360-degrees around the limbus into a three-dimensional representation (Fig. 11.2) showed that SC had segmental anatomy with wider or narrower regions [36]. In various live species including humans, pilocarpine [37], rho-kinase (ROCK) inhibitors [38], and laser trabeculoplasty [39] have been reported to increase SC size. In contrast, IOP elevation has been shown to do the opposite [40].

Despite being able to study AHO structure in live subjects, OCT has limitations that in some cases are unique to the anterior segment. For example, compared to the posterior segment of the eye where clinical OCT imaging covers ~5–6 mm and where ~50–100 scans can guide surgical decisions, the distance traveled in the anterior segment for AHO is much larger. For 3D reconstruction of circumferential AHO pathways, over 5000 B-scans was utilized in one case [36]. This was true as to complete comprehensive AHO OCT imaging, the entire circumference along the limbus must be covered (2 X π X radius [average 6 mm] = 37.68 mm which is ~6–7 times the distance compared to retina OCT). Relevant structures such as CCs are also small, and ground-truth validation of OCT structures are not always present. Typical commercial OCTs have a B-scan to B-scan distance of ~35 microns and can miss CCs that are ~10 microns in size. Posterior to SC and CC, hypo-reflective OCT lumens are not always necessarily AHO-related because arteries, lymphatics, and non-AHO veins exist as well. Most importantly, unlike posterior-segment OCT which has tracking and reference functions that allow imaging of the same retina location longitudinally over time [41], in anterior segment OCT this functionality does not exist. Therefore, it becomes difficult for investigators to know if AHO pathway imaging across two sessions are really imaging the same structures at the same orientation. All it takes is a shift in the image acquisition angle to make a single SC appear bigger of smaller across different image acquisition sessions.

Finally, despite being able to visualize AHO structure, the relationship between structural characteristics and actual fluid flow is unclear. For example, it is not clear whether complex vs. simple CC orifices or larger vs. smaller OCT outflow lumens necessarily equate to easier or more difficult AHO. In the case of OCT AHO lumens, a large pathway could represent a low-resistance pathway that facilitates AHO or a stagnant pocket of fluid that is trapped in an outflow cul-du-sac. Therefore, while anterior segment OCT imaging of AHO pathways has the enormous advantage of being non-invasive, in the future, significantly more anterior segment OCT research on AHO structural mapping coupled with technological advances are needed. In the meantime, functional assessment of fluid flow may be easier to understand.

Functional AHO Assessment

In functional AHO assessment, tracers are introduced into the eye and followed as a proxy for AHO. Therefore, tracer-based studies are an alternative approach that simply asks "where is the fluid going" regardless of anatomic detail. The difference between static and real-time methods have to do with the choice of tracer and method of visualization.

Static Functional AHO Assessment

Static functional AHO assessment usually employs tracers such as gold particles, fluorescent microspheres, or quantum dots that could range in size from (0.01 to 20 micons) [15, 25, 42–45]. Since water (the primary constituent of aqueous humor) has a molecular weight of 18 g/mol or daltons (Da), these larger tracers ($\sim 10^3$–10^7 Da) were usually caught in the TM which then required ocular dissection with visualization of tracer location either by whole-mount with exposed TM or as fixed histological section containing AHO pathways. Due to tracer accumulation at filtration points, static AHO imaging was quite useful in visualizing flow at the TM or CCs. Unfortunately, these methods were not compatible with live subjects.

Static methods were one of the first to suggest the idea of segmental AHO. Using post-mortem cow and human eyes, early work using isolated anterior segment organ culture allowed quantification of fluorescent TM uptake. Percent effective filtration length (PEFL) was determined in histological section by dividing the length (L) over which tracers were observed by the total length (TL) of TM sectioned (PEFL = L/TL) [25]. It was found that AHO did not occur uniformly circumferential around the limbus but instead arose in focused segmental areas.

Static method have also been useful in studying basic TM/SC biology and segmental AHO. Rho-kinase inhibitors were found to abolish AHO segmentalization as seen by gold particle distribution during electron microscopic analyses of SC cells [42]. In fluorescent microsphere studies, segmental TM uptake in wild-type mice became more homogeneous in a Secreted Protein Acidic and Rich in Cysteine (SPARC) mutant [43].

To probe the underlying biological difference between high- and low-flow TM regions, said regions were identified by fluorescent microbead accumulation and isolated to enrich for biological differences. An increase in versican (a large extracellular matrix proteoglycan) was seen at the RNA and protein level in low-flow human TM [44]. Gene expression analyses with some immunofluorescence confirmation revealed increases in collagen and matrix metalloproteinases in high-flow regions [45]. Structurally, low-flow regions were noted to be biomechanically stiffer with an elevated elastic modulus [14].

For TM cells and at an electron microscopic level, micron-sized pores (I-pores: intracellular pores for fluid flow across a cell; B-pores: border pores for paracellular flow between cells) have been hypothesized to move fluid past the contiguous border between the inner-wall of SC and the juxtacanalicular TM [15]. Segmental tracer accumulation positively correlated with total pore and B-pore density, suggesting that the paracellular pores represented the dominant pathway for transendothelial filtration across the SC inner-wall [15].

Real-Time Functional AHO Assessment

Since static functional AHO assessment methods were not compatible with live subjects, to move in a clinical direction, real-time methods were developed. Here, tracers were soluble and methods utilized clinical instrumentation found in clinics and operating rooms. Overall, 3 major methods exist to visualize real-time AHO in living subjects: the episcleral venous fluid wave, canalography, and aqueous angiography.

Episcleral Venous Fluid Wave

The episcleral venous fluid wave (EVFW) was developed in the operating room using standard cataract surgery perfusion equipment [46]. By delivering a clear perfusate into the anterior chamber, AHO pathways were identified on the ocular surface in live patients by looking for the disappearance of blood from episcleral veins viewed through a surgical microscope. When studied retrospectively, a statistically significant correlation was seen between patients with observable episcleral fluid waves and better surgical success using trabecular ablation [47]. The advantage of this technique was that it was easily accessible and familiar to anterior segment ophthalmic surgeons. However, several disadvantages were present as well. First, irrigation of perfusate into the eye using commercial phacoemulsification units occurred at high and supra-physiologic pressures. Second, relying on a loss of signal or disappearance of episcleral veins could be a challenge. Loss-of-signal approaches require surgeons to recognize, record, and remember the episcleral venous pattern before the perfusate is pushed forward in order to identify what was lost.

Canalography

Canalography (sometimes termed channelography) is another real-time method that relied on direct introduction of fluorescent tracers (fluorescein, indocyanine green [ICG], or trypan blue) into SC [48–50]. This could occur as direct tracer injection into SC during deep sclerectomy or canaloplasty surgeries. Alternatively, during the canaloplasty step where the fiber-optic catheter is backed out of the eye with delivery of viscoelastic to achieve a viscocanulostomy, a fluorescent tracer could be substituted for the viscoelastic instead. While showing distal AHO anatomy, canalograms didn't show physiologic AHO since tracer introduction occurred after the TM (in the SC). Therefore, the result was more akin to what AHO could look like after 360-degree trabeculotomy. Also, direct injection of tracer into SC or via the canaloplasty catheter would be at high (supra-physiologic) pressure, and introducing the tracer while the canaloplasty catheter was being backed out of the eye would not achieve delivery of tracer to all portions of the circumferential outflow pathways simultaneously.

Aqueous Angiography

To complement canalograms, aqueous angiography was devised. Aqueous angiography was developed in a bedside to bench to bedside approach by starting in the clinic and operating room [16, 51, 52]. Clinical equipment (such as the Spectralis HRA + OCT [Heidelberg Engineering, Heidelberg, Germany] and operating room blades and tubing) was brought into the laboratory to develop aqueous angiography. Using post-mortem eyes, fluorescein or ICG was delivered into pig [52], bovine [53], cat [54], and human eyes [52, 55] (Fig. 11.3) at physiologic pressures, and AHO was imaged utilizing the angiographic function on the Spectralis. This was akin to using the Spectralis to visualize retinal blood flow [56] after intravenous tracer delivery except here the tracer was delivered in the anterior chamber and the angiographic camera pointed at the ocular surface.

Regardless of species tested, segmental AHO patterns were seen [52–55]. Angiographic patterns were validated as AHO by using concurrent anterior segment OCT. Regions with (but not without) angiographic signal demonstrated instrascleral lumens capable of carrying AHO [52–55] (Fig. 11.4). Fixable fluorescent dextrans also provided aqueous angiographic signal and could be trapped by post-angiography

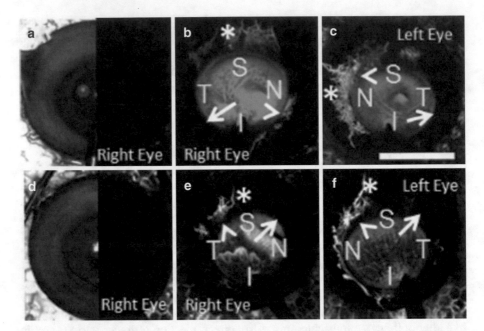

Fig. 11.3 Aqueous angiography in enucleated human eyes. Aqueous angiography was performed on enucleated eyes from two female subjects not known to have glaucoma at 10 mm Hg (subject 1 = **a–c** and subject 2 = **d–f**). Both right and left eyes from each subject were investigated and shown at 10–25 s. **a/d**) Composite cSLO infrared (left-side) and pre-injection background images (right-side) are shown from the right eyes of these two subjects. S = superior; T = temporal, N = nasal; I = inferior. AC = anterior chamber, TM = trabecular meshwork, SC = Schlemm's Canal. Scale bars = 1 cm. Adapted from Saraswathy et al. (2016) PLoS One Jan 25;11 (1):e0147176.doi: https://doi.org/10.1371/journal.pone.0147176. eCollection 2016 [52]

fixation. Here, regions with (but not without) angiographic signal showed fluorescent dextrans trapped in AHO pathways [52–55] (Fig. 11.5).

Aqueous angiography was also useful in the laboratory to study fundamental outflow concepts. After performing aqueous angiography on post-mortem human eyes, TM near-adjacent high- and low-flow angiographic regions were identified and dissected, thereby enriching biological differences. Immunofluorescence and biochemical testing showed increased levels of versican and TGF-β pathway proteins [57]. This supported the role of TGF-β in regulating outflow and "Static Functional AHO Assessment" results above. Additionally, given that aqueous angiography was viewed from the ocular surface (the only view that a surgeon would see because surgeons could not possibly see intraocular TM trapping of larger tracers without opening the eye and looking internally), these results confirmed that clinical and external aqueous angiographic patterns were reflective of underlying TM biology within the eye.

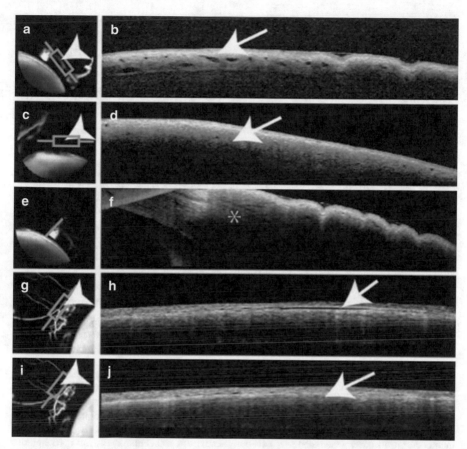

Fig. 11.4 Aqueous angiography and optical coherence tomography (OCT). Aqueous angiography was conducted in pig eyes in parallel with anterior segment OCT. (**a/g**) Angiographically positive areas (arrowheads) correlated with (**b/h**) intrascleral lumens on OCT (arrows). (**c/i**) In contrast, angiographically lacking areas (arrowheads) were (**d/j**) devoid of intrascleral lumens on OCT (arrows). (**e**) Angiographically positive areas could be associated with a classical "side-ways Y" aqueous vein (asterisk). Adapted from Saraswathy et al. (2016) PLoS One Jan 25;11 (1):e0147176. doi: https://doi.org/10.1371/journal.pone.0147176. eCollection 2016 [52]

To bring aqueous angiography to live testing, the FLEX module (Heidelberg Engineering) was developed. The FLEX module was a modified surgical boom arm upon which the Spectralis was installed for angiographic or OCT imaging in any body position. Using the FLEX module, aqueous angiography was performed in live non-human primates [58] and humans [59] using fluorescein and ICG in the operating room (Fig. 11.6). Results continued to demonstrate segmental AHO patterns. Again, to validate the angiographic signal as compatible for outflow, using multi-modal imaging, concurrent OCT on (but not off) angiographic structures showed intrascleral lumens capable of carrying aqueous [58, 59]. Concurrent to

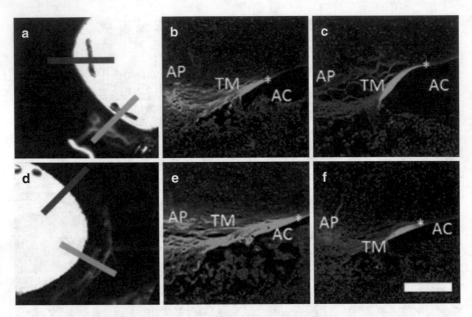

Fig. 11.5 Aqueous angiography localizes to AHO pathways. Aqueous angiography was conducted with 3 kD fixable fluorescent dextrans in pig eyes. Two representative eyes (**a–c** and **d–f**) are shown here. Angiographically positive (**a/d**; green lines) or diminished (**a/d**; red lines) regions were identified with aqueous angiography and then sectioned. In the first eye (**a–c**), angiographically positive (green line in **a** corresponds to panel **b**) but not angiographically negative (red line in **a** corresponds to panel **c**) regions showed trapping of dextrans within outflow pathways. In the second eye (**d–f**), angiographically positive (green line in **d** corresponds to panel **e**) but not angiographically negative (red line in **d** corresponds to panel **f**) regions also showed trapping of dextrans within outflow pathways. Note similar degree of non-specific fluorescence seen in Descemet's membrane in all cases (asterisks). *AP* aqueous plexus; *TM* trabecular meshwork; *AC* anterior chamber. Scale bar = 100 microns. Adapted from Saraswathy et al. (2016) PLoS One Jan 25;11 (1):e0147176.doi: https://doi.org/10.1371/journal.pone.0147176. eCollection 2016 [52]

aqueous angiography, infrared (IR) imaging showed overlap of aqueous angiographic vessels with episcleral veins [58, 59]. In addition to segmental patterns, a pulsatile behavior similar to ph-OCT [32, 33] results was seen. Rare dynamic behaviors were also documented as regions with or without aqueous angiographic signal had the ability to lose or develop signal [58, 59], respectively. This showed for the first time that AHO was not static but could move across the eye, thereby unveiling new points of potential regulation.

Since the Spectralis HRA could detect both fluorescein and ICG, sequential angiography was additionally developed in single eyes with ICG followed by fluorescein. Results showed similar patterns between the two tracers [53, 55]. This established a method where a baseline ICG angiographic pattern for a particular eye could be determined followed by an intervention and then fluorescein aqueous angiography to test the impact of the intervention. This approach was first tested in the lab using post-mortem bovine [53] and human eyes [55], and it showed that

Fig. 11.6 Aqueous angiography in a live normal human subject. Aqueous angiography was performed on a 75-year old Asian female during routine cataract surgery. Indocyanine green was introduced into the anterior chamber at 20 mm Hg and the patient asked to look temporal, exposing the post-limbal nasal portion of the eye. Arrows point out Y-shaped angiographic aqueous and episcleral veins

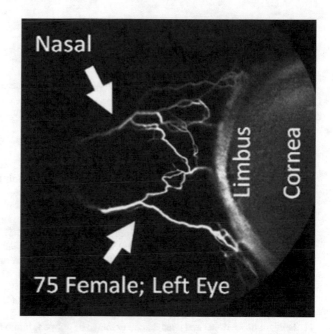

trabecular bypass (iStent Inject; Glaukos Corporation) had the capability to rescue regions of initially low angiographic signal. This method was further modified for live humans where experiments have shown a similar result. In glaucoma patients, initially poor ICG angiographic regions could be improved after trabecular bypass stenting as assessed by fluorescein aqueous angiography [23].

Conclusion

In conclusion, AHO is critically important to stable vision as evidenced by its role in tissue nourishment and optics. However, dis-regulation of AHO can occur resulting in elevated IOP and the largest risk factor for glaucomatous optic neuropathy. AHO has many determinants and seminal work has long-established the crucial role of the TM in outflow resistance although there is emerging evidence regarding the importance of the distal AHO pathways and segmental AHO as well. Essential to studying AHO as an entire unit (both TM and distal) better structural and functional tools are needed and under development in both the laboratory and clinical space.

Acknowledgements Funding for this work came from National Institutes of Health, Bethesda, MD (R01EY030501 [ASH]); Research to Prevent Blindness Career Development Award 2016 [ASH]; and an unrestricted grant from Research to Prevent Blindness (New York, NY).

References

1. Brubaker RF. Goldmann's equation and clinical measures of aqueous dynamics. Exp Eye Res. 2004;78(3):633–7.
2. Goel M, Picciani RG, Lee RK, Bhattacharya SK. Aqueous humor dynamics: a review. Open Ophthalmol J. 2010;4:52–9.
3. Civan MM, Macknight AD. The ins and outs of aqueous humour secretion. Exp Eye Res. 2004;78(3):625–31.
4. Ruskell GL. An ocular parasympathetic nerve pathway of facial nerve origin and its influence on intraocular pressure. Exp Eye Res. 1970;10(2):319–30.
5. Phelps CD, Thompson HS, Ossoinig KC. The diagnosis and prognosis of atypical carotid-cavernous fistula (red-eyed shunt syndrome). Am J Ophthalmol. 1982;93(4):423–36.
6. Johnson M, McLaren JW, Overby DR. Unconventional aqueous humor outflow: a review. Exp Eye Res. 2017;158:94–111.
7. S HA, Structure NWR. Mechanism of uveoscleral outflow. In: Francis BA, Sarkisian SR, Tan JC, editors. Minimally invasive glaucoma surgery. New York: Thieme; 2017.
8. Yucel YH, Johnston MG, Ly T, et al. Identification of lymphatics in the ciliary body of the human eye: a novel "uveolymphatic" outflow pathway. Exp Eye Res. 2009;89(5):810–9.
9. Toris CB, Yablonski ME, Wang YL, Camras CB. Aqueous humor dynamics in the aging human eye. Am J Ophthalmol. 1999;127(4):407–12.
10. Bill A, Phillips CI. Uveoscleral drainage of aqueous humour in human eyes. Exp Eye Res. 1971;12(3):275–81.
11. Bill A. Conventional and uveo-scleral drainage of aqueous humour in the cynomolgus monkey (Macaca irus) at normal and high intraocular pressures. Exp Eye Res. 1966;5(1):45–54.
12. Grant WM. Experimental aqueous perfusion in enucleated human eyes. Arch Ophthalmol. 1963;69:783–801.
13. Johnson M. What controls aqueous humour outflow resistance? Exp Eye Res. 2006;82(4):545–57.
14. Vranka JA, Staverosky JA, Reddy AP, et al. Biomechanical rigidity and quantitative proteomics analysis of segmental regions of the trabecular meshwork at physiologic and elevated pressures. Invest Ophthalmol Vis Sci. 2018;59(1):246–59.
15. Braakman ST, Read AT, Chan DW, et al. Colocalization of outflow segmentation and pores along the inner wall of Schlemm's canal. Exp Eye Res. 2015;130:87–96.
16. Huang AS, Mohindroo C, Weinreb RN. Aqueous humor outflow structure and function imaging at the bench and bedside: a review. J Clin Exp Ophthalmol. 2016;7(4)
17. Tandon A, Tovey JC, Sharma A, et al. Role of transforming growth factor Beta in corneal function, biology and pathology. Curr Mol Med. 2010;10(6):565–78.
18. Tripathi RC, Li J, Chan WF, Tripathi BJ. Aqueous humor in glaucomatous eyes contains an increased level of TGF-beta 2. Exp Eye Res. 1994;59(6):723–7.
19. Tamm ER, Fuchshofer R. What increases outflow resistance in primary open-angle glaucoma? Surv Ophthalmol. 2007;52(Suppl 2):S101–4.
20. Ochiai Y, Ochiai H. Higher concentration of transforming growth factor-beta in aqueous humor of glaucomatous eyes and diabetic eyes. Jpn J Ophthalmol. 2002;46(3):249–53.
21. Inatani M, Tanihara H, Katsuta H, et al. Transforming growth factor-beta 2 levels in aqueous humor of glaucomatous eyes. Graefes Arch Clin Exp Ophthalmol. 2001;239(2):109–13.
22. Quigley HA. The contribution of the sclera and lamina cribrosa to the pathogenesis of glaucoma: diagnostic and treatment implications. Prog Brain Res. 2015;220:59–86.
23. Huang AS, Penteado RC, Papoyan V, Voskanyan L, Weinreb RN. Aqueous angiographic outflow improvement after trabecular microbypass in glaucoma patients. Ophthalmol Glaucoma. 2019;2(1):11–21.
24. Dvorak-Theobald G, Kirk HQ. Aqueous pathways in some cases of glaucoma. Am J Ophthalmol. 1956;41(1):11–21.

25. Battista SA, Lu Z, Hofmann S, et al. Reduction of the available area for aqueous humor outflow and increase in meshwork herniations into collector channels following acute IOP elevation in bovine eyes. Invest Ophthalmol Vis Sci. 2008;49(12):5346–52.
26. Bentley MD, Hann CR, Fautsch MP. Anatomical variation of human collector channel orifices. Invest Ophthalmol Vis Sci. 2016;57(3):1153–9.
27. Ashton N. Anatomical study of Schlemm's canal and aqueous veins by means of neoprene casts. Part I. Aqueous veins. Br J Ophthalmol. 1951;35(5):291–303.
28. Van Buskirk EM. The canine eye: the vessels of aqueous drainage. Invest Ophthalmol Vis Sci. 1979;18(3):223–30.
29. Hann CR, Bentley MD, Vercnocke A, et al. Imaging the aqueous humor outflow pathway in human eyes by three-dimensional micro-computed tomography (3D micro-CT). Exp Eye Res. 2011;92(2):104–11.
30. Chen RI, Barbosa DT, Hsu CH, et al. Ethnic differences in trabecular meshwork height by optical coherence tomography. JAMA Ophthalmol. 2015;133(4):437–41.
31. Gold ME, Kansara S, Nagi KS, et al. Age-related changes in trabecular meshwork imaging. Biomed Res Int. 2013;2013:295204.
32. Hariri S, Johnstone M, Jiang Y, et al. Platform to investigate aqueous outflow system structure and pressure-dependent motion using high-resolution spectral domain optical coherence tomography. J Biomed Opt. 2014;19(10):106013.
33. Li P, Shen TT, Johnstone M, Wang RK. Pulsatile motion of the trabecular meshwork in healthy human subjects quantified by phase-sensitive optical coherence tomography. Biomed Opt Express. 2013;4(10):2051–65.
34. Kagemann L, Wollstein G, Ishikawa H, et al. Visualization of the conventional outflow pathway in the living human eye. Ophthalmology. 2012;119(8):1563–8.
35. Kagemann L, Wollstein G, Ishikawa H, et al. Identification and assessment of Schlemm's canal by spectral-domain optical coherence tomography. Invest Ophthalmol Vis Sci. 2010;51(8):4054–9.
36. Huang AS, Belghith A, Dastiridou A, et al. Automated circumferential construction of first-order aqueous humor outflow pathways using spectral-domain optical coherence tomography. J Biomed Opt. 2017;22(6):66010.
37. Li G, Farsiu S, Chiu SJ, et al. Pilocarpine-induced dilation of Schlemm's canal and prevention of lumen collapse at elevated intraocular pressures in living mice visualized by OCT. Invest Ophthalmol Vis Sci. 2014;55(6):3737–46.
38. Li G, Mukherjee D, Navarro I, et al. Visualization of conventional outflow tissue responses to netarsudil in living mouse eyes. Eur J Pharmacol. 2016;787:20–31.
39. Skaat A, Rosman MS, Chien JL, et al. Microarchitecture of Schlemm Canal before and after selective laser trabeculoplasty in enhanced depth imaging optical coherence tomography. J Glaucoma. 2017;26(4):361–6.
40. Kagemann L, Wang B, Wollstein G, et al. IOP elevation reduces Schlemm's canal cross-sectional area. Invest Ophthalmol Vis Sci. 2014;55(3):1805–9.
41. Huang AS, Kim LA, Fawzi AA. Clinical characteristics of a large choroideremia pedigree carrying a novel CHM mutation. Arch Ophthalmol. 2012;130(9):1184–9.
42. Sabanay I, Gabelt BT, Tian B, et al. H-7 effects on the structure and fluid conductance of monkey trabecular meshwork. Arch Ophthalmol. 2000;118(7):955–62.
43. Swaminathan SS, Oh DJ, Kang MH, et al. Secreted protein acidic and rich in cysteine (SPARC)-null mice exhibit more uniform outflow. Invest Ophthalmol Vis Sci. 2013;54(3):2035–47.
44. Keller KE, Bradley JM, Vranka JA, Acott TS. Segmental versican expression in the trabecular meshwork and involvement in outflow facility. Invest Ophthalmol Vis Sci. 2011;52(8):5049–57.
45. Vranka JA, Bradley JM, Yang YF, et al. Mapping molecular differences and extracellular matrix gene expression in segmental outflow pathways of the human ocular trabecular meshwork. PLoS One. 2015;10(3):e0122483.
46. Fellman RL, Grover DS. Episcleral venous fluid wave: intraoperative evidence for patency of the conventional outflow system. J Glaucoma. 2014;23(6):347–50.

47. Fellman RL, Feuer WJ, Grover DS. Episcleral venous fluid wave correlates with trabectome outcomes: intraoperative evaluation of the trabecular outflow pathway. Ophthalmology. 2015;122(12):2385–91.e1.
48. Grieshaber MC. Ab externo Schlemm's canal surgery: viscocanalostomy and canaloplasty. Dev Ophthalmol. 2012;50:109–24.
49. Zeppa L, Ambrosone L, Guerra G, et al. Using canalography to visualize the in vivo aqueous humor outflow conventional pathway in humans. JAMA Ophthalmol. 2014;132(11):1281.
50. Grieshaber MC, Pienaar A, Olivier J, Stegmann R. Clinical evaluation of the aqueous outflow system in primary open-angle glaucoma for canaloplasty. Invest Ophthalmol Vis Sci. 2010;51(3):1498–504.
51. Huang AS, Francis BA, Weinreb RN. Structural and functional imaging of aqueous humour outflow: a review. Clin Exp Ophthalmol. 2018;46(2):158–68.
52. Saraswathy S, Tan JC, Yu F, et al. Aqueous angiography: real-time and physiologic aqueous humor outflow imaging. PLoS One. 2016;11(1):e0147176.
53. Huang AS, Saraswathy S, Dastiridou A, et al. Aqueous angiography with fluorescein and indocyanine green in bovine eyes. Transl Vis Sci Technol. 2016;5(6):5.
54. Snyder KC, Oikawa K, Williams J, Kiland JA, Gehrke S, Teixeira LBC, Huang AS, McLellan GJ. Imaging distal aqueous outflow pathways in a spontaneous model of congenital glaucoma. Transl Vis Sci Technol. 2019;8(5):22.
55. Huang AS, Saraswathy S, Dastiridou A, et al. Aqueous angiography-mediated guidance of trabecular bypass improves angiographic outflow in human enucleated eyes. Invest Ophthalmol Vis Sci. 2016;57(11):4558–65.
56. Keane PA, Sadda SR. Imaging chorioretinal vascular disease. Eye (Lond). 2010;24(3):422–7.
57. Saraswathy S, Bogarin T, Barron E, Francis BA, Tan JCH, Weinreb RN, Huang AS. Segmental differences found in aqueous angiographic-determined high – and low-flow regions of human trabecular meshwork. Exp Eye Res. 2020;196:108064.
58. Huang AS, Li M, Yang D, et al. Aqueous angiography in living nonhuman primates shows segmental, pulsatile, and dynamic angiographic aqueous humor outflow. Ophthalmology. 2017;124(6):793–803.
59. Huang AS, Camp A, Xu BY, et al. Aqueous angiography: aqueous humor outflow imaging in live human subjects. Ophthalmology. 2017;124(8):1249–51.

Chapter 12
Ocular Rigidity and Tonometry

Jibran Mohamed-Noriega and Keith Barton

Introduction

In the current management of patients with glaucoma, the only modifiable factor that has been proven to reduce the rate of progression is IOP. It can be evaluated by digital palpation, invasive manometry inside the eye, or tonometry through the coating layers of the eye. In this chapter, we will explore the mechanisms of action of different tonometers and how they are affected by OR and by changes in OR induced by surgery.

What Is Tonometry, and Description of Different Tonometers?

Applanation Tonometers

Goldmann Applanation Tonometer (GAT)

The current reference standard for tonometry is the Goldmann Applanation Tonometer (GAT), introduced by Hans Goldmann and Theo Schmidt in 1957 [1]. Since then, a variety of instruments have been developed for the same purpose but

J. Mohamed-Noriega
Department of Ophthalmology, Faculty of Medicine and University Hospital, Universidad Autónoma de Nuevo León (U.A.N.L.), Monterrey, Mexico

NIHR Biomedical Research Centre at Moorfields Eye Hospital NHS Foundation Trust and UCL Institute of Ophthalmology, London, UK
e-mail: jibran.mohamednrg@uanl.mx

K. Barton (✉)
NIHR Biomedical Research Centre at Moorfields Eye Hospital NHS Foundation Trust and UCL Institute of Ophthalmology, London, UK
e-mail: keith@keithbarton.co.uk

© Springer Nature Switzerland AG 2021
I. Pallikaris et al. (eds.), *Ocular Rigidity, Biomechanics and Hydrodynamics of the Eye*, https://doi.org/10.1007/978-3-030-64422-2_12

utilising different mechanisms. The continuing development of new instruments reflects the dissatisfaction of clinicians with some aspects of each of the currently available tonometers. An ideal tonometer for clinical use should be an inexpensive, easy to use instrument that exposes the patient to no risk of harm, while accurately measuring the true IOP in a precise way and capturing all of the IOP characteristics that are relevant for glaucoma management. Unfortunately, all current tonometers fail to satisfy these requirements. A problem with GAT, which is common to many tonometers, is that they rely on the so-called Imbert-Fick law. This law has been described predominantly in the ophthalmic literature and has been found to have little validity in modelling exercises [2]. It postulates that the pressure inside a sphere (P) that is filled with a liquid and is surrounded by a dry, extremely thin, and perfectly flexible membrane is proportional to the force (W) required to flatten an area (A) of the membrane.

$$W = P * A$$

However, the layers comprising the wall of the eye (cornea or sclera) are neither extremely thin nor perfectly flexible. In addition, the cornea is covered by a tear film layer that creates surface tension that attracts the tip of the GAT. To overcome these violations of the assumptions required in the previous formula, Goldmann included corneal resistance to applanation (b) and the surface tension created by the tear film (s).

$$W + s = P * A + b$$

GAT flattens an area of the cornea of 7.35 mm^2 that was defined based on two theoretical advantages: (1) at this area the surface tension (s) and the resistance to applanation (b) forces cancel each other, so that an equilibrium between the forces is theoretically reached, and (2) the force in grams (W) required to flatten the cornea multiplied by 10 is equivalent to the IOP in mmHg (Fig. 12.1c).

Non-contact Tonometer (NCT)

The requirement of topical anaesthesia and trained staff to use GAT has encouraged companies to produce tonometers that can be operated with minimal training, without direct contact with the cornea, and without the need for topical anaesthesia. In 1972 Grollman reported the principles of the first NCT to measure the IOP [3].

NCT is a type of applanation tonometry, based on a similar principle to GAT. A fixed area of the cornea is flattened (10.18 mm^2), but instead of touching the cornea, as in GAT, NCT uses a jet of air. A sensor measures the force of the air required to flatten the cornea over a predefined area. The instrument recognises that the desired flattening of the cornea has been reached when the flattened cornea acts as a plane mirror to light emitted by the instrument and recorded by an optical sensor.

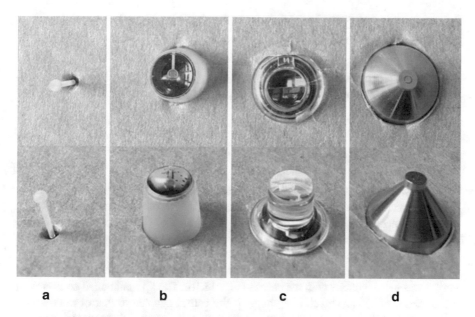

a   b   c   d

Fig. 12.1 Shows the tips of some of the most commonly used tonometers, both side and end on. (**a**) iCare, (**b**) DCT, (**c**) disposable GAT, and (**d**) Tonopen

Pneumotonometer

In 1965, when many clinicians considered IOP to be almost the only factor involved in glaucoma pathogenesis, Durham et al. [4] reported an instrument that was able to measure the IOP continuously. This new instrument was called pneumatic applanation tonometry because it was based on a similar principle to GAT but, used a flow of gas to move a 5 mm (area of 19.6 mm^2) diameter silicone membrane toward the cornea, until it flattened an area equal to that of the silicone membrane. A transducer measured the force required by the gas to flatten 19.6 mm^2 of the corneal surface. The pulsatile characteristics of the IOP measurements were continuously plotted on a moving chart.

Shiotz Indentation Tonometer

Before the development of GAT, the most extensively used instrument was the indentation tonometer designed by Hjalmar Shiotzin 1905. It was used with the patient in the supine position, and the IOP was measured, based on the degree of indentation of the globe produced by a plunger with different weights. The main principle was that a known force (the weight of the plunger and weights) indented the eye more or less if the IOP was low or high, respectively.

Instruments Designed to Measure the IOP Less Influenced by the Corneal Biomechanics

New tonometers have attempted to circumnavigate corneal biomechanics in order to obtain IOP measurements that are less influenced by these characteristics and closer to the true IOP.

Pascal Dynamic Contour Tonometer (DCT)

In 2002, Kanngiesser [5] described a completely new approach to tonometry. The aim was to reduce the influence of corneal thickness and radius of curvature. They designed a 7 mm diameter Goldmann-like tip with a concave surface (10.5 mm radius of curvature) based on the ideal shape that would continuously and directly record the pressure. A piezoelectric pressure sensor was built into the centre of the concave surface. This Goldmann-like tip is mounted on a slit-lamp, and the operator moved the tip forward until it was just in contact with the cornea (Fig. 12.1b). The tip maintained contact with the cornea for 5–10 s. The convex shape of the cornea adapted to that of the tip with minimal deformation allowed the piezoelectric sensor to constantly recorded the pressure. The ability to continuously measure the IOP permitted the recording of diastolic and systolic IOP readings. The difference between these was reported as the ocular pulse amplitude (OPA), and the diastolic reading was reported as the IOP value.

Applanation Resonance Tonometer (ART)

In 2000 a new piezoelectric sensor, based on vibration technology, was developed to measure IOP [6, 7]. This tonometer is available as a portable instrument or mounted in a slit-lamp. It has a Goldmann-like tip, 4 mm in diameter that touches the cornea with a constant force, measuring the change in frequency of vibration on contact with the cornea. From the shift in the frequency, the software calculates the area of the cornea that has been flattened and reports the IOP following the same Imbert-Fick law as GAT. Continuous contact with the cornea (2 s) allows the device to produce multiple IOP readings and calculate a single final result.

Instruments Designed to Measure the IOP and Aspects of the Corneal Biomechanics

Some instruments have taken a different approach to reduce the influence of corneal biomechanics. Instead of creating a device that is less affected by corneal biomechanics, this group of instruments measure some characteristics of the corneal biomechanics that are likely to be a source of error in the IOP estimation. These devices produce metrics for corneal biomechanical characteristics and finally, report an IOP value that is analogous to applanation tonometry or corrected, based on the identified corneal biomechanics.

Ocular Response Analyzer (ORA)

This instrument is described in detail as a surrogate for the measurement of OR in Sect. "Applanation Tonometer". Briefly, it was the first instrument with the ability to measure some of the biomechanical characteristics of the cornea. In 2005 Reichert Inc. published the first results of their new instrument that combined a jet of air, similar to NCT, with an electro-optical collimation detector system that measures the changes in the curvature of the eye in the central 3.0 mm of the cornea during the 20 ms measurement [8]. The company coined the terms corneal hysteresis (CH) to refer to the difference in the two IOP measurement recorded when the cornea is flattened (CH = P1-P2) and corneal resistance factor (CRF) to refer to the difference of P1 and P2 and a constant (k) that considers the relationship between pressure and CCT (CRF = P1-kP2). The jet of air pushes the cornea and changes it from a convex to a concave curvature during the 20 ms measurement. During this change in corneal curvature, the cornea is flattened twice, during its inward and outward trajectory. The difference in the IOP values from the inward and outward flattenings is mostly due to the energy absorbed due to the corneal tissue's viscoelastic properties.

Corneal Visualization Scheimpflug Technology (Corvis ST)

In 2011, in an effort to characterise the biomechanical characteristics of the cornea better, OCULUS (Optikgeräte GmbH) presented the first results from an instrument that is designed to combine the principles of non-contact tonometry with an ultra-high-speed Scheimpflug camera [9]. The sensor measures the force in the jet of air required for the first applanation of the cornea and produces an IOP reading that is similar to NCT. A single Scheimpflug image is used to measure the central corneal thickness. The video output, with 4330 images per second, is used to measure diversity of parameters such as length and velocity of the first and second applanation, and the amplitude and time to reach the highest concavity. The clinical report displays many of these biomechanical characteristics including IOP both uncorrected and corrected for CCT.

Instruments Designed to Be Portable

Hand-Held Applanation Tonometer (Perkins Tonometer)

In an effort to stretch the potential use of GAT into screening programmes, supine position, and animal research, E. S. Perkins published in 1965 the characteristics of a hand-held tonometer that was based on the same principles as GAT [10]. It weighs around 1 kg, is fully portable, and can also be used in the supine position.

Tonopen

In 1959 Mackay and Marg described possible types of tonometers that could be faster, automatic, accurate, repeatable, gentle, and able to produce a direct-reading. They reported a new tonometer that combined characteristics of applanation and indentation tonometry [10]. Similarly to GAT, it used an approximate applanation area of 7 mm^2 but was combined with a small plunger of approximately 1.5 mm in diameter that measured the pressure electronically in a similar manner to indentation tonometry [11]. The reduction in the size of the plunger that directly measured the IOP from the flattened cornea was postulated to reduce the influence of corneal biomechanical characteristics. The original Mackay-Marg tonometer is no longer commercially available, but the Tonopen, a portable tonometer, simple to use and unaffected by position, is based on a similar principle [12] (Fig. 12.1d).

iCare

In the 1930s the concept of ballistic tonometry was used to refer to a new type of tonometer that measured the IOP based on the dynamic response of a small hammer striking the cornea at a constant and known speed [13]. Over the years this type of tonometry was renamed "rebound tonometry" and was translated into a commercially available portable device [14]. This instrument was designed to be used without local anaesthesia, be fully portable, and based on a principle of tonometry other than applanation or indentation. It uses a 1 mm diameter probe that strikes the cornea at a known speed, and the instrument measures the deceleration of the probe when it rebounds after the impact (Fig. 12.1a).

ART

The ART tonometer, described above (Sect. "Applanation Resonance Tonometry"), can be used with a handheld adapter as a portable tonometer. As the tip of the tonometer moves towards the cornea automatically, when handheld, it can obtain IOP measurement in any position.

Portable Non-contact Tonometer

Portable NCT technology has been available since the late 1980s when the Pulsair tonometer became commercially available [15]. More recently the PT-100 tonometer, using the same NCT technology, is a newer, lighter, and more portable version [16].

Table 12.1 briefly summarises the mechanism that each tonometer uses to measure IOP, advantages, disadvantages, IOP results in comparison to GAT, and how much is influenced by OR. Unfortunately, all the available instruments are affected to a certain extent by other forces in addition to the true IOP and the results should be interpreted with care.

Table 12.1 Summary table of available tonometers, along with their advantages, disadvantages and relation to GAT readings and OR

Mechanism of action	Tonometer	Advantages	Disadvantages	IOP results in comparison to GAT (17)[a]	Degree of influence by ocular rigidity
Indentation	Shiotz	Very affordable Easy to use	Direct contact Supine position	−0.24 (−6.6 to 6.1)[a]	Significant
Applanation	GAT	Affordable Most widely used Reference for clinical use	Direct contact Training required	Reference	Moderate
	NCT	Easy to use No contact	Expensive	0.2 (−3.8 to 4.3)[a]	Moderate
	Perkins	Affordable Same mechanism as reference GAT	Direct contact Training required	−1.2 (−5.2 to 2.8)[a]	Moderate
	Pneumotonometer	Can be used for tonography Reports the ocular pulse waveform	Direct contact Training required	5.5 (0.8–10.2)[b]	Minimal
Mixed	Tonopen	Portable Not affected by the position Easy to use	Expensive Requires a new tip cover per patient	−0.2 (−6.2 to 5.9)[a]	Moderate
Rebound	iCare	Portable One version is not affected by the position Easy to use No anaesthesia required	Expensive Requires a new probe per patient	0.9 (−4.3 to 6.1)[a]	Moderate

(continued)

Table 12.1 (continued)

Mechanism of action	Tonometer	Advantages	Disadvantages	IOP results in comparison to GAT (17)[a]	Degree of influence by ocular rigidity
Less influenced by corneal biomechanics	DCT	Reports ocular pulse amplitude	Direct contact Requires a new tip cover per patient	1.8 (−2.9 to 6.5)[a]	Minimal
	ART	Portable or slit-lamp based Not affected by the position Easy to use	Direct contact	1.7 (−4.3 to 7.6)[b]	Moderate
NCT + evaluation of corneal biomechanics	ORA	Easy to use No contact	Expensive	1.5 (−3.9 to 7.0)[a]	Moderate[c]
	Corvis ST	Easy to use No contact	Very expensive	−3.8 (−7.5 to −0.2)[b]	Moderate[c]

[a]Data from pooled estimates presented as mean difference compared to GAT (mean IOP from the comparator tonometer minus mean GAT IOP) and the 95% limits of agreement [17]
[b]Data from a single publication [18–21]
[c]Could be minimal if corrections based on biomechanical variables are used to improve the accuracy

The Relationship Between Ocular Rigidity and Tonometry

OR is an ophthalmic concept that was initially introduced by Friedenwald in an attempt to understand the reason that IOP readings vary so much among different tonometers [22]. OR was defined as a measure of the resistance which the eye exerts to distending forces, and it is the result of a combination of the morphological characteristics and material properties of the eyeball. On the other hand, the most appropriate engineering term to describe the eye pressure-volume relationship is elasticity, as measured by Young's modulus, and utilising Pascals (Pa) as the units of measurement. Elasticity has the ability to investigate the independent contributions of the material properties and morphological characteristics of the eye [23]. Young's modulus, or modulus of elasticity, is defined as the ratio of the stress (load per unit area) and strain (displacement per unit length). Mathematical modelling of the effect of changes in corneal characteristics on GAT, e.g. thickness, curvature, and Young's modulus, demonstrate that all affect GAT tonometry but, the greatest impact is from changes in Young's modulus [24].

Irrespective of the terminology used to explain the pressure-volume relationship in the eye, OR or Young's modulus, these have been identified as the variables with the greatest influence on IOP readings [25, 26]. However, in clinical practice, the most common variable that is investigated is central corneal thickness (CCT), even though it only represents one aspect of the morphological characteristics of the eye and does not measure the material properties. In addition, mathematical modelling has shown that variation in CCT only explains a difference of 2.87 mmHg in the predicted IOP readings [24].

The ORA is described in more detail in Sect. "Applanation Tonometers", but is important to mention, as it has been extensively studied, and the biomechanical variables that are reported (CH = corneal hysteresis, and CRF = corneal resistance factor) are sometimes used as surrogates of OR or elasticity. However, these variables seem to represent only a small portion of the biomechanical properties of the eye and not the full elasticity or OR. For instance, in patients with keratoconus who have undergone corneal cross-linking (CXL) and who have had their CH and CRS measured before and after the intervention, no change in these variables was demonstrated [27], even though corneas after CXL have been found to have a fourfold increase in Young's modulus [28]. It seems that CH and CRS represent the viscoelastic properties of the cornea and not the full OR or Young's modulus of elasticity.

Effect of Ocular Rigidity on the IOP Readings from Different Tonometers

As previously discussed, OR affects tonometry, but the magnitude of this influence varies among different tonometers (Table 12.1). In the following section, we will broadly classify, by mechanism of action, the most widely used and novel tonometers, and discuss how OR can affect the IOP readings.

Applanation Tonometers

Differences in the material properties or morphological characteristics of the eye such as CCT, corneal astigmatism, corneal curvature, and axial length produce changes in OR and influence IOP readings compared with the IOP as measured by manometry [29]. For instance, the area that needs to be flattened with the tip of the tonometer or with a jet of air (7.35 mm², 10.18 mm², 19.6 mm² for GAT, NCT, or pneumotonometer) will be influenced by OR and hence, if the OR is higher or lower, the pressure required to produce the same applanation will be correspondingly greater or lesser. Also, the amount of aqueous humour displaced by the indentation will vary, depending on morphological characteristics such as corneal curvature [30].

One influence of OR on IOP, that is unique to NCT, is the effect of the time taken to flatten the cornea. It is possible that, in situations where other biomechanical characteristics are similar, the applanation created by a jet of air in NCT is influenced more by changes in OR because of the rapidity of the applanation (8–20 ms) in comparison with the slower manual applanation in GAT [31].

The ORA and the Corvis ST that measure IOP with an NCT tonometer are influenced similarly to other NCT equipment. However, they have the advantage that they measure some of the biomechanical characteristics of the eye that are responsible for inaccuracies in applanation tonometry [32]. Newer methods of postprocessing data help to identify corneal parameters that better represent Young's modulus of elasticity [27, 33, 34]. Adjustments for these newer biomechanical parameters that better represent OR might produce a better estimate of the true IOP. However, further studies are required to compare these new IOP-corrected readings with manometry and confirm if they are more accurate.

Indentation Tonometers

The Shiotz tonometer assumes an average scleral rigidity and produces unexpected IOP readings in individuals with higher or lower OR such as hyperopes and myopes respectively. This type of tonometry is significantly affected by OR because it measures the IOP by directly gauging how much the plunger sinks (pushes the cornea inwards) in comparison to the footplate [35]. In addition, this technique displaces more aqueous humour than any other tonometer, which can further affect the IOP reading.

Mixed Indentation and Applanation Tonometers

The combined mechanism of action and the very small area of indentation of Tonopen result in this tonometer being less influenced by CCT than applanation tonometry [32]. It also seems to be less affected by the expected ageing increase in OR compared to applanation tonometry [31].

Rebound Tonometers

One variable that is critical to this tonometer is the distance from the probe to the eye before it is triggered (recommended 3–5 mm) and the angle of contact between the probe and the cornea (recommended <25°). These variables will influence the effect that different parameters involved in OR will have on the final IOP readings.

This method of tonometry seems to be particularly affected by CCT [36], as has been demonstrated in healthy individuals and more dramatically in children with glaucoma and thick corneas [37]. The limits of agreement, when compared with GAT in children with IOP readings over 21 mmHg and thick corneas, were from −21.08 to 10.04 mmHg. This discrepancy could be partially explained by CCT, but some other variables must be involved to create these very broad limits of agreement. For instance, it has been reported that corneal hysteresis is significantly correlated with IOP readings taken using the iCare rebound tonometer [38]. This could reflect the greater influence that some biomechanical characteristics might have on this tonometer.

Dynamic Contour Tonometer

The Dynamic Contour Tonometer was manufactured with the aim of reducing the influence of corneal biomechanics by creating minimal distortion of the cornea when measuring the IOP. It has proved to be less influenced by corneal biomechanics and more accurate when compared to other tonometers in cadaveric or in vivo manometry. DCT was shown to be more accurate in comparison to GAT and pneumotonometer [39, 40] and it has been investigated in patients with corneal pathology and found to be less influenced by CCT compared to GAT [41].

ART

ART measures the flattened area of the cornea with a resonance sensor, based on the acoustic impedance of the eye. It has been suggested that the slow reduction in anterior chamber volume associated with ageing, could affect impedance in the eye and potentially underestimate the IOP readings of elderly individuals [42]. A study with healthy young and healthy elderly participants found higher GAT-IOP in elderly while ART-IOP readings were the same in both age groups. The acoustic impedance could also be increased and underestimate IOP readings if the corneal epithelium is damaged and the probe is in direct contact with deeper layers of the cornea. It could also be decreased and overestimate the IOP readings if the cornea is not sufficiently moist. Another characteristic of this tonometer is that it requires very good tip centration on the cornea. Failure to achieve good centration has been considered a possible explanation for the lower precision compared to GAT when measurements are repeated in the same individuals [43]. This tonometer significantly overestimates the results when the IOP is higher than 21 mmHg, which could be due to the effect of high IOP on OR, independent of CCT.

Effect of Post-surgical Changes in Ocular Rigidity on Different Tonometers

Investigation of the changes in IOP readings after surgery is complicated due to different reasons (1) the possibility that the surgical intervention itself might have produced a real change in the IOP, (2) the complex and non-homogeneous healing process between and within individuals, and (3) the variability in the surgical technique that causes different morphological changes after the same procedure in different individuals and also in each eye of the same individual. Chapter 16 explores in more detail the relationship between OR and surgery. In this section, we will briefly describe some of the possible reasons why some surgical interventions have been reported to affect tonometry.

Refractive Surgery

The constant development of surgical options to modify the cornea for refractive purposes, reflects the continued effort to find options that have less effect on the corneal biomechanics, are less likely to produce corneal ectasia, and therefore would also have less effect on tonometry. Unfortunately, recent surgical techniques (e.g. SMILE compared to LASIK [44]) have not been shown to reduce the impact on corneal biomechanics [45], and most tonometers seem to be affected [46].

All refractive procedures influence some of the variables that comprise OR to some extent. The morphology of the cornea is modified by a reduction in its thickness, curvature, topography, and selective change in specific layers. The material properties of the cornea may also be affected by the wound healing process. The more dependent the tonometer on corneal biomechanical properties, the greater the influence will be. For that reason, tonometers less influenced by corneal biomechanics, like the DCT, produce IOP readings after refractive surgery that are closer to the pre-operative values than those that are more influenced by corneal biomechanics. It has therefore been suggested that the DCT is a more accurate tonometer in such patients [47]. Another approach in overcoming the changes in GAT IOP readings after surgery has been the use of correction formulae based on preoperative data, surgical data, postoperative changes, age, or a combination of variables [48]. This approach works statistically, but unfortunately, when the results are individualised, they are not sufficiently accurate to be of clinical use.

Cross-Linking

The influence of corneal cross-linking on tonometric measurements is difficult to assess because it is performed in patients with progressive keratoconus that will have, by definition, corneas that are far from the ideal assumed by the Imbert-Fick law for applanation tonometry. Cross-linking modifies corneal curvature, thickness, topography, and microarchitecture of the collagen fibrils but, in the few studies that have reported IOP, the changes seem to be minimal [49].

Corneal Transplantation

The increased risk of developing glaucoma after different types of corneal transplantation and the prolonged use of steroids makes the recording of accurate IOP essential to avoid serious and irreversible glaucomatous damage. The expected variation in IOP after the surgery itself and the significant alteration of corneal architecture renders estimation of the most accurate form of tonometry, extremely difficult. Even if we assume that the true postoperative IOP is the same as that before the transplant, the material and the morphological characteristics of the cornea will have been modified, and all types of tonometers will be affected. Different tonometers will be influenced to different degrees, depending on the type of transplant [50–53]. For instance, lamellar transplants, which are becoming more common, significantly increase CCT and tonometers that are heavily influenced by this parameter, have been shown to underperform [53]. Finally, it is important to emphasise that publications that have compared different tonometers during the postoperative follow-up after corneal transplantation have reported results with significantly different IOP measurements and very wide limits of agreement [54].

Vitrectomy

The removal of the vitreous, replacing it with gas or silicone oil affects corneal biomechanics measured by ORA. Although other components of OR, that have not been measured, may also be altered. The architectural changes induced by pars plana incisions, the change in choroidal thickness and circulation [55], and the direct effect of silicone oil or gas [56, 57] could affect OR by different mechanisms. For example, IOP readings change when measured with different tonometers in eyes after silicone oil exchange [58].

Scleral Buckling

It has been shown in the past, that tonometers are differentially affected by buckling procedures [59], which influence multiple components of OR. The anterior chamber angle and depth [60], the pulsatile ocular blood flow [61], and the ocular pulse amplitude [62] decreased significantly after buckling and could be responsible for the changes in IOP readings.

Keratoprosthesis

After this operation, severe morphological changes in the anterior segment of the eye and the absence of a cornea, render accurate IOP measurement almost impossible. Given that recalcitrant glaucoma is extremely common after this type of surgery, the inability to measure IOP accurately is one of the obstacles to success in keratoprosthesis surgery. Scleral tonometry with indentation methods, tonopen, pneumotonometer, or rebound tonometer have been suggested as options to monitor IOP [63, 64] but overall, IOP measurement is extremely challenging in these eyes.

Glaucoma Surgery

Trabeculectomy, deep sclerectomy, and glaucoma drainage devices produce changes in OR that affect tonometry, in addition to the real reduction in IOP. Changes in corneal curvature, reduction in axial length, and increased in corneal hysteresis have been reported, and these will affect tonometers differently [65].

Clinical Implications

OR influences all tonometric IOP readings, but the magnitude of the effect varies between individuals and between eyes in the same person. The effect of OR on the measurements produced by different tonometers depends on numerous factors that can be roughly divided into changes in morphology of specific structures in the eye or changes in the materials that comprise the tissues of the eye. In clinical practices, what eye care professionals face, is variability between tonometers and poor accuracy in IOP readings. It is important to remember that abnormal IOP readings have a different impact on the management of patients depending on the clinical scenario.

The following four scenarios cover most of the management dilemmas faced by clinicians:

1. *Incidental discovery of high IOP in an otherwise healthy eye:* A typical example is a high IOP with NCT on routine optometric examination. In this scenario, it is important to repeat the measurement and confirm the IOP level using a different tonometer (usually GAT). For example, the UK NICE guidelines for glaucoma in 2017, changed the recommendation on identification of patients that require referral to an ophthalmologist, based on IOP elevation. They increased the threshold IOP for referral from 21 to 24 mmHg and recommended that it should be recorded on two different visits [66].

2. *Unexpectedly low IOP in an individual with glaucomatous neuropathy:* After pathological causes for hypotony have been excluded (cyclodialysis cleft, uveitis, retinal detachment, etc.), it is important to search for reasons that could reduce OR (thin CCT, low CH, previous refractive surgery, etc.)

3. *Unexpectedly high IOP in an individual with glaucomatous neuropathy:* After confirming good compliance with medication; factors that overestimate the IOP should be considered (thick CCT, high CH, etc). Finally, the clinician should carefully remember that IOP is only one part of the examination and clinical decisions should be supported by other important parameters such as visual fields, optic nerve topographic assessment, or retinal nerve fibre layer measurement.

4. *Unexpectedly abnormal IOP after ophthalmic surgery:* In the early postoperative period it is important to consider high or low IOP as a direct consequence of surgery, until proven otherwise. It is common to develop hypotony or IOP spikes after surgery, but it is impossible to fully predict when this will happen. Later in the postoperative period, if unexpected IOP readings are encountered, the following ocular changes induced by surgery that could over or underestimate the true IOP should be considered: increased CCT due to transient corneal oedema, changes in corneal curvature induced by sutures, shortening or elongation of AL after glaucoma surgery or scleral buckling, changes in choroidal thickness or circulation after intraocular surgery.

The following points emphasise frequently discussed topics, and clinical considerations with relevance to daily practice:

1. *Correction of IOP based on CCT:* The well-known relationship between CCT and IOP has driven some researchers to develop regression models to account for the influence of CCT on the true IOP. Although this could be a useful method to analyse data from populations, regression models and equations that have been popularised are insufficiently accurate to use in individual patients. To correct for CCT in clinical practice is safer to categorise patients in groups of thin, normal, and thick and consider this as a rough guide to the possible over or underestimation of the true IOP.

2. *Automatic corrections of IOP from instruments that measure other ocular parameters:* ORA and Corvis ST measure multiple ocular parameters that influence OR and can be used to correct the recorded IOP based on the NCT technology that those instruments use. It is important to emphasise that any correction has risks of over or underestimating IOP and should not be considered as a direct recording of the true IOP but a post-acquisition correction.

3. *Use of IOP readings from different tonometers interchangeably:* Even when mean IOP readings are similar in studies comparing two types of tonometer, the readings can still not be considered interchangeable. When IOP readings from single participants are compared, the limits of agreements can be extremely wide and the reporting of similar means over larger numbers of patients can be misleading with respect to the individual patient.

References

1. Goldmann H, Schmidt T. Applanation tonometry. Ophthalmologica. 1957;134(4):221–42.
2. GGl C, Fitt AD, Sweeney J. On the validity of the Imbert-Fick Law: mathematical modelling of eye pressure measurement. World J Mech. 2016;06(03):17.
3. Grolman B. A new tonometer system. Am J Optom Arch Am Acad Optom. 1972;49(8):646–60.
4. Durham DG, Bigliano RP, Masino JA. Pneumatic applanation tonometer. Trans Am Acad Ophthalmol Otolaryngol. 1965;69(6):1029–47.
5. Kanngiesser HE, Robert YA. Dynamic contour tonometry. Invest Ophthalmol Vis Sci. 2002;43(13):301.
6. Eklund A, Backlund T, Lindahl OA. A resonator sensor for measurement of intraocular pressure–evaluation in an in vitro pig-eye model. Physiol Meas. 2000;21(3):355–67.
7. Eklund A, Hallberg P, Linden C, Lindahl OA. An applanation resonator sensor for measuring intraocular pressure using combined continuous force and area measurement. Invest Ophthalmol Vis Sci. 2003;44(7):3017–24.
8. Luce DA. Determining in vivo biomechanical properties of the cornea with an ocular response analyzer. J Cataract Refract Surg. 2005;31(1):156–62.
9. Roberts CJ, Mahmoud AM, Ramos I, Caldas D, Silva RSD. Factors influencing corneal deformation and estimation of intraocular pressure. Invest Ophthalmol Vis Sci. 2011;52(14):4384.
10. Mackay RS, Marg E. Fast, automatic, electronic tonometers based on an exact theory. Acta Ophthalmol. 1959;37:495–507.
11. Moses RA. The Mackay-Marg tonometer. A report to the committee on standardization of tonometers. Trans Am Acad Ophthalmol Otolaryngol. 1962;66:88–95.
12. Hessemer V, Rossler R, Jacobi KW. Comparison of intraocular pressure measurements with the Oculab Tono-Pen vs manometry in humans shortly after death. Am J Ophthalmol. 1988;105(6):678–82.
13. Dekking HM, Coster HD. Dynamic tonometry. Ophthalmologica. 1967;154(1):59–74.
14. Kontiola A. A new electromechanical method for measuring intraocular pressure. Doc Ophthalmol. 1996;93(3):265–76.
15. Fisher JH, Watson PG, Spaeth G. A new handheld air impulse tonometer. Eye (Lond). 1988;2(Pt 3):238–42.
16. Muller A, Godenschweger L, Lang GE, Kampmeier J. Prospective comparison of the new indentation tonometer TGdC-01, the non-contact tonometer PT100 and the conventional Goldmann applanation tonometer. Klin Monatsbl Augenheilkd. 2004;221(9):762–8.
17. Cook JA, Botello AP, Elders A, Fathi Ali A, Azuara-Blanco A, Fraser C, et al. Systematic review of the agreement of tonometers with Goldmann applanation tonometry. Ophthalmology. 2012;119(8):1552–7.
18. Barkana Y, Gutfreund S. Measurement of the difference in intraocular pressure between the sitting and lying body positions in healthy subjects: direct comparison of the iCare pro with the Goldmann applanation tonometer, Pneumatonometer and Tonopen XL. Clin Exp Ophthalmol. 2014;42(7):608–14.
19. Ottobelli L, Fogagnolo P, Frezzotti P, De Cilla S, Vallenzasca E, Digiuni M, et al. Repeatability and reproducibility of applanation resonance tonometry: a cross-sectional study. BMC Ophthalmol. 2015;15:36.
20. Nakao Y, Kiuchi Y, Okimoto SA. Comparison of the corrected intraocular pressure obtained by the Corvis ST and Reichert 7CR Tonometers in Glaucoma patients. PLoS One. 2017;12(1):e0170206.
21. Jain AK, Saini JS, Gupta R. Tonometry in normal and scarred corneas, and inpostkeratoplasty eyes: a comparative study of the Goldmann, the ProTon and the Schiotz tonometers. Indian J Ophthalmol. 2000;48(1):25–32.
22. Friedenwald J. Contribution to the theory and practice of tonometry. Am J Ophthalmol. 1937;20(10):985–1024.
23. Young WC, Budynas RG. Roark's formulas for stress and strain. New York: McGraw-Hill; 2001.

24. Liu J, Roberts CJ. Influence of corneal biomechanical properties on intraocular pressure measurement: quantitative analysis. J Cataract Refract Surg. 2005;31(1):146–55.
25. Sit AJ, Lin SC, Kazemi A, McLaren JW, Pruet CM, Zhang X. In vivo noninvasive measurement of Young's Modulus of elasticity in human eyes: a feasibility study. J Glaucoma. 2017;26(11):967–73.
26. Eisenlohr JE, Langham ME, Maumenee AE. Manometric studies of the pressure-volume relationship in living and enucleated eyes of individual human subjects. Br J Ophthalmol. 1962;46(9):536–48.
27. Spoerl E, Terai N, Scholz F, Raiskup F, Pillunat LE. Detection of biomechanical changes after corneal cross-linking using ocular response analyzer software. J Refract Surg (Thorofare, NJ 1995). 2011;27(6):452–7.
28. Wollensak G, Spoerl E, Seiler T. Stress-strain measurements of human and porcine corneas after riboflavin-ultraviolet-A-induced cross-linking. J Cataract Refract Surg. 2003;29(9):1780–5.
29. Whitacre MM, Stein R. Sources of error with use of Goldmann-type tonometers. Surv Ophthalmol. 1993;38(1):1–30.
30. Abdalla MI, Hamdi M. Applanation ocular tension in myopia and emmetropia. Br J Ophthalmol. 1970;54(2):122–5.
31. Tonnu PA, Ho T, Newson T, El Sheikh A, Sharma K, White E, et al. The influence of central corneal thickness and age on intraocular pressure measured by pneumotonometry, non-contact tonometry, the Tono-Pen XL, and Goldmann applanation tonometry. Br J Ophthalmol. 2005;89(7):851–4.
32. Mollan SP, Wolffsohn JS, Nessim M, Laiquzzaman M, Sivakumar S, Hartley S, et al. Accuracy of Goldmann, ocular response analyser, Pascal and TonoPen XL tonometry in keratoconic and normal eyes. Br J Ophthalmol. 2008;92(12):1661–5.
33. Matalia J, Francis M, Tejwani S, Dudeja G, Rajappa N, Sinha Roy A. Role of age and myopia in simultaneous assessment of corneal and extraocular tissue stiffness by air-puff applanation. J Refract Surg (Thorofare, NJ 1995). 2016;32(7):486–93.
34. Shih PJ, Huang CJ, Huang TH, Lin HC, Yen JY, Wang IJ, et al. Estimation of the corneal Young's modulus in vivo based on a fluid-filled spherical-Shell model with Scheimpflug imaging. J Ophthalmol. 2017;2017:5410143.
35. Patel H, Gilmartin B, Cubbidge RP, Logan NS. In vivo measurement of regional variation in anterior scleral resistance to Schiotz indentation. Ophthalmic Physiol Opt. 2011;31(5):437–43.
36. Dey A, David RL, Asokan R, George R. Can corneal biomechanical properties explain difference in tonometric measurement in normal eyes? Optometry Vis Sci. 2018;95(2):120–8.
37. Dahlmann-Noor AH, Puertas R, Tabasa-Lim S, El-Karmouty A, Kadhim M, Wride NK, et al. Comparison of handheld rebound tonometry with Goldmann applanation tonometry in children with glaucoma: a cohort study. BMJ Open. 2013;3(4)
38. Chui W-S, Lam A, Chen D, Chiu R. The influence of corneal properties on rebound tonometry. Ophthalmology. 2008;115(1):80–4.
39. Kniestedt C, Nee M, Stamper RL. Accuracy of dynamic contour tonometry compared with applanation tonometry in human cadaver eyes of different hydration states. Graefes Arch Clin Exp Ophthalmol. 2005;243(4):359–66.
40. Boehm AG, Weber A, Pillunat LE, Koch R, Spoerl E. Dynamic contour tonometry in comparison to intracameral IOP measurements. Invest Ophthalmol Vis Sci. 2008;49(6):2472–7.
41. Ozbek Z, Cohen EJ, Hammersmith KM, Rapuano CJ. Dynamic contour tonometry: a new way to assess intraocular pressure in ectatic corneas. Cornea. 2006;25(8):890–4.
42. Johannesson G, Hallberg P, Ambarki K, Eklund A, Linden C. Age-dependency of ocular parameters: a cross sectional study of young and elderly healthy subjects. Graefes Arch Clin Exp Ophthalmol. 2015;253(11):1979–83.
43. Salvetat ML, Zeppieri M, Tosoni C, Brusini P. Repeatability and accuracy of applanation resonance tonometry in healthy subjects and patients with glaucoma. Acta Ophthalmol. 2014;92(1):e66–73.
44. Sefat SM, Wiltfang R, Bechmann M, Mayer WJ, Kampik A, Kook D. Evaluation of changes in human corneas after femtosecond laser-assisted LASIK and Small-Incision Lenticule

Extraction (SMILE) using non-contact tonometry and ultra-high-speed camera (Corvis ST). Curr Eye Res. 2016;41(7):917–22.

45. Fernandez J, Rodriguez-Vallejo M, Martinez J, Tauste A, Pinero DP. Corneal biomechanics after laser refractive surgery: unmasking differences between techniques. J Cataract Refract Surg. 2018;44(3):390–8.

46. Yao WJ, Crossan AS. An update on postrefractive surgery intraocular pressure determination. Curr Opin Ophthalmol. 2014;25(4):258–63.

47. Aristeidou AP, Labiris G, Katsanos A, Fanariotis M, Foudoulakis NC, Kozobolis VP. Comparison between Pascal dynamic contour tonometer and Goldmann applanation tonometer after different types of refractive surgery. Graefes Arch Clin Exp Ophthalmol. 2011;249(5):767–73.

48. De Bernardo M, Capasso L, Caliendo L, Vosa Y, Rosa N. Intraocular pressure evaluation after myopic refractive surgery: a comparison of methods in 121 eyes. Semin Ophthalmol. 2016;31(3):233–42.

49. Meiri Z, Keren S, Rosenblatt A, Sarig T, Shenhav L, Varssano D. Efficacy of corneal collagen cross-linking for the treatment of Keratoconus: a systematic review and meta-analysis. Cornea. 2016;35(3):417–28.

50. Murugesan V, Bypareddy R, Kumar M, Tanuj D, Anita P. Evaluation of corneal biomechanical properties following penetrating keratoplasty using ocular response analyzer. Indian J Ophthalmol. 2014;62(4):454–60.

51. Faramarzi A, Feizi S, Najdi D, Ghiasian L, Karimian F. Changes in corneal biomechanical properties after Descemet stripping automated endothelial keratoplasty for pseudophakic bullous keratopathy. Cornea. 2016;35(1):20–4.

52. Clemmensen K, Hjortdal J. Intraocular pressure and corneal biomechanics in Fuchs' endothelial dystrophy and after posterior lamellar keratoplasty. Acta Ophthalmol. 2014;92(4):350–4.

53. Achiron A, Blumenfeld O, Avizemer H, Karmona L, Leybowich G, Man V, et al. Intraocular pressure measurement after DSAEK by iCare, Goldmann applanation and dynamic contour tonometry: a comparative study. J Fr Ophtalmol. 2016;39(10):822–8.

54. Salvetat ML, Zeppieri M, Miani F, Tosoni C, Parisi L, Brusini P. Comparison of iCare tonometer and Goldmann applanation tonometry in normal corneas and in eyes with automated lamellar and penetrating keratoplasty. Eye (Lond). 2011;25(5):642–50.

55. Ahn SJ, Woo SJ, Park KH. Choroidal thickness change following vitrectomy in idiopathic epiretinal membrane and macular hole. Graefes Arch Clin Exp Ophthalmol. 2016;254(6):1059–67.

56. Teke MY, Elgin U, Sen E, Ozdal P, Ozturk F. Early effects of pars plana vitrectomy combined with intravitreal gas tamponade on corneal biomechanics. Ophthalmologica. 2013;229(3):137–41.

57. Teke MY, Elgin U, Sen E, Ozdal P, Ozturk F. Intravitreal silicone oil induced changes in corneal biomechanics. Int Ophthalmol. 2014;34(3):457–63.

58. Zhang Y, Zheng L, Bian A, Zhou Q. IOP measurement in silicone oil tamponade eyes by Corvis ST tonometer, Goldmann applanation tonometry and non-contact tonometry. Int Ophthalmol. 2017;38(2):697–703.

59. Harbin TS Jr, Laikam SE, Lipsitt K, Jarrett WH 2nd, Hagler WS. Applanation-Schiotz disparity after retinal detachment surgery utilizing cryopexy. Ophthalmology. 1979;86(9):1609–12.

60. Khanduja S, Bansal N, Arora V, Sobti A, Garg S, Dada T. Evaluation of the effect of scleral buckling on the anterior chamber angle using ASOCT. J Glaucoma. 2015;24(4):267–71.

61. Yokota H, Mori F, Nagaoka T, Sugawara R, Yoshida A. Pulsatile ocular blood flow: changes associated with scleral buckling procedures. Jpn J Ophthalmol. 2005;49(2):162–5.

62. Katsimpris JM, Petropoulos IK, Pournaras CJ. Ocular pulse amplitude measurement after retinal detachment surgery. Klin Monatsbl Augenheilkd. 2003;220(3):127–30.

63. Lin CC, Chen A, Jeng BH, Porco TC, Ou Y, Han Y. Scleral intraocular pressure measurement in cadaver eyes pre- and postkeratoprosthesis implantation. Invest Ophthalmol Vis Sci. 2014;55(4):2244–50.

64. Estrovich IE, Shen C, Chu Y, Downs JC, Gardiner S, Straiko M, et al. Schiotz tonometry accurately measures intraocular pressure in Boston type 1 keratoprosthesis eyes. Cornea. 2015;34(6):682–5.
65. Pakravan M, Afroozifar M, Yazdani S. Corneal biomechanical changes following trabeculectomy, phaco-trabeculectomy, Ahmed glaucoma valve implantation and phacoemulsification. J Ophthal Vis Res. 2014;9(1):7–13.
66. Gulland A. Patients with low risk of developing glaucoma should not be referred to specialist care, says NICE. BMJ. 2017;j5100:359.

Chapter 13
Tonography and Ocular Rigidity

Eric Chan and Carol B. Toris

Introduction

Aqueous Humor Dynamics

Aqueous humor production, circulation and drainage (aqueous humor dynamics) maintain the intraocular pressure (IOP) in the eye. This pressure is maintained under careful homeostasis to preserve optic nerve health and clear vision. Aqueous humor is produced by the ciliary processes of the ciliary body, then is secreted into the posterior chamber where it flows mainly through the pupil into the anterior chamber. Drainage from the anterior chamber occurs through one of two outflow pathways: uveoscleral and trabecular. Abnormal changes to drainage can lead to elevated IOP and an increased risk of glaucoma. Treatments for glaucoma target aqueous humor production or its drainage pathways. Uveoscleral outflow is an unconventional pathway with less resistance. This pathway includes drainage from the anterior chamber into the ciliary muscle. From there the fluid flows in multiple directions including the supraciliary and suprachoroidal spaces, across the sclera, through emisarial canals, and into choroidal vessels. Trabecular outflow is a conventional, pressure dependent pathway that includes the trabecular meshwork, Schlemm's canal, and a series of channels and veins. Resistance in this pathway is ten times that

E. Chan
Department of Ophthalmology and Visual Sciences, Case Western Reserve University, Cleveland, OH, USA

C. B. Toris (✉)
Department of Ophthalmology and Visual Sciences, Case Western Reserve University, Cleveland, OH, USA

Department of Ophthalmology and Visual Sciences, University of Nebraska Medical Center, Omaha, NE, USA
e-mail: ctoris@unmc.edu

© Springer Nature Switzerland AG 2021
I. Pallikaris et al. (eds.), *Ocular Rigidity, Biomechanics and Hydrodynamics of the Eye*, https://doi.org/10.1007/978-3-030-64422-2_13

of the uveoscleral outflow pathway. The resistance is mainly in the proximal drainage system beginning in the layers of the trabecular meshwork. The juxtacanicular layer, which precedes Schlemm's canal along the pathway, offers the highest resistance to outflow in the trabecular meshwork system. The next areas of resistance are the endothelial membrane surrounding Schlemm's canal and the canal itself, the dimensions of which can vary dynamically due to ocular pulse amplitude. The distal outflow pathway lies beyond Schlemm's canal starting at the collector channel entrance, followed by the intrascleral collector channels of the deep scleral plexus, and then the episcleral and aqueous veins superficially. Choroidal vascular volume, ocular pulsation and scleral rigidity are some of the factors that affect the distal outflow resistance in the collector channels in addition to the scleral and episcleral venous drainage system [1, 2]. Reduction in outflow resistance lowers IOP and is a treatment modality for glaucoma. Assessment of this resistance is difficult but important. An accessible assessment of outflow facility in humans is by tonography.

To further understand the pathophysiology of glaucoma from the perspective of outflow facility decline, tonography serves a key role in research studies with a more limited role in clinical diagnostics. Accurate determination of outflow facility values is important in glaucomatous eyes. Additionally, ocular wall biomechanics, which includes the elastic properties of the sclera, cornea and choroid, behave differently in glaucoma and thus will influence the results of tonography.

Practice of Tonography

Tonography Instruments

Tonography is a method of measuring outflow facility, the inverse of outflow resistance. Tonography has been fundamentally unchanged since its inception many decades ago. It was designed initially to serve as a tool to diagnose glaucoma. Two instruments to access outflow facility are the Schiøtz tonometer (Fig. 13.1) and the pneumatonometer (Fig. 13.2).

The Schiøtz tonometer consists of a foot plate with a 15 mm radius of curvature connected to a plunger with variable applied weights (usually 5.5, 7.5, 10, or 15 g). The carrier portion containing the footplate weighs 11.0 g. With the subject in a supine position and eyes gazing at the ceiling, the tonometer is applied to the cornea which becomes indented by the weight of the footplate and plunger. The indentation does not cause an immediate change in total intraocular volume since intraocular fluid, composed primarily of water, is non-compressible. Instead, the cornea deforms and ocular tissues distend, while intraocular pressure increases as dictated by the pressure-volume inverse relationship in an enclosed chamber. The Schiøtz tonometer provides a reading correlated to the intraocular pressure when the weight is applied (Table 13.1). Based on the nomogram curve generated by Jonas Friedenwald [4] (Fig. 13.3), the intraocular pressure before the weight is applied, or

Fig. 13.1 Schiøtz
tonometer with different
weight attachments

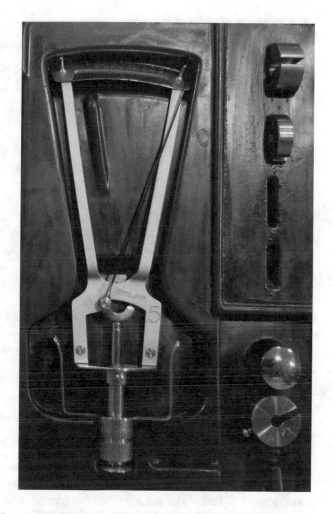

the steady state pressure P_0, can be determined by tracing the nomogram curve back
to the corresponding value when no weight is applied and the indentation volume is
zero. P_0 is needed to determine the outflow facility coefficient (see Eq. 13.1 below).
An electronic Schiøtz tonometer is a similar device but with the reading scale
replaced with an electronic amplifier and recording galvanometer such that measurements can be recorded continuously on a paper strip and can facilitate tonography measurements [3, 5].

The pneumatonometer uses a near frictionless applanation surface generated by
flowing gas. A cylinder probe with a plastic sensor tip covered with a thin porous
silicone membrane contacts the cornea. Gas flows through a valve into the system
through the porous membrane to create an air bearing. The tip of the probe contacts
the cornea and impedes gas flow through the membrane, which causes gas pressure
within the system to rise. Once the internal intraocular pressure and gas pressure
within the system are in balance, an electronic signal output is converted into a

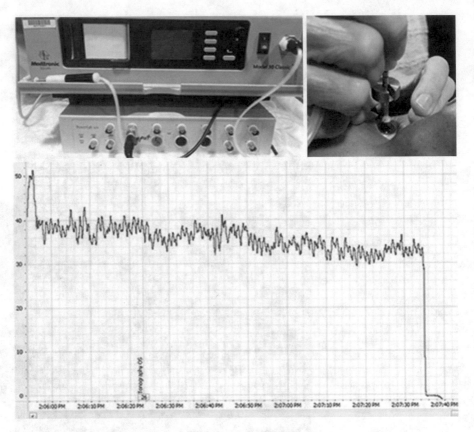

Fig. 13.2 Pneumatonography. The pneumatonometer with probe (top-left). Placement over the eye of the tonometer probe with attached 10 g weight (top-right). Example of a two-minute recorded tonography tracing of a human subject with ocular hypertension

measurement of intraocular pressure. This instrument allows for IOP measurement in both the supine and sitting positions. For tonography, a 10 g weight is attached to a small platform on the shaft of the hand piece and the probe is placed on the cornea for 2 or 4 min while the subject is in a supine position.

There have been documented differences between the pneumatonometer and the Schiøtz tonometer [6]. The Schiøtz tonometer has fewer issues with probe movement during timed tonography intervals compared to the pneumatonometer. The Schiøtz tonometer probe tip has a large concave diameter, whereas, the pneumatonometer probe tip is flat with a small diameter which predisposes it to a higher incidence of probe movement when held by the user. Consequently, the pneumatonometer has higher inter-subject and inter-observer measurement variability in comparison to the Schiøtz tonometer, although the calculated outflow facility values from the two instruments are similar [7, 8]. Each of these instruments have numerous assumptions and limitations leaving open the need for improved methods to assess outflow facility in humans.

Table 13.1 Schiøtz tonometer calibration scale for four different weights on the probe [3]

Schiøtz Scale Reading	Intraocular pressure (mm Hg)			
	5.5 g	7.5 g	10 g	15 g
0.0	41.5	59.1	81.7	127.5
0.5	37.8	54.2	75.1	117.9
1.0	34.5	49.8	69.3	109.3
1.5	31.6	45.8	64.0	101.4
2.0	29.0	42.1	59.1	94.3
2.5	26.6	38.8	54.7	88.0
3.0	24.4	35.8	50.6	81.8
3.5	22.4	33.0	46.9	76.2
4.0	20.6	30.4	43.4	71.0
4.5	18.9	28.0	40.2	66.2
5.0	17.3	25.8	37.2	61.8
5.5	15.9	23.8	34.4	57.6
6.0	14.6	21.9	31.8	53.6
6.5	13.4	20.1	29.4	49.9
7.0	12.2	18.5	27.2	46.5
7.5	11.2	17.0	25.1	43.2
8.0	10.2	15.6	23.1	40.2
8.5	9.4	14.3	21.3	38.1
9.0	8.5	13.1	19.6	34.6
9.5	7.8	12.0	18.0	32.0
10.0	7.1	10.9	16.5	29.6
10.5	6.5	10.0	15.1	27.4
11.0	5.9	9.0	13.8	25.3
11.5	5.3	8.3	12.6	23.3
12.0	4.9	7.5	11.5	21.4
12.5	4.4	6.8	10.5	19.7
13.0	4.0	6.2	9.5	18.1
13.5		5.6	8.6	16.5
14.0		5.0	7.8	15.1
14.5		4.5	7.1	13.7
15.0		4.0	6.4	12.6
15.5			5.8	11.4
16.0			5.2	10.4
16.5			4.7	9.4
17.0			4.2	8.5
17.5				7.7
18.0				6.9
18.5				6.2
19.0				5.6
19.5				4.9
20.0				4.5

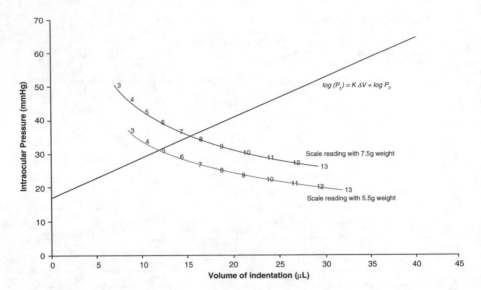

Fig. 13.3 The Friedenwald nomogram for the Schiøtz tonometer showing the relationship between indentation volume ΔV and intraocular pressure P_t. With two measurements at different weights applied to the eye, the steady state pressure P_0 and ocular rigidity K of the eye can be determined [3, 4]

Principle of Tonography

The concept of tonography is based on the principle that at different intraocular pressures, fluid will be filtered out of the anterior chamber at a constant rate (Fig. 13.4). If a weight is placed on the eye, a certain amount of fluid inside the eye will be displaced over a set amount of time. The intraocular pressure change from the added weight can be measured concurrently, and thus outflow facility can be determined as a unit of cubic millimeters of fluid (or microliters of fluid, µL) per minute per millimeter mercury of pressure (mm³/min/mm Hg). Tonographic outflow facility is a variable that is derived from other measurements including intraocular volume change and intraocular pressure. In addition, tonography is based on several theoretical assumptions and relies on calculated reference values gathered from experimental data.

Several assumptions are inherent in tonography. (1) There is continuous aqueous humor outflow. (2) Aqueous humor production is constant and is not impacted by changes in intraocular pressure. Specifically, the change in ocular volume equals the formation of aqueous humor minus the loss of aqueous humor. Thus, if aqueous humor production is held constant, then any change in ocular volume is due to aqueous humor outflow only. However, it has been shown that the production rate of aqueous humor is affected by pressure. With an increase in IOP, there is a corresponding decrease in production, which has been termed pseudofacility [10]. (3) Intraocular pressure itself is an independent variable of outflow resistance such that

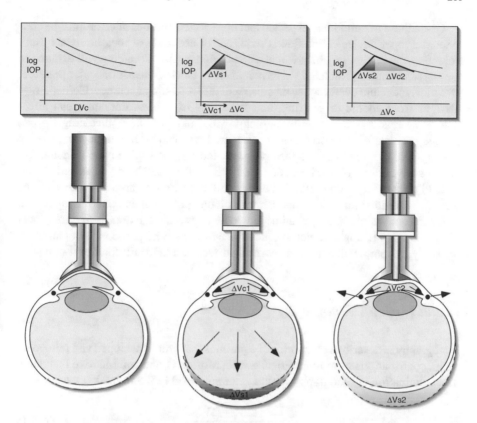

Fig. 13.4 Theory behind tonography. The figure and graph on the left summarize the effect of the tonometer probe applied to the eye without a set weight on the probe. The figure and graph in the middle show initial corneal deformation ΔV_{C_I} and scleral distention ΔV_{S_I} with immediate application of the weighted probe and subsequent intraocular pressure rise. The figure and graph on the right summarize changes during tonography, in which the weighted tonometer probe has forced fluid through the trabecular meshwork and subsequently changed the corneal deformation volume ΔV_{C2} and scleral contraction volume ΔV_{S2}. Combined, ΔV_{C2} and ΔV_{S2} represent the volume of fluid lost through the outflow system during tonography (Modified from Choplin, N., and Lundy, D. Atlas of Glaucoma. Ed. 1, London, 1998, Martin Dunitz Ltd., with permission) [9]

changing pressure within the eye does not affect how easily fluid exits the eye. (4) The uveal intravascular volume is constant during tonography. (5) Outflow facility by tonography measures facility through the trabecular meshwork, canal of Schlemm, and scleral venous network. (6) The eye maintains a steady state IOP before tonography without any ongoing IOP fluctuations [3]. (7) Tonography can vary based on ocular rigidity, which includes both scleral rigidity and corneal hysteresis (a viscoelastic property of the cornea). An average standardized value of ocular rigidity is presumed for the outflow facility calculation. It is assumed that ocular rigidity adds only a small correction factor to outflow facility values in most cases.

Given these assumptions, expected and unexpected sources of error must be considered. Proper device calibration is required for accuracy of measurements. Both voluntary and involuntary behavior can affect tonography. Coughing will disturb the measurement and a prolonged Valsalva maneuver can increase intraocular pressure. Eye movement and eyelid squeezing also will affect reading accuracy. Cornea irregularities from edema or scarring, and variations in corneal curvature can affect tonometry readings and thus tonography. Movement of the applanating tip can change the area of the cornea being measured and can alter intraocular pressure readings due to variation in applied pressure. Ideally, the supine patient should fixate on a target directly overhead, and the eyelids of the eye being measured should be held wide open without blinking during the test. Fingers can be used to keep the lids open provided that additional pressure on the globe is not applied. Evaporation of tears from the fixating eye can be slowed by covering the area with a thin sheet of plastic wrap taking care not to touch the eye itself. The probe is then placed on the study eye perpendicular to the corneal surface and held still for 2 or 4 min [3].

Initial Work on Tonography

Tonography is described by a series of equations that were developed and refined by major contributions from Jonas Friedenwald, Morton Grant, and Maurice Langham. The culmination of tonography studies is summarized in the following equation.

$$C = \frac{\Delta V_s + \Delta V_c}{\left[P_{avg} - \left(P_0 + P_s \right) \right] t} \tag{13.1}$$

C is the outflow facility, ΔV_s is the change in intraocular volume during tonography from scleral distention due to the pressure change, ΔV_c is the change in intraocular volume from corneal indentation, P_0 is the intraocular pressure before tonography, P_s is the correction of steady state pressure to account for episcleral venous pressure change during tonography, P_{avg} is the average of the initial and final intraocular pressures during the test, and t is the tonography test's time duration. Current calculations for outflow facility use an initial applanation pressure before tonography as P_0. In 1950, Morton Grant developed a simplified formula of Eq. (13.1) in which the total volume change, ΔV, is represented by a single variable and the episcleral vein pressure P_s is not taken into consideration:

$$C = \frac{\Delta V}{\left[P_{avg} - P_0 \right] t} \tag{13.2}$$

Additionally, scleral rigidity can be calculated as follows:

$$K = \frac{\log P_1 - \log P_0}{V_1 - V_0} \qquad (13.3)$$

In this equation, K is the scleral rigidity coefficient; P_0 and V_0 respectively represent the steady state pressure and volume before a weight is applied to the cornea; and P_1 and V_1 respectively represent the pressure and volume when the weight is applied. These equations were established and refined by contributions from Friedenwald, Grant, and Langham, and are discussed in the following section [4, 5, 11].

Friedenwald initially studied intraocular pressure in enucleated rabbit eyes with the Schiøtz tonometer. The eyes were connected to an open manometer and readings from the Schiøtz tonometer were correlated with co-existing intraocular pressure measurements at different applied weights. Friedenwald then developed a nomogram of intraocular pressures based on average scleral rigidity, which he calculated as 0.0215 μL^{-1}. Specifically, the key equations assumed that there was a proportional constant between corneal indentation volume and intraocular pressure represented as the coefficient of ocular rigidity. Rearranging Eq. (13.3) to:

$$\log P_1 = K \triangle V + \log P_0, \qquad (13.4)$$

a linear plot equivalent to $y = ax + b$ can be drawn with volume of indentation on the x-axis and intraocular pressure on the y-axis. The Schiøtz tonometer scale readings with different applied weights also can be plotted as an overlay (Fig. 13.3). Intraocular pressure values at two different weights are plotted to form a straight line with the y-intercept, P_0, representing the intraocular pressure before any weight is applied (i.e. steady state pressure) and with the slope of the line, K, representing the scleral rigidity. Outflow facility can be calculated now that P_0 is known. Friedenwald accounted only for intraocular volume change from cornea indentation from the tonometer probe. He did not include a variable for volume change due to other factors such as posterior globe indentation from orbital tissue compression or changes in choroidal vascular volume [4]. Ocular rigidity is higher in enucleated eyes than live eyes, which is mostly due to the absence of active choroidal blood flow in enucleated eyes [12].

Grant studied tonography in greater depth with the electronic Schiøtz tonometer, which at the time allowed for continuous graphical recording of Schiøtz scale measurements. He performed 5-min tonography tests with four different weights (5.5, 7.5, 10, and 15 g) in normal living human eyes. In this test, P_{avg}, was taken as the average pressure changes in half-minute intervals. From his results, Grant developed his own table of the estimated volume displacement for different weights and the corresponding measurement on the Schiøtz scale (Table 13.2). This table was derived with an average scleral rigidity in mind. As mentioned previously, Grant's equation represented the total change in intraocular volume in a single variable in the numerator. Using a similar equation, he found, in normal eyes, a mean outflow facility of 0.243 μl^{-1} with a range of 0.15 to 0.34 μl^{-1} [5].

Table 13.2 Grant's table showing intraocular volume change (μL) for different weights at different tonometer scale readings [5]

Schiøtz Scale Reading	Intraocular volume change (μL)			
	5.5 g	7.5 g	10 g	15 g
0	0.0	0.0	0.0	0.0
1	3.1	2.6	2.4	2.0
2	6.3	5.4	4.8	4.1
3	9.5	8.2	7.2	6.1
4	12.7	11.0	9.6	8.3
5	16.0	13.8	12.1	10.4
6	19.5	16.7	14.6	12.5
7	22.8	19.7	17.3	14.8
8	26.3	22.9	20.1	17.2
9	29.9	26.1	22.8	19.6
10	33.7	29.8	25.7	22.2
11	37.3	32.6	28.7	24.8
12	41.2	36.0	31.7	27.6
13	45.3	39.6	34.7	30.5
14	49.4	43.4	38.2	33.5
15	53.7	47.3	41.5	36.7

Langham's studies focused on pneumatonometer-based tonography in normal and glaucomatous eyes of human volunteers. His measurements were performed with the subject in the supine position with a 10 g weight applied to the cornea for either 2 or 4 min. Seated pressures were taken before tonography with the Goldmann applanation tonometer and the pneumatonometer to determine P_0. Using empirical data which he collected, he developed tables for the intraocular volume change V_s from scleral distention due to intraocular pressure change (Table 13.3) and V_c from corneal deformation during tonography (Table 13.4). He also compared intraocular pressure measurements in the supine position with the Schiøtz tonometer and pneumatonometer. In both normal and glaucomatous eyes, he consistently found that the Schiøtz tonometer measured lower pressures with the difference in measurements twice as large in glaucomatous eyes versus healthy eyes. Using the pneumatonometer, he calculated a mean outflow facility value of 0.28 ± 0.01 μL/min/mm Hg in healthy eyes versus 0.16 ± 0.01 μl/min/mmHg in glaucomatous eyes. The means were statistically significantly different [11].

Ocular Rigidity and Tonography

Ocular rigidity significantly impacts tonography measurement of intraocular pressure [13–16]. It includes scleral rigidity and corneal biomechanics. The sclera's biomechanical properties vary by anatomic eye regions, age, and disease state. In a study [17] of human sclera specimens, scleral thickness ranged from 1062 μm at the posterior pole, to 716 μm in the anterior sclera and to 767 μm at the cornea-scleral

Table 13.3 Langham's table showing the intraocular volume change V_s (µL) required to increase intraocular pressure P (mm Hg) from 10 to 50 mm Hg with incremental steps of 0.5 mm Hg [11]

P	Vs	P	Vs	P	Vs
10.0	0.0	23.5	28.2	37.0	45.3
10.5	1.7	24.0	29.0	37.5	45.8
11.0	3.1	24.5	29.5	38.0	46.4
11.5	4.5	25.0	30.2	38.5	46.8
12.0	5.8	25.5	30.9	39.0	47.3
12.5	7.0	26.0	31.8	39.5	47.8
13.0	8.2	26.5	32.2	40.0	48.4
13.5	9.4	27.0	32.9	40.5	49.0
14.0	10.5	27.5	33.6	41.0	49.6
14.5	11.7	28.0	34.2	41.5	50.1
15.0	12.5	28.5	34.7	42.0	50.6
15.5	13.8	29.0	35.5	42.5	51.3
16.0	14.7	29.5	36.1	43.0	51.8
16.5	15.8	30.0	36.6	43.5	52.5
17.0	16.8	30.5	37.2	44.0	53.0
17.5	17.8	31.0	37.9	44.5	53.5
18.0	18.8	31.5	38.5	45.0	54.0
18.5	19.7	32.0	39.2	45.5	54.7
19.0	20.6	32.5	39.9	46.0	55.3
19.5	21.5	33.0	40.5	46.5	56.0
20.0	22.5	33.5	41.1	47.0	56.6
20.5	23.3	34.0	41.7	47.5	57.0
21.0	24.2	34.5	42.3	48.0	57.6
21.5	25.0	35.0	42.8	48.5	58.3
22.0	25.8	35.5	43.4	49.0	58.9
22.5	26.7	36.0	44.0	49.5	59.5
23.0	27.5	36.5	44.6	50.0	59.9

border at the limbus. When mechanical stress was applied to the sclera, the anterior sclera was stiffer than the posterior sclera. The thicker posterior sclera may provide additional resistance to stress loading to compensate for reduced mechanical stiffness. Similarly, the sclera thins with age but develops increased mechanical stiffness [18]. With changes to intraocular volume and pressure, the sclera also demonstrates a viscoelastic property: with increased stress load, whether by volume or pressure, the sclera shows linear stretching with a return to its original state once the stress is removed (as when standing on one's head for a short time). However, with prolonged constant stress load (as in primary open angle glaucoma), the sclera shows slow gradual mechanical creep with permanent stretching and deformation from its original state [19]. Creep rates were less in non-glaucomatous versus glaucomatous eyes [18]. The microscopic properties which govern these dynamic and chronic changes are likely due to the interaction of type 1 collagen, collagenase enzymes such as matrix metalloproteinases in the extracellular matrix, and contractile myofibroblast cells such as alpha smooth muscle actin. These are some of the factors

Table 13.4 Langham's table showing the relationship between intraocular pressure P and corneal deformation volume V_c with a 10 g weight applied to the eye [11]

P	Vc
15	26.5
16	25.0
17	23.5
18	22.0
19	20.7
20	19.5
21	18.2
22	17.0
23	16.0
24	15.0
25	14.3
26	13.7
27	13.0
28	12.4
29	11.8
30	11.2
31	10.5
32	9.9
33	9.3
34	8.7
35	8.2
36	7.8
37	7.4
38	7.0
39	6.7
40	6.4
41	6.1
42	5.8

affecting scleral rigidity that need to be considered in tonography and in interpreting calculated outflow facility values [19].

Differences in IOP due to cornea biomechanics are best noted when comparing indentation versus applanation methods of IOP measurement [20]. The preferred applanation tonometer is the Goldmann applanation tonometer. It is considered the gold standard against which all other tonometers are evaluated. With a diameter of 3.06 mm, the Goldmann applanation tip has minimal corneal indentation and displaces about 0.45 µL of intraocular fluid, which raises the IOP by about 0.5 mm Hg.

The suspicion of ocular rigidity impacting IOP and outflow facility measurements was initially suggested by comparison of Schiøtz and applanation tonometer values since the Schiøtz tonometer was larger in diameter and displaced a much larger intraocular volume. A higher IOP with a Schiøtz tonometer compared to the applanation tonometer implied greater ocular rigidity with the inverse implying lower ocular rigidity. More generalized, ocular rigidity is inversely related to

217

intraocular volume and proportional to intraocular pressure. The impact of ocular rigidity on outflow facility calculation was seen mainly in the change in intraocular volume due to scleral distention [21]. The outflow facility equation assumes an average ocular rigidity constant, which Friedenwald, Grant, and Langham have incorporated into their tables for the expected change in intraocular volume during tonography. Thus, for calculated outflow facility values based on the average ocular rigidity constant, higher ocular rigidity is associated with a lower actual outflow facility and lower ocular rigidity is associated with a higher actual outflow facility. Mathematically, the correction factor would modify Eq. (13.1) as follows:

$$C = \frac{\Delta V_s \times \dfrac{K_N}{K} + \Delta V_c}{\left[P_{avg} - \left(P_0 + P_s\right)\right]t}$$ (13.5)

where $\dfrac{K_N}{K}$ is the ocular rigidity correction factor with K_N representing the normal ocular rigidity coefficient and K representing the actual ocular rigidity coefficient of the eye. This volume-pressure relationship has been refined into a more accurate constant based on empirical data [22]. Using all published data collected from in vivo tonography studies, a best fit curve was created to determine the intraocular volume change equation for a certain intraocular pressure:

$$\Delta V = V\left(C + C_0 x \ln P + C_1 xP\right)$$ (13.6)

where C, C_0 and C_1 are constants derived from the best fit curve, V is the steady state intraocular volume, P is the intraocular pressure, and ΔV is the expected intraocular volume change. By extrapolation, the predicted intraocular volume change due to the effects of ocular rigidity and pressure change is larger than Friedenwald's original estimate in enucleated eyes [22]. In vivo data and measurements provide a more realistic calculation as the effect of intravascular and extravascular fluid in the eye wall is included as a determinant of the eye's ocular rigidity [22].

Summary

Tonography provides an important tool to analyze outflow facility and study the dynamics of aqueous flow. This is especially important in understanding the pathogenesis of glaucoma. Intraocular pressure is a modifiable therapeutic target which is manipulated in order to prevent or slow the progression of glaucoma. Studying outflow facility provides a methodology of examining resistance pathways that can increase intraocular pressure due to insufficient drainage. Although tonography relies on several assumptions and there can be variability of measurements due to ocular rigidity differences in the population, the method has shown that there is a difference in outflow facility between glaucomatous and normal eyes. The data from tonography provides a general measurement of overall outflow resistance including the proximal trabecular meshwork to the distal scleral and episcleral venous pathways. Further methods which can isolate areas of resistance to distal, trabecular or uveoscleral pathways when combined with tonography has the potential to generate a more definitive mapping of aqueous humor flow dynamics out of the anterior chamber.

Acknowledgments This work was supported by an unrestricted departmental grant to Case Western Reserve University from Research to Prevent Blindness.

References

1. Carreon T, van der Merwe E, Fellman RL, Johnstone M, Bhattacharya SK. Aqueous outflow - a continuum from trabecular meshwork to episcleral veins. Prog Retin Eye Res. 2017;57:108–33.
2. Xin C, Wang RK, Song S, Shen T, Wen J, Martin E, et al. Aqueous outflow regulation: optical coherence tomography implicates pressure-dependent tissue motion. Exp Eye Res. 2017;158:171–86.
3. Drews R. Manual of tonography. St. Louis, MO: The C. V. Mosby Company; 1971.
4. Friedenwald J. Contribution to the theory and practice of tonometry. Am J Ophthalmol. 1937;20:985–1024.
5. Grant WM. Tonographic method for measuring the facility and rate of aqueous flow in human eyes. Arch Ophthalmol. 1950;44(2):204–14.
6. Jain MR, Marmion VJ. A clinical evaluation of the applanation pneumatonograph. Br J Ophthalmol. 1976;60(2):107–10.
7. Feghali JG, Azar DT, Kaufman PL. Comparative aqueous outflow facility measurements by pneumatonography and Schiotz tonography. Invest Ophthalmol Vis Sci. 1986;27(12):1776–80.
8. Wheeler NC, Lee DA, Cheng Q, Ross WF, Hadjiaghai L. Reproducibility of intraocular pressure and outflow facility measured by pneumatic tonography and Schiotz tonography. J Ocul Pharmacol Ther. 1998;14(1):5–13.
9. Choplin NT, Lundy DC. Atlas of glaucoma. 1st ed. London: Martin Dunitz; 1998.
10. Toris CB, Yablonski ME, Wang YL, Camras CB. Aqueous humor dynamics in the aging human eye. Am J Ophthalmol. 1999;127(4):407–12.
11. Langham ME, Leydhecker W, Krieglstein G, Waller W. Pneumatonographic studies on normal and glaucomatus eyes. Adv Ophthalmol. 1976;32:108–33.
12. Ebneter A, Wagels B, Zinkernagel MS. Non-invasive biometric assessment of ocular rigidity in glaucoma patients and controls. Eye (Lond). 2009;23(3):606–11.
13. Moses RA, Becker B. Clinical tonography; the scleral rigidity correction. Am J Ophthalmol. 1958;45(2):196–208.
14. Dastiridou AI, Ginis HS, De Brouwere D, Tsilimbaris MK, Pallikaris IG. Ocular rigidity, ocular pulse amplitude, and pulsatile ocular blood flow: the effect of intraocular pressure. Invest Ophthalmol Vis Sci. 2009;50(12):5718–22.
15. Detorakis ET, Pallikaris IG. Ocular rigidity: biomechanical role, in vivo measurements and clinical significance. Clin Exp Ophthalmol. 2013;41(1):73–81.
16. Moses RA. Constant-pressure tonography. AMA Arch Ophthalmol. 1958;59(4):527–31.
17. Elsheikh A, Geraghty B, Alhasso D, Knappett J, Campanelli M, Rama P. Regional variation in the biomechanical properties of the human sclera. Exp Eye Res. 2010;90(5):624–33.
18. Coudrillier B, Tian J, Alexander S, Myers KM, Quigley HA, Nguyen TD. Biomechanics of the human posterior sclera: age- and glaucoma-related changes measured using inflation testing. Invest Ophthalmol Vis Sci. 2012;53(4):1714–28.

19. McBrien NA, Jobling AI, Gentle A. Biomechanics of the sclera in myopia: extracellular and cellular factors. Optom Vis Sci. 2009;86(1):E23–30.
20. Becker B, Gay AJ. Applanation tonometry in the diagnosis and treatment of glaucoma: an evaluation of decreased scleral rigidity. AMA Arch Ophthalmol. 1959;62(2):211–5.
21. Drance SM. The coefficient of scleral rigidity in normal and glaucomatous eyes. Arch Ophthalmol. 1960;63:668–74.
22. Silver DM, Geyer O. Pressure-volume relation for the living human eye. Curr Eye Res. 2000;20(2):115–20.

Chapter 14
Age Related Changes in Ocular Rigidity

George Kontadakis and George Kymionis

Introduction

Ocular rigidity is a feature of ocular physiology that is involved is many pathophysiologic mechanisms and the clinical course of several diseases. Although it solely refers to the mathematical relationship between pressure and volume changes in the eyeball, due to the complexity of the eyeball structure it is separately affected by the response to pressure changes of each different element of the ocular anatomy [1]. Consequently, any change in each of these anatomical elements would also effect ocular rigidity itself.

The effect of age in ocular physiology is evident in all structures of the eye. Numerous anatomic changes occur in the eye with age. These changes generally comprise cell loss, such as the corneal endothelium, degenerative processes, such as vitreous liquefaction, and accumulations of materials, such as drusen [2, 3].

Molecular changes in the extracellular matrix that happen in aging, and structural and functional changes in vasculature have also been detected. Such changes happen throughout the body and contribute in the altered behavior of various tissues during physiological aging.

Ocular consequences of those changes are the increase of corneal and scleral rigidity, and also the changes in biomechanical properties of the choroid [4–6]. All

G. Kontadakis (✉)
Laboratory of Vision and Optics and Department of Ophthalmology, University of Crete, Heraklion, Greece

Whipps Cross University Hospital, London, UK

G. Kymionis
Department of Ophthalmology, University of Lausanne, Jules-Gonin Eye Hospital, Fondation Asile des Aveugles, Lausanne, Switzerland

Department of Ophthalmology, University of Athens, Athens, Greece
e-mail: kymionis@med.uoc.gr

© Springer Nature Switzerland AG 2021
I. Pallikaris et al. (eds.), *Ocular Rigidity, Biomechanics and Hydrodynamics of the Eye*, https://doi.org/10.1007/978-3-030-64422-2_14

these alterations in total contribute in the changes of ocular rigidity that have been described in the literature. Changes in ocular rigidity have been considered as part of the normal aging process. Scleral and corneal stiffness is known to increase with age and also choroidal compressibility is altered [4–6]. All those parameters naturally would lead to a change in ocular rigidity with age, which has been experimentally studied by many authors.

Reports of Ocular Rigidity Modification with Age

The relationship of age with ocular rigidity has been described in several reports in the literature since the very early studies on tonometry and rigidity. As early as 1872, a study by Pfluger [7] on cadaver eyes suggested that difference on calibration of tonometers in older eyes is attributed to increased rigidity. Müller [8] reached the same conclusion in post mortem eyes. Kalfa [9] constructed an elastometric curve and found a steeper rise in older eyes due to the increase in rigidity.

In his landmark study of rigidity, Friedenwald [10] reported results of 500 eyes over 15 years old measured in vivo. In this study, the author used a set of tonometric measurements with the employment of two or more different tonometric weights in a Schiotz tonometer. The distribution of the calculated rigidity in the population of the study as a function of age was positively skewed due to the increased rigidity in the elderly population. When plotted in separate age groups rigidity was normally distributed and similar in subjects under 30 years old and between 30 and 50 years old, but started to increase and demonstrate skewness in the groups of over 60 years old. Despite that, there was a wide range of rigidity within the older age groups, which demonstrated that even among senior subjects a low rigidity similar to younger ages could have been measured. Among healthy eyes the variations of rigidity were relatively low, thus stretching out the significance of variations found in older ages. Consequently Friedenwald in vivo acknowledged rigidity as one of the parameters of ocular physiology effected by aging.

Other studies using similar methods as Friedenwald reached the same conclusion. A number of other studies based on his methods have appeared in recent years. Kiritoshi [11], Leydhecker [12], and Goodside [13] all found that rigidity coefficient increased with age, although the results in the latter two studies were not totally conclusive.

Gaasterland et al. [14] evaluated rigidity with paired electronic indentation tonometer readings in healthy eyes of a young age group ranging from 18 to 26 years and an old aged group from 49 to 81 years old. The authors sought to evaluate the effect of age on IOP parameters and concluded that among others, rigidity is also affected by age since it significantly increased in the older age group.

Other studies that used paired indentation tonometry also demonstrated the increased rigidity with age. Singh et al. [15] in a study from India found a definite increase of rigidity in patients over 50 years of age. Wong and Yap [16], studied a Chinese population divided in a young group ranging from 19 to 30 years old and an older group ranging 57–90 years. The authors found an increased rigidity in the elderly that was not statistically significant though. Lam et al. [17] more recently used linear regression in a population of 118 healthy subjects to demonstrate significant increase in scleral rigidity with age. The authors in this study had excluded high myopes to eliminate the effect of axial length.

Furthermore, the effect of age has been assessed with studies using manometry. Perkins [18] used post mortem enucleated eyes unsuitable for transplantation and uncovered a significant correlation between the coefficient of rigidity and age.

More recently, Pallikaris et al. published a manometry study of ocular rigidity performed in 79 living eyes [19]. Patients undergoing cataract surgery were enrolled in this study and the ocular rigidity was manometrically determined in anesthetised eyes trough a specially developed hydraulic system directly communicating with the anterior chamber. Eyes with glaucoma, ocular hypertension and previous surgery were excluded. The ocular rigidity was measured within a range of clinically encountered IOPs in this study (pressure range 10–35 mmHg). The authors investigated the correlation of the result with other parameters such as age, axial length, central corneal thickness and presence of diabetes, hypertention and age related macular degeneration. Age range in this study was 27–91 years with an average age of 65 years. The age of the patients was positively correlated with the measured rigidity, thus confirming the previous findings of post mortem and indirect in vivo studies. Other correlations were not found, apart from a trend of decreased rigidity in correlation with axial length that marginaly did not reach statistical significance. This was the largest manometric in vivo study dealing with the correlation or rigidity with age in human eyes.

Additionally, the overall effect of age on ocular rigidity has been confirmed in vitro, in scleral rigidity studies of human and other primates. Girard et al. [20] studied the inhomogeneous, anisotropic, non-linear biomechanical properties of posterior sclera of monkeys as function of age. Authors found that posterior sclera of older monkeys was significantly stiffer than that of young monkeys, possibly affecting the optic nerve head. Friberg and Lace [21] evaluated the modulus of elasticity of scleral strips from human eye-bank eyes and also found an increase in stiffness with age.

Changes of scleral stiffness with age may result from several parameters of scleral physiology that are affected by the aging process [4]. The mechanical properties of cornea and sclera are controlled by the extracellular matrix which is comprised from connective tissue fibres. The biomechanical properties of the extracellular matrix are strongly dependent on the specific composition and concentration of matrix components, and also by post-translational modifications, such as glycosylation and cross-linking [22, 23]. The ageing process has an intense effect alterations in extracellular matrix microstructure and subsequent cross-linking. Aged scleral elastic fibres exhibit larger constituent fibril diameters in the outer region and altered electron density within the fibres' central area, indicative of elastin molecular alterations and fibrillary degeneration [24]. Cornea demonstrates decreased collagen interfibrillar distance, collagen fibril breakdown and the presence of small collagen-free spaces in the posterior stroma of older specimens has been found to happen with increasing age in electron microscopy studies [23]. Brown et al. [25] reported that human sclera loses, on average, approximately 1% of its water content per decade, and that tissue dehydration is correlated with the progressive loss of hydrophilic sulphated glycosaminoglycans. Changes in proteoglycans, another major extacellular matrix (ECM) component, have also been demonstrated with age in the human ocular tissues. One of the most important metabolic processes that may be associated with the correlation of increased tissue stiffening with age is non-enzymatic glycosylation of macromolecules [26]. Lipid and Calcium levels also increase significantly with age in both cornea and sclera [27]. Choroid also undergoes changes with choriocapillary vascular dropout and changes to choroidal thickness with age [5]. Investigators are recognizing the increasing importance of the role of age-related alterations in ECM composition and microstructure and the resulting altered ocular tissue stiffness which are likely to contribute to pathologically modified glaucomatous conditions [27].

Despite the theoretical background and the plethora of experimental data supporting the increase of ocular rigidity with age, there are also some studies that do not confirm this or even confer contradicting results.

Leydhecker [12] found in 1497 eyes, that increase with age was minimal, and in both his and Goodside's [13] investigations certain age groups show a lower rigidity coefficient than the age group below. Armaly [28] found a maximum at 40–50 years of age in an investigation of 519 patients. Lavergne et al. [29] found no significant age variation, and Schneider et al. [30] found no increased rigidity coefficient on investigating 770 patients between the ages of 62–98 years.

Ytteborg et al. [31] performed a large in vivo study in 166 eyes using differential tonometry. A Goldmann applanation tonometer and a Mueller electronic tonometer with a 5.5 g plunger weight were used in the study. The age range of subjects included in the study was 12–92 years and authors divided them into 4 age groups. There was a trend of rigidity to decrease from one group to the other that did not reach statistical significance when comparing adjacent groups, but was significant when comparing the younger with the older group. In the same study a postmortem manometric study was performed in 50 eyes, that demonstrated a slight but not significant increase of rigidity with age.

Drance et al. [32] approached rigidity by measuring the applanation tonometry in sitting positon and them the indentation tonometry with a Shchiotz tonometer with the 10 g weight. Seven hundred ninety eyes were analyzed with regard to age, ranging from 10 to more than 70 years old. The subjects were divided in age groups covering a span of 10 years each and no difference was found between the average rigidity in each group, although the values of rigidity were similar to those calculated by Friedenwald [33]. Schneider et al. [30] also used differential tonometry and found no significant difference with age.

Despite the contradicting results, it is predominatly considered that ocular rigidity is affected by age and that it participates in the evolution of age-related ocular pathology, such as glaucoma and age-related macular degeneration. Regarding the latter, the group of Pallikaris executed a manometric study in patients with AMD [34]. This study comprised patients with dry or neovascular AMD and age matched control subjects. The macular health status of patients was determined by clinical examination and fluorescein angiography. All patients were scheduled for cataract surgery and rigidity was manometrically measured in theater prior to the operation as described previously [19]. The authors did not find any differences between AMD patients and controls, but is a subgroup analysis they found a significant difference between neovascular and non-neovascular or control patients. Authors consider that this implicates a participation of increased rigidity in the development of neovascular AMD.

In another study with the same method in open angle glaucoma patients and controls, ocular rigidity was not found to be different between patients and controls [35]. In this study patients and controls were matched in terms of age and axial length and no other ocular comorbidities apart from cataract were accepted. Despite failing to provide evidence of altered scleral distensibility in OAG, this study demonstrated the statistically significant difference though in outflow facility.

Conclusion

Ocular rigidity as measured by various methods is a factor that has been shown to increase with age since the early studies of ocular rigidity. Changes of ocular physiology with age support this result. Despite this, not all studies confirm the correlation of age with rigidity, although the disparity in findings among studies might be attributed to the method of measurements. Nevertheless, rigidity remains a significant parameter of ocular physiology which is possibly contributing to development of ocular age-related disease.

References

1. Detorakis ET, Pallikaris IG. Ocular rigidity: biomechanical role, in vivo measurements and clinical significance. Clin Exp Ophthalmol. 2013;41:73–81.
2. Lin JB, Tsubota K, Apte RS. A glimpse at the aging eye. NPJ Aging Mech Dis. 2016;2:16003.
3. Grossniklaus HE, Nickerson JM, Edelhauser HF, et al. Anatomic alterations in aging and age-related diseases of the eye. Investig Ophthalmol Vis Sci. 2012;54:7378.
4. Geraghty B, Whitford C, Boote C, et al. Age-related variation in the biomechanical and structural properties of the corneo-scleral tunic. Cham: Springer; 2015. p. 207–35.
5. Chirco KR, Sohn EH, Stone EM, et al. Structural and molecular changes in the aging choroid: implications for age-related macular degeneration. Eye. 2017;31:10–25.
6. Ravalico G, Toffoli G, Pastori G, et al. Age-related ocular blood flow changes. Investig Ophthalmol Vis Sci. 1996;37:2645–50.
7. Pfluger E. Beiträge zur Ophthalmo Tonometrie. Arch Augen- und Ohren. 1872;2:1.
8. Müller HK. Augendruck und Lebensalter. Arch Augenh. 1942;105:504.
9. Kalfa S. Über den Innenaugendruck regulierenden Gefässreflex und seine Bedeutung für die Pathogenese des Glaukoms. Arch Augenh. 1932;106:271.

10. Friedenwald JS. Contribution to the theory and practice of tonometry. Am J Ophthalmol. 1937;20:985–1024.
11. Kiritoshi Y. Rigidity of ocular coat II. Acta Soc Ophth Jap. 1955;59:1719.
12. Leydhecker W. Die Schwierigkeiten der Rigiditätsbestimmung mit dem Schiötz-Tonometer. Klin Monatsbl Augenh 1959;669.
13. Goodside V. Ocular rigidity: a clinical study. AMA Arch Ophthalmol. 1959;62:839.
14. Gaasterland D, Kupfer C, Milton R, et al. Studies of aqueous humour dynamics in man. VI. Effect of age upon parameters of intraocular pressure in normal human eyes. Exp Eye Res. 1978;26:651–6.
15. Singh YP, Goel SK, Misra RN. Scleral rigidity in emmetropes. J All India Ophthalmol Soc. 1970;18:167–9.
16. Wong E, Yap MKH. Factors affecting ocular rigidity in the Chinese. Clin Exp Optom. 1991;74:156–9.
17. Lam AKC, Chan ST, Chan H, Chan B. The effect of age on ocular blood supply determined by pulsatile ocular blood flow and color Doppler ultrasonography. Optom Vis Sci. 2003;80:305–11.
18. Perkins ES. Ocular volume and ocular rigidity. Exp Eye Res. 1981;33:141–5.
19. Pallikaris IG, Kymionis GD, Ginis HS, et al. Ocular rigidity in living human eyes. Investig Ophthalmol Vis Sci. 2005;46:409–14.
20. Girard MJA, JKF S, Bottlang M, et al. Scleral biomechanics in the aging monkey eye. Invest Ophthalmol Vis Sci. 2009;50:5226–37.
21. Friberg TR, Lace JW. A comparison of the elastic properties of human choroid and sclera. Exp Eye Res. 1988;47:429–36.
22. Reiser KM. Minireview: nonenzymatic glycation of collagen in aging and diabetes. Proc Soc Exp Biol Med. 1991;196:17.
23. Malik NS, Moss SJ, Ahmed N, et al. Ageing of the human corneal stroma: structural and biochemical changes. Biochim Biophys Acta. 1992;1138:222–8.
24. Coudrillier B, Pijanka J, Jefferys J, et al. Collagen structure and mechanical properties of the human sclera: analysis for the effects of age. J Biomech Eng. 2015;137:0410061.
25. Brown CT, Vural M, Johnson M, Trinkaus-Randall V. Age-related changes of scleral hydration and sulfated glycosaminoglycans. Mech Ageing Dev. 1994;77:97–107.
26. Tezel G, Luo C, Yang X. Accelerated aging in glaucoma: immunohistochemical assessment of advanced glycation end products in the human retina and optic nerve head. Investig Ophthalmol Vis Sci. 2007;48:1201–11.
27. Liu B, McNally S, Kilpatrick JI, et al. Aging and ocular tissue stiffness in glaucoma. Surv Ophthalmol. 2018;63:56–74.
28. Armaly MF. The consistency of the 1955 calibration for various tonometer weights. Am J Ophthalmol. 1959;48(5):602–11.
29. Anon. Acquisitions récentes en tonométrie. Arch Ophtalmol. 1957:256–70.
30. Schneider J, Feldstein M, Kornzweig AL. Scleral rigidity and tonometry in the aged. Am J Ophthalmol. 1959;48:643–7.
31. Ytteborg J. Further investigations of factors influencing size of rigidity coefficient. Acta Ophthalmol. 1960;38:643–57.
32. Drance SM. The coefficient of scleral rigidity in normal and glaucomatous eyes. Arch Ophthalmol (Chicago Ill 1960). 1960;63:668–74.
33. Friedenwald JS. Clinical significance of ocular rigidity in relation to the tonometric measurement. Trans Am Acad Ophthalmol Otolaryngol. 1949;53:262–4.
34. Pallikaris IG, Kymionis GD, Ginis HS, et al. Ocular rigidity in patients with age-related macular degeneration. Am J Ophthalmol. 2006;141:611–5.
35. Dastiridou AI, Tsironi EE, Tsilimbaris MK, et al. Ocular rigidity, outflow facility, ocular pulse amplitude, and pulsatile ocular blood flow in open-angle glaucoma: a manometric study. Investig Ophthalmol Vis Sci. 2013;54:4571–7.

Chapter 15
Ocular Rigidity and Axial Length

Anna I. Dastiridou

Introduction-Rationale for the Association Between Axial Length and Ocular Rigidity

Based on the various mathematical expressions, mainly the one by Friedenwald, but also by other researchers as well throughout the years, that have been proposed to characterize ocular rigidity (OR) and its coefficient, it is evident that OR is affected by ocular volume [1–8]. In Friedenwald's original paper, K is assumed to represent a (more fundamental) parameter k divided by the ocular volume V [1]. In clinical practice, the best surrogate marker for volume is axial length. In a normal eye with a clear crystalline lens, this could also mean that ocular rigidity is associated with refractive error. This is becoming more relevant in fact with the increasing prevalence of myopia which already is affecting 1 billion people worldwide (see Chap. 21) [9].

Ocular Rigidity, Axial Length and Refraction

The first report of the dependence of ocular rigidity on refraction was evidenced in Friedenwald's original studies in young individuals. For this analysis, he excluded patients aged more than 50 years, in order to exclude the effects of cataract and the myopic shifts that often occurs with it, and the effects of age. These measurements were in line with the theoretical predictions, with the exception of the case of very high myopic eyes where OR coefficient K would take an increased value. This may suggest that these pathologic myopia eyes may have been stretched up to their

A. I. Dastiridou (✉)
2nd Ophthalmology Department, Aristotle University of Thessaloniki, Thessaloniki, Greece

School of Medicine, University of Thessalia, Larissa, Greece

© Springer Nature Switzerland AG 2021
I. Pallikaris et al. (eds.), *Ocular Rigidity, Biomechanics and Hydrodynamics of the Eye*, https://doi.org/10.1007/978-3-030-64422-2_15

elasticity limit. Furthermore, an association was reported by Friedenwald between rigidity coefficient K and mean keratometry [1]. Naturally, it is expected that this is mainly due to the strong correlation between the cornea curvature and axial length that exists in the population during the course of emmetropisation [10]. Moreover, in his original studies, Friedenwald found no correlation between K and cornea astigmatism [1]. This finding may further support that cornea properties, and their variability at least in normal eyes, do not play a major role in the final OR coefficient, compared to other factors.

In the first half of the twentieth century, other researchers also investigated the relationship between OR and axial length and their findings generally agreed to the ones by Friedenwald. Goldmann [11] also reported that rigidity was low in myopia. This has been again demonstrated in several studies and the OR coefficient is reported to vary in myopia between 0.0060 and 0.0214, while in hyperopia, Draeger reported values >0.021 [12–15].

Castrem and Pohjola [16] set out to characterize the relationship between refraction and rigidity using applanation and Schiotz tonometry with the 10 g weight in young individuals aged up to 40 years old and found again that myopes as a group had lower OR compared to either the controls or the hyperopic group, but the hyperopic and emmetropic group did not manifest statistically significant difference in OR. However, it was again interesting to see that some myopic eyes would exhibit OR coefficients that were much higher than the average value or even the mean value found in the hyperopic refraction group. They measured a mean OR coefficient of 0.0162 ± 0.0005 (0.0108–0.0255) in myopia, 0.0184 ± 0.0002 (0.0128–0.0282) in emmteropia and 0.0189 ± 0.0003 (0.0115–0.0270) in hyperopia.

Silver and Geyer, in their original paper, have proposed a mathematical expression that incorporates the volume of the eye for use in calculations of volume changes from pressure changes, after analysis of the then available data from living human eyes [2, 3]. It is evident, in their study, that the pressure volume relationship is affected by the eye volume and also by other material properties of the tissue.

Finally, in a study conducted by our group [17], we explored the association between OR and axial length and showed that the OR coefficient measured intraoperatively in a large number of human eyes is inversely correlated to axial length. We also found in that study that ocular pulse amplitude and pulsatile ocular blood flow also decrease with increasing axial length. The participants' median axial length was 23.69 mm (interquartile range 3.53 mm) and the measured OR coefficient was $0.0218 \pm 0.0053 \, \mu l^{-1}$ (see Fig. 15.1). These measurements suggest decreased pulsatility in eyes with longer axial length and might also be important in the tonographic and pneumotonometry measurements. In that study we did not analyse data for refraction since the eyes examined had cataracts which would have artificially modified their refraction.

However, it is important to acknowledge that in myopia not only volume, but also the biomechanical properties of the sclera (and the choroid) may vary (see Chap. 5). So which parameter is more important? Perkins conducted a study to test whether it is mainly the larger volume in myopic eyes that is responsible for the

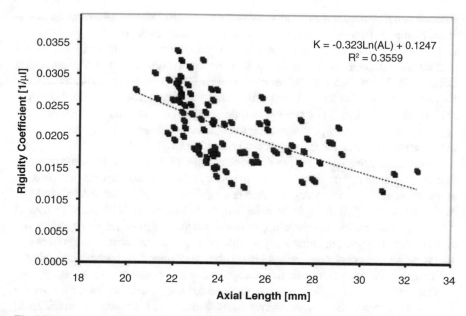

Fig. 15.1 Scatter-plot of the ocular rigidity coefficient versus axial length measurements from the manometric study by our group [17] using the relationship proposed by Kotliar et al. [18]

difference in OR. He used enucleated eyes 1–16 days postmortem and concluded that most of the variability in OR can be directly attributed to a difference in ocular volume, rather that alterations in the biomechanical properties of the sclera [19].

Ocular Rigidity and Shape of the Eye

The volume of the eye is also related to its shape. The shape of the eye is not spherical, and in fact this may be more pronounced in highly myopic or highly hyperopic eyes. Therefore, the ocular volume may not be well approximated by the antero-posterior diameter, which we measure in clinical practice as the axial length. An interesting study in enucleated eyes has provided indirect evidence that the shape of the globe influences the measured OR. In that study, Friberg et al. [20] measured OR in 14 enucleated eyes before and after scleral buckling and found that OR was lower after the procedure. This difference was attributed to the distortion in the shape of the eye caused by the buckling procedure and also implied that greater volumes of gases, antibiotics etc. can be injected in those eyes before causing an extensive IOP rise. This effect was also tested in another study in enucleated eyes [21], with a marked reduction in OR measured upon placement of the buckle and reversibility of the effect after its removal. Interestingly, it is proposed that elastic silicone banding material produces greater changes in OR compared to the influence of altered shape and wall stress that occurred with metal banding [22].

If the eye dimensions vary considerably relative to axial length, this would explain a percentage of the variance seen in the relation between the latter and OR. In a study conducted by Silver et al. (Silver DM, et al. IOVS 2010; 51: ARVO E-Abstract 5019), the authors proposed a formula that relates the volume to the axial length of the eye. They studied human eyes postmortem and reported that this approximation generally provides acceptable accuracy. However, it remains uncertain whether large deviations may occur in highly myopic eyes.

Tabernero and Schaeffel [23], analyzed peripheral refraction profiles and concluded that the peripheral retinal shape is more irregular in cases of low myopia compared to emmetropic eyes. This may signify that large differences in ocular volume and OR may occur with small changes in axial length. Furthermore, imaging with optical coherence tomography and three-dimensional magnetic resonance tomography has revealed that irregular curvature in eyes with myopia is found more often in eyes that also manifest retinochoroidal lesions [24]. This is very important because it highlights again the link between biomechanical factors and specific disease phenotypes.

Therefore, the association between OR and axial length is not linear across the range of axial length. Eyes with staphylomas for instance are expected to manifest an altered response to an increase in volume. In fact, the relationship between myopia and low OR coefficient may also be influenced by concurrent changes in the properties of the sclera. During the course of a volume increase in the eyes of animal models, researchers have found changes in the distensibility and the thickness of the scleral wall [25–28]. These correspond to alterations in the cellular level and in the exracellular matrix, as well as at the level of the choroid and lead to changes in ocular blood flow [25–27, 29–31]. In the human eye, the increase in the volume of the eye in the case of pathological myopia is accompanied with changes in both the anterior and the posterior segment [32, 33]. However, the anterior segment is more consistent geometrically. The dimensions of the posterior segment can vary considerably (see Fig. 15.2). It is well known that high myopia can cause severe complications from the posterior segment, including chorioretinal atrophy, retinal detachment, myopic maculopathy and choroidal neovascularisation [33]. Some of these complications may also be causing changes in ocular rigidity. Moreover, the issue can be complicated even more, since pressure measurements can be inaccurate, especially in cases after refractive surgery or in thin corneas and also, eyes with myopia are more prone to developing open angle glaucoma, compared to the general population [34]. Finally, there are theories that support that the mechanical load of IOP drives the process of eye elongation. It is however generally believed that matrix and cellular factors contribute to the biomechanically weakened sclera and eye elongation that occurs in myopia [35].

Fig. 15.2 Magnetic
resonance imaging in a case
of nanophthalmos (above)
and high myopia (below)

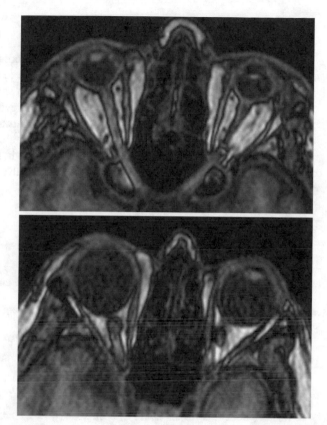

Additional Considerations

The negative correlation between OR coefficient K and axial length underlies the difference in the effect of a fixed volume intravitreal injection on the IOP rise in different eyes. The intravitreal injection produces a volume change and results to a pressure change that is more pronounced in hyperopic eyes with a short axial length compared to long myopic eyes. This was reported in a very interesting study by Kotliar et al. [18], where the authors used Schiotz tonometry to measure intraocular pressure before and after injection of 0.1 ml of triamcinolone. This is also important to take into consideration when injecting any drug in the vitreous in a smaller eye.

The relationship between axial length or refraction and ocular rigidity is also important to consider when using formulas where pressure changes are used to calculate volume changes. Therefore, by assuming a mean ocular rigidity value, pulsatile ocular blood flow can be estimated with pneumotonometry and outflow facility can also be calculated with tonography. Interestingly there are reports of altered POBF in myopic eyes compared to controls and the possible confounder in these results is that ocular rigidity in those eyes may vary as well compared to the control group [36–38].

Conclusion

Ocular rigidity measured either manometrically or by indentation tonometry varies according to the axial length of the eye. Eyes with longer axial length and/or myopia manifest lower values of ocular rigidity, while eyes with smaller axial length and/or hyperopia show higher values of the coefficient. However, some eyes with high myopia may show a high ocular rigidity coefficient, contrary to the aforementioned association. This relation with axial length may be important to consider in the pathophysiology of myopia. This may also be important in tonography, ocular pulse amplitude and pulsatile ocular blood flow studies and also when performing intra-vitreal injections.

References

1. Friedenwald JS. Contribution to the theory and practice of tonometry. Am J Ophthalmol. 1937;20:985–1024.
2. Silver DM, Geyer O. Pressure-volume relation for the living human eye. Curr Eye Res. 2000;20:115–20.
3. Mc Bain E. Tonometer calibration. II. Ocular rigidity. AMA Arch Ophthalmol. 1958;60:1080–91.
4. Holland MG, Madison J, Bean W. The ocular rigidity function. Am J Ophthalmol. 1960;50:958–74.
5. McEwen WK, St Helen R. Rheology of the human sclera. Unifying formulation of ocular rigidity. Ophthalmologica. 1965;150:321–46.
6. Woo SL, Kobayashi AS, Lawrence C, et al. Mathematical model of the corneo–scleral shell as applied to intraocular pressure–volume relations and applanation tonometry. Ann Biomed Eng. 1972;1:87–98.
7. Hibbard RR, Lyon CS, Shepherd MD, et al. Immediate rigidity of an eye. I. Whole, segments and strips. Exp Eye Res. 1970;9:137–43.
8. van der Werff TJA. New single-parameter ocular rigidity function. Am J Ophthalmol. 1981;92:391–5.
9. Holden BA, Fricke TR, Wilson DA, Jong M, Naidoo KS, Sankaridurg P, Wong TY, Naduvilath TJ, Resnikoff S. Global prevalence of myopia and high myopia and temporal trends from 2000 through 2050. Ophthalmology. 2016;123:1036–42.
10. Mutti DO, Mitchell GL, Jones LA, Friedman NE, Frane SL, Lin WK, Moeschberger ML, Zadnik K. Axial growth and changes in lenticular and corneal power during emmetropization in infants. Invest Ophthalmol Vis Sci. 2005;46:3074–80.
11. Goldmann H. Un nouveau tonometre applanation. Bull Soc Franc Ophthalmol. 1955;67:474.
12. Goldmann HR, Schmidt T. Der Rigiditatskoeffizient (Friedenwald). Ophthalmologica. 1957;233:330.
13. Lavergne G, Weekers R, Prijot E. Etude clinique de la rigiditkoculaire. Bull Soc Belge Ophtalmol. 1957;116:298.
14. Draeger I. Untersuchungeniiber den Rigidittskoeffizienten. Documenta Ophthalmol. 1959;13:431.
15. Heinzen HR Luder P, Muller A. Untersuchungen zum Rigiditatsfaktor. Ophthalmologica. 1958;135:649.
16. Castren JA, Pohjola S. Refraction and scleral rigidity. Acta Ophthalmol (Copenh). 1961;39:1011–4.

17. Dastiridou AI, Ginis H, Tsilimbaris M, Karyotakis N, Detorakis E, Siganos C, Cholevas P, Tsironi EE, Pallikaris IG. Ocular rigidity, ocular pulse amplitude, and pulsatile ocular blood flow: the effect of axial length. Invest Ophthalmol Vis Sci. 2013;54:2087–92.
18. Kotliar K, Maier M, Bauer S, Feucht N, Lohmann C, Lanzl I. Effect of intravitreal injections and volume changes on intraocular pressure: clinical results and biomechanical model. Acta Ophthalmol Scand. 2007;85:777–81.
19. Perkins ES. Ocular volume and ocular rigidity. Exp Eye Res. 1981;33:141–5.
20. Friberg TR, Fourman SB. Scleral buckling and ocular rigidity. Clinical ramifications. Arch Ophthalmol. 1990;108:1622–7.
21. Johnson MW, Han DP, Hoffman KE. The effect of scleral buckling on ocular rigidity. Ophthalmology. 1990 Feb;97(2):190–5.
22. Whitacre MM, Emig MD, Hassanein K. Effect of buckling material on ocular rigidity. Ophthalmology. 1992;99:498–502.
23. Tabernero J, Schaeffel F. More irregular eye shape in low myopia than in emmetropia. Invest Ophthalmol Vis Sci. 2009;50:4516–22.
24. Ohno-Matsui K, Akiba M, Modegi T, et al. Association between shape of sclera and myopic retinochoroidal lesions in patients with pathologic myopia. Invest Ophthalmol Vis Sci. 2012;53:6046–61.
25. Gottlieb MD, Joshi HB, Nickla DL. Scleral changes in chicks with form deprivation myopia. Curr Eye Res. 1990;9:1157–65.
26. Norton TT. Experimental myopia in tree shrews. Ciba Found Symp. 1990;155:178–94. discussion 194–199
27. Tokoro T, Funata M, Akazawa Y. Influence of intraocular pressure on axial elongation. J Ocul Pharmacol. 1990;6:285–91.
28. Phillips JR, McBrien NA. Form deprivation myopia: elastic properties of sclera. Ophthalmic Physiol Opt. 1995;15:357–62.
29. Reiner A, Shih YF, Fitzgerald ME. The relationship of choroidal blood flow and accommodation to the control of ocular growth. Vis Res. 1995;35:1227–45.
30. Wallman J, Wildsoet C, Xu A, Gottlieb MD, Nickla DL, Marran L, et al. Moving the retina: choroidal modulation of refractive state. Vis Res. 1995;35:37–50.
31. Nickla DL, Wallman J. The multifunctional choroid. Prog Retin Eye Res. 2010;29:144–68.
32. Chang SW, Tsai IL, Hu FR, Lin LL, Shih YF. The cornea in young myopic adults. Br J Ophthalmol. 2001;85:916–20.
33. Grossniklaus HE, Green WR. Pathologic findings in pathologic myopia. Retina. 1992;12:127–33.
34. Marcus MW, de Vries MM, JunoyMontolio FG, Jansonius NM. Myopia as a risk factor for open-angle glaucoma: a systematic review and meta-analysis. Ophthalmology. 2011;118:1989–94.
35. McBrien NA, Jobling AI, Gentle A. Biomechanics of the sclera in myopia: extracellular and cellular factors. Optom Vis Sci. 2009;86:E23–30.
36. James CB, Trew DR, Clark K, et al. Factors influencing the ocular pulse-axial length. Graefes Arch Clin Exp Ophthalmol. 1991;229:341–4.
37. Mori F, Konno S, Hikichi T, et al. Factors affecting pulsatile ocular blood flow in normal subjects. Br J Ophthalmol. 2001;85:529–30.
38. Lam AK, Chan ST, Chan B, et al. The effect of axial length on ocular blood flow assessment in anisometropes. Ophthalmic Physiol Opt. 2003;23:315–20.

Chapter 16
Ocular Rigidity and Intraocular Pressure

Anna I. Dastiridou

Introduction

Intraocular pressure (IOP) corresponds to the tissue pressure of the eye. It is also the most important risk factor for the development and progression of glaucoma. Based on the description of ocular rigidity (OR), it is expected that IOP should play an important role in the biomechanics of the eye [1]. Interestingly, measurements in the living human eye suggest that the pressure volume relationship is non linear and that the ocular rigidity, i.e. the slope of the change in pressure with a change in volume, increases with increasing intraocular pressure [2–11]. However, there is disagreement in the literature as to the influence of IOP on the rigidity coefficient K.

The Effect of Intraocular Pressure on Ocular Rigidity

The association between OR an IOP was an important matter of investigation in the middle of twentieth century. It was especially important since Schiotz tonometry was an important tool commonly used in tonometry and OR and its variability was another source of error in the measurement of IOP. However, in the twenty-first century, this relationship may in fact have more important implications as to the calculation of pulsatile ocular blood flow (POBF) with pneumotonometry or outflow facility with tonography, since these techniques are based on measurement of pressure changes [8, 12].

It is generally accepted that the rate of pressure change versus volume change increases with increasing IOP. This was found in animal studies, enucleated human

A. I. Dastiridou (✉)
2nd Ophthalmology Department, Aristotle University of Thessaloniki, Thessaloniki, Greece

School of Medicine, University of Thessalia, Larissa, Greece

© Springer Nature Switzerland AG 2021
I. Pallikaris et al. (eds.), *Ocular Rigidity, Biomechanics and Hydrodynamics of the Eye*, https://doi.org/10.1007/978-3-030-64422-2_16

eye studies and living human eyes [2–11]. In a previous study published by our group [9], we explored the characteristics of the pressure volume relationship in the living human eye based on measurements performed with a manometric setup in the operating theater, prior to phacoemulsification surgery. This was performed under topical anesthesia with drops for a range of pressures between 15 and 40 mmHg, which is clinically relevant. We fitted the experimental data with an exponential curve, based on Friedenwald's approach [1], which was justified based on the R^2 values that were over 0.97. The average K in our set of measurements was 0.0224 μl^{-1} which is similar to the 0.0215 value used by Friedenwald. The slope of the pressure volume curve increases with increasing IOP suggesting that the eye becomes stiffer in higher IOP levels in agreement with the above investigations (Fig. 16.1). The association between K and IOP was not consistent in every eye in the subset of eyes where such an analysis was performed (unpublished data). Factors that may have somehow affected the results include the use of mydriatics, the fact that all measurements were performed in otherwise normal eyes with cataracts and that measurements were performed in the supine position. Nevertheless, the process of increasing the IOP could probably be regarded as more physiologic compared to the pharmacologic IOP modulation or application of a suction cup. This is also the largest series of measurements in the living human eye.

Previous research has focused on the association between the rigidity coefficient and IOP. Ytteborg performed his manometric measurements in 9 eyes scheduled for enucleation and stated that the OR coefficient was negatively correlated to IOP

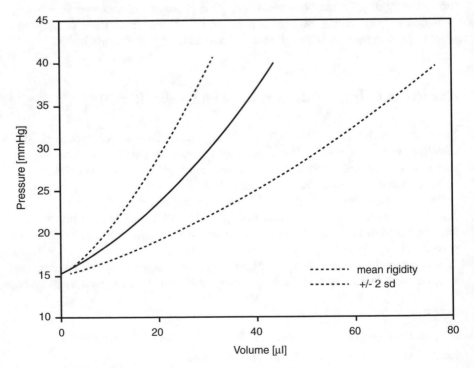

Fig. 16.1 Pressure volume relationship in the living human eye (Reproduced with permission from [9])

[4]. In his study in a larger number of enucleated human eyes, he again reported (using a different measurement setup) a fall in rigidity coefficient with rise in pressure [3]. In addition, he reported considerable individual variation between eyes. Prijot also suggested that OR is influenced by the level of IOP and it is not constant over the range of pressures [2, 13, 14]. Gloster and Perkins also set out to investigate the relation between K and IOP [15–17]. Initially, they performed manometric studies in rabbits [15], where they reported that K increases with increasing IOP, in both living and dead animals. A large variability in OR measurements between eyes was also found. However, experiments in the dead human eye found the exact opposite results, with K decreasing with increasing IOP, although there was a wide variation in the results between eyes [16, 17]. These measurements were performed in the dead eye in situ or in enucleated eyes. Grant and Trotter, finally, performed their measurements in enucleated human eyes and did not observe a dependence of K on IOP in the pressure range of 10–45 mmHg [18].

Mathematical expressions other than Friedenwald's also have also been suggested. The most recent analysis was by Silver and Geyer [19]. They analysed the data available in the literature by 5 researchers from pressure-volume measurements in 21 living human eyes that were scheduled for enucleation. The measurements were performed in a pressure range between 8 and 61 mmHg. The underlying pathology may have as well altered the results but the data analyzed were the only data available then for the human eye in vivo. Silver proposed a new mathematical expression for ocular rigidity based on these data, since the raw data suggest a smaller pressure rise for a given volume increment compared to the Friedenwald data, from enucleated eyes [2–7, 13, 14]. In fact, the initial part of the pressure volume relationship is thought to be affected by the blood supply, mainly from the choroid and in animal experiments, this was shown to be affected by systemic blood pressure [20]. It is also true that measurements differ in the living and dead eye and this is attributed to a large extent to the role of the blood supply in the measurement [3, 6]. Silver and Geyer in fact proposed that their equation may be more accurate for use in estimating volume change for both clinical and research purposes.

Finally, other metrics of the biomechanical properties of the eye also seem to be affected by the mechanical load that IOP exerts. Corneal deformation spatial and temporal profiles in air puff measurements seem to be largely affected by the IOP [21]. The deformation of the optic nerve tissue and lamina cribrosa is also affected by the IOP [22, 23]. The interrelation between biomechanics and glaucoma also becomes more complicated, since differences in biomechanical properties of the eye wall seem to influence tonometry readings [24].

Ocular Pulse Amplitude, Pulsatile Ocular Blood Flow and the Relationship with Intraocular Pressure

IOP flunctuates in relation to the heart beat. With each cardiac systole the heart pumps a bolus of blood in the vessels of the eye. The amplitude of this pulsation represents the ocular pulse amplitude (OPA). There are various ways to measure

OPA, but the main ones nowadays include dynamic contour tonometry with the Pascal tonometer and pneumotonometry.

Pulsatile ocular blood flow (POBF) is a parameter that measures a significant percentage of the total ocular blood flow that is related to the heart rate. It represents the amount of blood flow that enters the eye with each heartbeat. In order to quantify POBF, real time pressure recordings are transformed with the use of the pressure-volume relationship to volume changes [12, 25]. This is the principle behind pneumotonometry. POBF is a parameter that mainly characterizes the choroidal circulation, while the retinal contribution is regarded to account for only a small percentage of POBF. Age, axial length, posture and eye disease have been reported to affect OPA and POBF [26–34].

In a study published by our group [9], we explored the relationship between IOP (and ocular rigidity) with OPA and POBF. Since we were able to artificially modulate IOP and volume, and therefore measure the rigidity of each given eye, we were able to improve the accuracy in the calculation of POBF. Based on our results, both OPA and POBF were affected by IOP (Fig. 16.2a–c). This was later reported in a cohort of open angle glaucoma patients as well [10]. Increasing IOP led to an increase in OPA and decrease in POBF (Fig. 16.3a, b). In fact, increasing the IOP from 15 to 40 mmHg led to an increase in OPA by 91% and a decrease in POBF by 29%. A positive correlation was also found between the rigidity coefficient and OPA (Fig. 16.4). This remained significant after controlling for other variables, such as age, mean blood pressure and pulse rate.

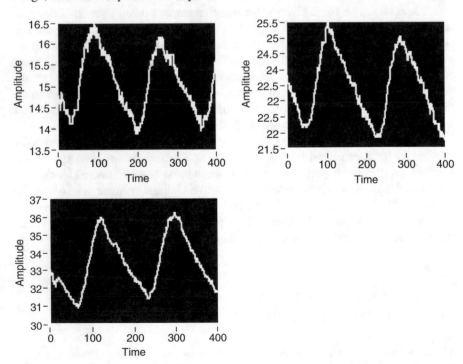

Fig. 16.2 (**a–c**) Real time pressure recordings after infusion of the anterior chamber with microvolumes in 3 different intraocular pressure levels

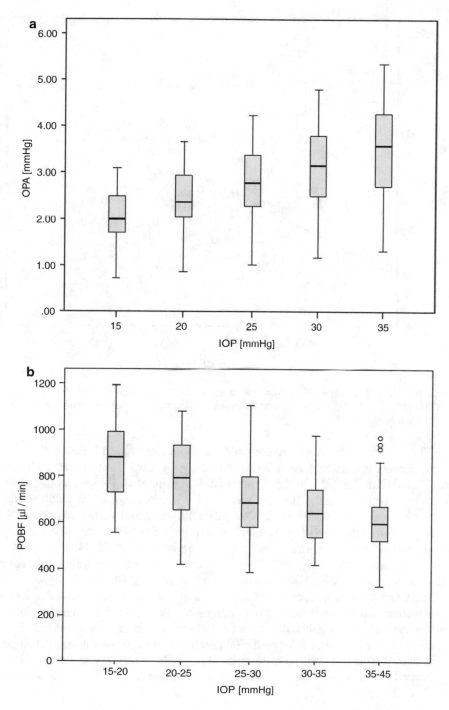

Fig. 16.3 (**a**, **b**) Boxplot diagram of the relation between ocular pulse amplitude (OPA) and pulsatile ocular blood flow (POBF) in 5 intraocular (IOP) pressure levels (Reproduced with permission from [9])

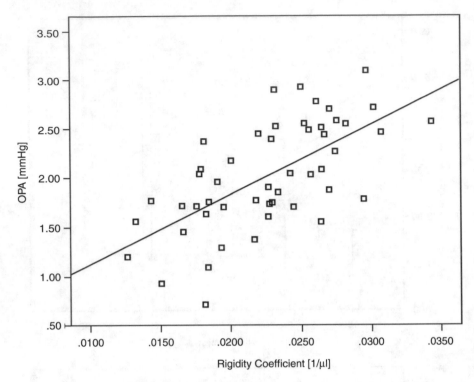

Fig. 16.4 Scatterplot of the relationship between the ocular pulse amplitude (OPA) at an intraocular pressure of 15 mmHg against the ocular rigidity coefficient K (r = 0.650) (Reproduced under permission from [9])

The association between IOP and OPA has been investigated before with some disagreement in the literature. In an animal study, OPA was found to be positively correlated with IOP [35]. In the human eye, Langham et al. [36] found that OPA decreased with increasing IOP, by means of a suction cup, while studies with dynamic contour tonometry concluded that OPA increased with increasing IOP [37–39]. POBF has also been reported to vary with IOP in patients with primary open angle glaucoma, normal tension glaucoma and in controls [40–43]. In our study, this association was found both in normal eyes and eyes with open angle glaucoma with increasing IOP between 15 and 40 mmHg [10].

Interestingly, during the course of the measurement a series of events take place. The increased IOP means that a given change in volume will lead to an even more pronounced change in IOP and a larger OPA. In the same time, the increase in IOP leads to a decrease in the ocular perfusion pressure in the eye and a decreased blood flow or even a different pattern of pulsatile to steady flow. Meanwhile, the increased pressure leads to an increasing amount of aqueous that is leaving the eye with the outflow channels.

Conclusion

Although some evidence exists that the rigidity coefficient may vary with intraocular pressure, this has not been confirmed in other studies. There is however considerable body of evidence suggesting that the pressure volume relationship in the living human eye is affected by the level of IOP and that the ocular pulse amplitude and pulsatile ocular blood flow are affected by the level of IOP in normal and glaucomatous eyes.

References

1. Friedenwald JS. Contribution to the theory and practice of tonometry. Am J Opthalmol. 1937;20:985.
2. Prijot E, Contribution à. l'étude de la tonométrie et de la tonographie en ophtalmologie. Docum Ophthamol. 1961;15:1–225.
3. Ytteborg J. The effect of intraocular pressure on rigidity coefficient in the human eye. Acta Ophthalmol. 1960;38:548–61.
4. Ytteborg J. Further investigations of factors influencing size of rigidity coefficient. Acta Ophthalmol. 1960;38:643–57.
5. Ytteborg J. Influence of bulbar compression on rigidity coefficient of human eyes, in vivo and enucleated. Acta Ophthalmol. 1960;38:562–77.
6. Ytteborg J. The role of intraocular blood volume in rigidity measurements on human eyes. Acta Ophthalmol. 1960;38:410–35.
7. Eisenlohr JE, Langham ME, Maumenee AE. Manometric studies of the pressure-volume relationship in living and enucleated eyes of individual human subjects. Br J Ophthalmol. 1962;46:536–48.
8. Karyotakis NG, Ginis HS, Dastiridou AI, Tsilimbaris MK, Pallikaris IG. Manometric measurement of the outflow facility in the living human eye and its dependence on intraocular pressure. Acta Ophthalmol. 2015;93:e343–8.
9. Dastiridou AI, Ginis HS, De Brouwere D, Tsilimbaris MK, Pallikaris IG. Ocular rigidity, ocular pulse amplitude, and pulsatile ocular blood flow: the effect of intraocular pressure. Invest Ophthalmol Vis Sci. 2009;50:5718–22.
10. Dastiridou AI, Tsironi EE, Tsilimbaris MK, Ginis H, Karyotakis N, Cholevas P, Androudi S, Pallikaris IG. Ocular rigidity, outflow facility, ocular pulse amplitude, and pulsatile ocular blood flow in open-angle glaucoma: a manometric study. Invest Ophthalmol Vis Sci. 2013;54:4571–7.
11. Dastiridou AI, Ginis H, Tsilimbaris M, Karyotakis N, Detorakis E, Siganos C, Cholevas P, Tsironi EE, Pallikaris IG. Ocular rigidity, ocular pulse amplitude, and pulsatile ocular blood flow: the effect of axial length. Invest Ophthalmol Vis Sci. 2013;54:2087–92.
12. Silver DM, Farrell RA. Validity of pulsatile ocular blood flow measurements. Surv Ophthalmol. 1994;38(suppl):S72–80.
13. Prijot E. La rigidité de l'oeil humain. Acta Ophthalmol. 1958;36:865–73.
14. Prijot E, Weekers R. Contribution à l'étude de la rigidité de l'oeil humain normal. Ophthalmologica. 1959;138:1–9.
15. Gloster J, Perkins ES. Distensibility of the eye. Br J Ophthalmol. 1957;41:93–102.
16. Gloster J, Perkins ES. Ocular rigidity and tonometry. Proc R Soc Med. 1957;50:667–74.
17. Gloster J, Perkins ES. Distensibility of the human eye. Br J Ophthalmol. 1959;43:97–101.

18. Grant WM, Trotter RR. Tonographic measurements in enucleated eyes. AMA Arch Ophthalmol. 1955;53:191–200.
19. Silver DM, Geyer O. Pressure-volume relation for the living human eye. Curr Eye Res. 2000;20:115–20.
20. Kiel JW. The effect of arterial pressure on the ocular pressure volume relationship in the rabbit. Exp Eye Res. 1995;60(3):267–78.
21. Kling S, Marcos S. Contributing factors to corneal deformation in air puff measurements. Invest Ophthalmol Vis Sci. 2013;54:5078–85.
22. Beotra MR, Wang X, Tun TA, Zhang L, Baskaran M, Aung T, Strouthidis NG, Girard MJA. In vivo three-dimensional lamina cribrosa strains in healthy, ocular hypertensive, and glaucoma eyes following acute intraocular pressure elevation. Invest Ophthalmol Vis Sci. 2018;59:260–72.
23. Bedggood P, Tanabe F, McKendrick AM, Turpin A, Anderson AJ, Bui BV. Optic nerve tissue displacement during mild intraocular pressure elevation: its relationship to central corneal thickness and corneal hysteresis. Ophthalmic Physiol Opt. 2018;38:389–99.
24. Liu J, Roberts CJ. Influence of corneal biomechanical properties on intraocular pressure measurement: quantitative analysis. Cataract Refract Surg. 2005;31:146–55.
25. Silver DM, Farrell RA, Langham ME, et al. Estimation of pulsatile ocular blood flow from intraocular pressure. Acta Ophthalmol. 1989;191(suppl):25–9.
26. Geyer O, Silver DM, Mathalon N, et al. Gender and age effects on pulsatile ocular blood flow. Ophthalmic Res. 2003;35(5):247–50.
27. Ravalico G, Toffoli G, Pastori G, et al. Age-related ocular blood flow changes. Invest Ophthalmol Vis Sci. 1996;37(13):2645–50.
28. Kothe AC. The effect of posture on intraocular pressure and pulsatile ocular blood flow in normal and glaucomatous eyes. Surv Ophthalmol. 1994;38(suppl):S191–7.
29. Lam AK, Wong S, Lam CS, et al. The effect of myopic axial elongation and posture on the pulsatile ocular blood flow in young normal subjects. Optom Vis Sci. 2002;79(5):300–5.
30. James CB, Smith SE. Pulsatile ocular blood flow in patients with low tension glaucoma. Br J Ophthalmol. 1991;75(8):466–70.
31. Fontana L, Poinoosawmy D, Bunce CV, et al. Pulsatile ocular blood flow investigation in asymmetric normal tension glaucoma and normal subjects. Br J Ophthalmol. 1998;82(7):731–6.
32. Mori F, Konno S, Hicichi T, et al. Pulsatile ocular blood flow study: decreases in exudative age related macular degeneration. Br J Ophthalmol. 2001;85(5):531–3.
33. Chen SJ, Cheng CY, Lee FL, et al. Pulsatile ocular blood flow in asymmetric exudative age related macular degeneration. Br J Ophthalmol. 2001;85(12):1411–5.
34. MacKinnon JR, O'Brien C, Swa K, et al. Pulsatile ocular blood flow in untreated diabetic retinopathy. Acta Ophthalmol Scand. 1997;75(6):661–4.
35. Lawrence C, Schlegel WA. Ophthalmic pulse studies. I. Influence of intraocular pressure. Invest Ophthalmol. 1966;5(5):515–25.
36. Langham ME, To'Mey KF. A clinical procedure for the measurements of the ocular pulse-pressure relationship and the ophthalmic arterial pressure. Exp Eye Res. 1978;27:17–25.
37. Kaufmann C, Bachmann LM, Robert YC, et al. Ocular pulse amplitude in healthy subjects as measured by dynamic contour tonometry. Arch Ophthalmol. 2006;124:1104–8.
38. Stalmans I, Harris A, Vanbellinghen V, et al. Ocular pulse amplitude in normal tension and primary open angle glaucoma. J Glaucoma. 2008;17:403–7.
39. Knecht PB, Bosch MM, Michels S, Mannhardt S, Schmid U, Bosch MA, Menke MN. The ocular pulse amplitude at different intraocular pressure: a prospective study. Acta Ophthalmol. 2011;89:e466–71.
40. Quaranta L, Manni G, Donato F, et al. The effect of increased intraocular pressure on pulsatile ocular blood flow in low tension glaucoma. Surv Ophthalmol. 1994;38(suppl):S177–81. discussion S182
41. Aydin A, Wollstein G, Price LL, et al. Evaluating pulsatile ocular blood flow analysis in normal and treated glaucomatous eyes. Am J Ophthalmol. 2003;136(3):448–53.

42. Kerr J, Nelson P, O'Brien C. A comparison of ocular blood flow in untreated primary open-angle glaucoma and ocular hypertension. Am J Ophthalmol. 1998;126(1):42–51.
43. Kerr J, Nelson P, O'Brien C. Pulsatile ocular blood flow in primary open-angle glaucoma and ocular hypertension. Am J Ophthalmol. 2003;136(6):1106–13.

Chapter 17
Ocular Rigidity and Cornea Disease

Argyrios Tzamalis, Esmaeil Arbabi, and David A. Taylor

Introduction

In the past few decades there has been a constantly increasing interest in the biomechanical properties of the cornea. The cornea is comprised of tissue with elements of both elasticity and viscosity [1, 2]. Any elements that change the structure of the cornea may impact its biomechanical properties. The 3-dimensional meshwork of transversely oriented collagen fibers plays a dominant role in giving the corneal stroma its specific visco-elastic configuration and is a significant factor in the determination of corneal shape [3].

The optical properties of the eye can be affected by very slight alterations in corneal shape [2, 4]. Such changes can be induced either by corneal diseases, such as ectatic disorders, or by refractive surgery [5–8]. These conditions or procedures not only change corneal structure and its optical properties, but they also have a great impact on its mechanical properties [7, 8]. Therefore, it has become crucial to better understand corneal biomechanics, as these properties may contribute significantly to the development of pathologies, and may allow us to predict corneal behavior and improve the results of treatment modalities. Beyond refractive procedures and corneal pathologies, the assessment of corneal biomechanics is a factor to be considered in glaucoma diagnosis and management, as this variable significantly impacts the measurement of intraocular pressure (IOP), prompting inaccurate

A. Tzamalis (✉)
2nd Department of Ophthalmology, Faculty of Medicine, Papageorgiou General Hospital, Aristotle University of Thessaloniki, Thessaloniki, Greece

E. Arbabi
St. Paul's Eye Unit, Royal Liverpool University Hospital, Liverpool, UK

D. A. Taylor
Reichert Technologies, Buffalo, NY, USA
e-mail: dave.taylor@ametek.com

© Springer Nature Switzerland AG 2021
I. Pallikaris et al. (eds.), *Ocular Rigidity, Biomechanics and Hydrodynamics of the Eye*, https://doi.org/10.1007/978-3-030-64422-2_17

tonometry readings even within the limits of a normal population, but especially after refractive surgery [9–12].

The development of devices designed to assess corneal biomechanics has been an important step to bring theory from the lab into clinical practice. The Ocular Response Analyzer (ORA, Reichert, Buffalo, New York, USA) based on non-contact applanation tonometry in a bidirectional mode and CorVis ST (Oculus Optikgeräte GmbH, Wetzlar, Germany) using Scheimpflug imaging of corneal deformation are the main in-vivo technologies which are currently available for a clinical evaluation of corneal biomechanical properties. Further methods that are still under investigation include Brillouin microscopy, ultrasonic elastography, speckle pattern interferometry and high frequency ultrasonic analysis of corneal changes. Although, significant advancements have been made in recent years in the measurement and understanding of corneal biomechanics, the unique and complex variables involved in in-vivo assessment of ocular biomechanics, particularly the IOP, may prohibit the determination of "classical" biomechanical indices, such as elastic modulus. It is, therefore, very important to understand the measurement parameters provided by these devices and to be able to interpret the results that are provided.

Ocular Rigidity and Corneal Biomechanics

Ocular rigidity (OR) is a measure of the resistance that the eye exerts to distending forces describing the relationship between pressure and volume changes in the human eye, mainly referring to the elasticity of the sclera and the cornea [13]. Well before modern corneal biomechanical parameters, such as corneal hysteresis (CH) and corneal resistance factor (CRF), were involved in the analysis of corneal elasticity and viscosity, ocular rigidity was estimated as an attempt to assess biomechanical properties of the cornea, especially in keratoconic patients [14–17].

Although in their initial study in 1978, Foster et al. did not show any difference in ocular rigidity between normal and keratoconic eyes [14], several other authors reported a significantly reduced ocular rigidity in ectatic corneas [15–17]. Furthermore, corneal thinning was found to be correlated with OR in some of those studies [17]. On the other hand, investigating ocular rigidity in living human eyes Pallikaris et al. found no significant correlation between the ocular rigidity coefficient and central corneal thickness, advocating that variations in central corneal thickness may affect corneal rigidity but have less impact on ocular rigidity [18]. However, as pointed out by Kalenak et al., Friedenwald's concept of ocular rigidity [13] is empirically derived and thus ocular elasticity should be classified using fundamental engineering terms, such as Young's modulus [19].

The impact of refractive surgery on ocular rigidity has also been investigated in several studies leading to controversial results. Using an invasive manometric ocular rigidity measurement device in rabbit eyes, Kymionis et al. showed no differences in ocular rigidity between eyes that underwent photorefractive keratectomy (for −10.00 diopters (D) in a 5-mm optical zone) and their fellow control eyes, when measuring OR 5 weeks later [20]. In contrast, Cronenberger et al. utilizing differential tonometry in human eyes after LASIK, found a significant change in ocular rigidity, induced by the procedure [21].

In recent years, multiple methods have been developed to measure corneal biomechanical properties in vivo, producing new biomechanical variables such as CH and CRF. However, their relationship to ocular rigidity has not been fully clarified yet. Attempting to do so, Lin et al. demonstrated a significant negative correlation between CRF and OR in normal eyes, while CH and OR were not found to be correlated to each other [22]. Interpreting their results, the authors support that CRF is related to OR as it primarily reflects ocular tissue elasticity, while CH is not associated with ocular rigidity and likely reflects tissue viscosity [22].

Corneal Structure and Biomechanics

Corneal structure and anatomy strongly differ between layers of the cornea as collagen orientation and density varies. Each corneal layer plays a role, to a lesser or greater level, in the biomechanical resistance. Some layers have almost no contribution to the stiffness of the cornea as they are purely cellular.

The epithelium and the endothelium have been proven to contribute very little in comparison to the stroma, although they can indirectly impact corneal stiffness due to their ability to regulate its hydration status [23]. Bowman's membrane, with its densely packed collagen lamellae, has a substantial role in preserving corneal stability, especially after refractive surgery [24]. The majority, thus, of corneal biomechanical properties can be attributed to the corneal stroma, which also varies between its anterior and posterior part. Finally, the pre-Descemet membrane, that has recently been described by Dua et al. [25] is still under investigation regarding its biomechanical contribution, but it is thought to contribute significantly to corneal stiffness due to its surmised mechanical strength.

Corneal Biomechanics of the Epithelium

Corneal epithelium is a thin layer that represents the anterior 50 μm of the cornea and its role in corneal stiffness has been investigated lately with controversial results. Yoo et al., using creep tests in bovine eyes, have shown a higher intrinsic stiffness of the epithelium in comparison to the corneal stroma [26]. Their findings are opposed to those reported by Elsheik et al., who were the first to evaluate the contribution of the epithelium to the overall corneal stiffness by means of inflation test in human corneas, and found that it was much less than the one produced by the corneal stroma [23]. The above-mentioned discrepancy could be attributed to differences in the methods used and the measured modulus to define corneal biomechanics. Recently, atomic force microscopy (AFM) has been used on rabbit corneas by Thomasy et al. to evaluate epithelium biomechanical properties, concluding that epithelial biomechanical strength was lower in comparison to other corneal layers [27]. The same technique has also been used on human corneas, showing that the elastic modulus of the basement membrane reached a mean of 7.5 ± 4.2 kPa ranging from 2 to 15 kPa, much higher than that of rabbits [28].

Corneal Biomechanics of the Bowman's Membrane

Bowman's membrane is a smooth, acellular, non-regenerating layer, that is 8-12 μm thick in adults [29]. It is composed of a densely packed meshwork of randomly oriented collagen fibrils and its posterior surface merges with the collagen fibrils of the corneal stroma, thus possibly playing a significant role in stabilizing corneal curvature [24]. Regarding its biomechanical properties, it is not considered to contribute substantially to corneal stiffness, although its disruption represents a risk factor for corneal ectatic disorders [30–32]. By means of AFM, Bowman's layer elastic modulus was found to be higher than the one of the anterior stroma, while using the finite element method (FEM) one fifth of the overall bending corneal rigidity was attributed to the Bowman's layer and the Descemet's membrane [33, 34].

Corneal Biomechanics of the Stroma

The corneal stroma accounts for almost 90% of the overall corneal thickness and has a high density in collagen fibrils. It is, thus, considered to be the main contributor to the corneal stiffness and in general the biomechanical properties of the cornea. It is consisted of numerous collagen lamellae that have a preferred orientation in the vertical and horizontal directions [35].

Extracellular matrix components also play a key role in the structure and subsequently the biomechanical behavior of the cornea and its transparent status. The diameter of collagen fibrils is controlled by keratan sulfate proteoglycans (PGs), while interfibrillar spacing and lamellar adhesion is regulated by dermatan sulfate proteoglycans [36]. On the other hand, Gycosaminoglycans (GAGs) interfere with collagen fibrils only in an electrostatic level. However, they are essential to sulfate PG core proteins which, when found in reduced levels, are strongly associated with several ectatic disorders [37–39]. Moreover, it has been found that acidic GAGs correlate positively with the degree of collagen fiber organization in the human corneal stroma [40].

Many methods and techniques have been utilized so far attempting to define the stromal biomechanics, both destructive ex-vivo as well as non-destructive in vivo. There has also been a great debate regarding differences of corneal elastic modulus and other properties between the anterior and posterior stroma, as well as between the central and peripheral part of the stroma. Collagen lamellae demonstrate specific differences between the anterior and posterior stroma. Their density is shown to be considerably higher and their arrangement much more complicated with extensive interlamellar branching in the anterior stroma [41, 42].

The anterior stroma has been shown to have a higher elastic modulus when compared to the posterior one in various studies [27, 43–45]. This has been proven both by indentation testing as well as by AFM in human and rabbit corneas respectively, indicating an almost 3 times greater corneal stiffness in the anterior stroma [27, 43]. Furthermore, an association was found between the axial gradient in lamellar intertwining with an axial gradient in the effective elastic modulus of the cornea [43]. Focusing exclusively on human corneas by means of AFM Dias et al. have reported average values of elastic modulus that ranged between 281 kPa in the anterior and 89.5 kPa in the posterior stroma [44]. Investigating the depth-dependent mechanical anisotropy of the human corneal stroma, Labate et al. reported a unique anisotropic elastic behavior in a tissue level (with a steep decrease at 140 μm depth of stroma) as well as in a molecular level [45].

Mikula et al. took the investigation of stromal elastic modulus a step further trying to produce a map of corneal elasticity by means of acoustic radiation force elasticity microscope (ARFEM) [46]. Their results showed that the average elastic modulus was higher in the anterior stroma in the central (4.2 ± 1.2 kPa [anterior] vs 2.3 ± 0.7 kPa [posterior]) and middle regions (3.4 ± 0.7 kPa [anterior] vs 1.6 ± 0.3 kPa [posterior]); however it was significantly lower than the one of posterior stroma when examining regions in the corneal periphery (1.9 ± 0.7 kPa [anterior] vs 2.9 ± 1.2 kPa [posterior]). There is some evidence that the posterior peripheral cornea exhibits more interweaving as the inclination angles of collagen lamellae are higher in this region, which could explain these results [47].

Corneal Biomechanics of the Dua's Layer

The pre-Descemet's layer or Dua's layer that has recently been demonstrated by Dua et al. using electron microscopy is an acellular layer above Descemet's membrane, 10.15 ± 3.6 microns thick, that consists of 5 to 8 lamellae of predominantly type-1 collagen bundles arranged in transverse, longitudinal, and oblique directions [15]. As it has only been described 7 years ago, limited data exist in the literature regarding its biomechanical response and properties. However, it is considered as an important factor in corneal hydrops and it has been shown that its stabilization with sutures and intracameral air injection could faster restore the imperviousness of posterior stroma throughout the control of acute hydrops [48].

Investigating the microstructure of endothelial keratoplasty grafts by means of two-photon optical microscopy, Lombardo et al. found that the far posterior stroma demonstrates an alteration in its configuration at approximately 10 μm above the Descemet's membrane (DM). The collagen fibrils of this pre-Descemetic layer exhibit an intertwined complex with DM, that cannot be separated using hydrodissection [49]. Consequently, although Dua's layer seems to play a key role in corneal stiffness its contribution needs to be further examined in future studies.

Corneal Biomechanics of the Descemet's Membrane

Descemet's membrane is a basement membrane that acts as a barrier between corneal stroma and the endothelial layer. It is 8–10 µm thick in adults, starting from 3 µm at birth and its structure includes different kinds of collagen (Type IV and VIII) being secreted by the single layer of squamous epithelial cells that lies underneath [50]. There is a great variety in the results of studies aiming to evaluate the elastic modulus of DM depending on the method used. For example, Last et al. [33] using AFM have measured the elastic modulus of DM as high as 50 ± 17.8 kPa, while in other studies utilizing creep tests the elastic modulus was found to be significantly higher and DM showed to be 3.4- to 5.2-fold stiffer and to attain 2.7- to 4.6-fold higher stress at a strain value of 0.10 when compared with lens capsule [51]. As mentioned before, the collagen fibrils of Dua's layer form an intertwined complex with DM and possibly this could explain why DM and Bowman's membrane contribute almost 20% to the overall corneal rigidity [52]. The topography of the Descemet membrane has been shown to be similar to that of the anterior basal membrane, but with a smaller pore size resulting in more dense structure. This structural difference may be responsible for the observed differences in elasticity. Determining these values could assist to the design of a better cellular environment model as well as to the production of artificial corneas [52].

Corneal Biomechanics of the Endothelium

Corneal endothelium is the inner and probably most important monolayer of the cornea. It consists of unique hexagonal cells that function as a barrier to the movement of aqueous humor towards the stroma. The dynamic balance, between the barrier and the active pump, controls hydration of the cornea, keeping the cornea transparent and regulating thus corneal stiffness [53]. Corneal endothelial cells density in infants aged 2 months old has been reported to reach up to 5.624 cells/mm^2, with an average of 4.252 cells/mm^2 during the first year of life and decreases with age as endothelial cells have limited ability to proliferate in vivo [54]. Yoo et al. working on bovine eyes have reported very high values of stiffness for the complex of the endothelium with DM, greater than any other corneal layer [26], while when using AFM in rabbit eyes, the elastic modulus was assessed 4.1 ± 1.7 kPa, lower than that of the corneal stroma [27]. However these studies refer to animal models and should be evaluated critically as the anatomy and microstructure may differ between species.

In Vivo Measurement of Corneal Biomechanical Properties

Currently two devices are available to characterize biomechanical properties of the cornea in the clinical setting: Ocular Response Analyzer (ORA) (Reichert, Buffalo, New York, USA) and Corvis ST (Oculus Optikgeräte GmbH, Wetzlar, Germany). However, there are many other techniques which are currently being evaluated with potential application in clinical practice. Such devices and techniques include electronic speckle pattern interferometry, high-frequency ultrasonographic analysis, ultrasonic elastography, and Brillouin microscopy.

Brillouin Optical Microscopy is not yet clinically available, but is a promising technique for measuring biomechanical properties of the cornea. It performs non-contact Brillouin imaging of the cornea using a combination of a confocal microscope with an ultrahigh resolution spectrometer. Brillouin imaging allows visualization of the spatially heterogeneous biomechanical properties of the cornea [55]. This has the potential to visualize corneal elasticity and measure depth-dependent variations of elastic modulus within the cornea noninvasively with three-dimensional resolution. This device was firstly used in bovine corneas and is currently in development for use in human eyes with a new commercial device currently being developed for by Avedro, Inc. A more detailed discussion of this, and the other techniques mentioned above, is beyond the scope of this chapter and therefore we limit our discussions to the two devices that are currently commercially available for clinical use.

Reichert Ocular Response Analyzer

The Ocular Response Analyzer (ORA) was developed by Luce in the early 2000s and released commercially in 2005 as a device capable of measuring corneal biomechanical properties and IOP values that are less dependent on these properties than applanation tonometry. It was the first device to evaluate corneal biomechanics in-vivo [56]. The system consists of a solenoid-driven air pump, an infrared light emitter, a light intensity detector, and a pressure transducer inside the air plenum chamber. It analyses the response of the cornea during a "bidirectional applanation process"—a rapid in/out flexing of the cornea under the increasing and decreasing force of an air jet. The air pump delivers a collimated stream of air that causes the cornea to move posteriorly, passing through a state of flattening (inward applanation) as it deforms. The infrared light simultaneously shines on the cornea and the reflected IR light signal is recorded by the detector from an approximate 3 mm zone of the corneal apex [57]. The inward applanation is identified as a peak in reflected IR light intensity from the cornea. The applied force of the air jet begins to decrease milliseconds after the first applanation and the cornea passes through a second flattening (outward applanation) as it returns to its original curvature. The two applanation events occur within milliseconds of each other, thus ensuring that neither the position of eye nor the ocular pulse contaminate the results of the measurement.

The device records the pressures associated with the two applanation events, which are termed P1 and P2 respectively. These two pressures are not the same due to viscoelastic properties of the cornea. Specifically, the viscous properties of the cornea cause a damping effect, that results in an overestimation of the IOP on the way in, and an underestimation of the IOP on the way out. The difference between the inward applanation (P1) and the outward applanation (P2) is termed Corneal Hysteresis. The term hysteresis comes from the Greek word meaning 'lagging behind' and is commonly used in physics and engineering to describe materials or systems that do not respond instantly to applied forces, but respond slowly, or dissipate a portion of the applied energy. Materials or systems that exhibit hysteresis under in/out application of force always have a viscous component. Materials that are purely elastic in nature do not have hysteresis. As such, the Corneal Hysteresis is primarily indicative of the viscous damping characteristics of the corneal and ocular tissue and is not directly reflective of "stiffness", "resistance", or "rigidity" as these are terms associated with elasticity, not viscosity.

The maximal air pressure applied by the ORA air pump is not constant. Instead, it depends on the first applanation pressure (P1) which is a function of the true IOP and the biomechanical properties of individual corneas [56]. Therefore, eyes with lower pressure on first applanation receive a lower maximum applied force and eyes with higher IOP received a higher maximum applied force [57]. This is essential to measuring hysteresis as hysteresis is a *rate dependent phenomenon* and, as such, it is important to apply and remove the force at the same rate and to induce a *similar* deformation for eyes with a wide range of possible intraocular pressures. The corneal hysteresis measurement is presented in millimeters of mercury (mmHg).

In addition to Corneal hysteresis (CH) the ORA provides a parameter known as Corneal Resistance Factor (CRF). CRF is also derived from P1 and P2 but using a constant (k) in a linear equation (CRF = P1-kP2). The constant k is theoretically related to elasticity of the cornea and is derived through empirical evaluation of relation between P1, P2 and CCT. Finally, utilizing the information gleaned though the ORA measurement process, the device also displays an IOP measurement (called IOPcc) that effectively compensates for biomechanical variables in corneal thickness. The derivation and clinical interpretation of this measurement is beyond the scope of this chapter.

It should be noted that the ORA monitors the complete corneal deformation via its electo-optical system, recording 400 data samples of reflected light signal from the cornea during the approximately 25 ms long measurement. ORA PC software versions 2.0 and later calculate of 37 "waveform" parameters that describes the actual measurement signal from the in/out corneal deformation process. These parameters provide additional information that appears to be useful in the evaluation of the corneal biomechanics. To this point, a "keratoconus Match Index" software module was released by Reichert in 2009, compatible with Generation 1 (2005–2012) versions of the ORA instrument. While results appear promising, more studies are needed to explain the exact application and meaning of these parameters in clinical context [58, 59].

Oculus Corvis ST

The Corvis ST (CVS) was introduced in 2010 and, like the ORA, uses a jet of air to deform the cornea [60]. However, it provides information about the response of the cornea via dynamic Scheimpflug imaging analysis [61, 62]. The air-puff has a fixed maximum pressure of 25 kPa which forces the cornea through several distinct phases. During the first phase of measurement (inward) the air puff moves the cornea posteriorly until it reaches the highest concavity (HC) which is then followed by a period of corneal oscillations. As the applied force decreases, the cornea passes through a second applanation (outward phase) before finally returning to its natural state of rest. The Ultra high speed Scheimpflug camera is capable of 4430 frames per second (capturing approximately 140 frames during the 30-ms process) using an ultraviolet free 455 nm blue light with a single slit beam along an 8.5 mm horizontal corneal coverage before, during, and after the air-puff induced dynamic deformation, which provides a two-dimensional visualization of the deformation process [61, 62].

The Corvis system continuously records the time of the corresponding applied air pressure during the measurement so the corneal state is correlated with the air pressure at specific points of time and specific applied air pressure [61]. Zero value for time is marked a few milliseconds before the start of the air pulse from the pump. The camera starts taking images to calculate the corneal thickness and curvature data before initiation of the air pulse and setting the cornea into motion. From the corneal thickness measurements and characterization profile the system calculates the Ambrósio Relational Thickness through the horizontal meridian (ARTh) which is comparable to some extent to the tomographic relational thickness calculations available on the Pentacam [63]. The corneas' response to air pressure is characterized by multiple deformation parameters, some of which are reported to be correlated with the tissue's mechanical stiffness [57, 64]. The system displays a video of the corneal deformation process and plots results on 3 graphs; deformation amplitude, applanation length, and corneal velocity. The Corvis measurement process makes possible the capture of numerous unique parameters including, but not limited to, the applanation times, applanation deformation amplitudes, applanation deflection amplitudes, applanation velocities, applanation lengths (the length of the applanated corneal segment), applanation deflection lengths, maximum deformation amplitude, maximum deflection amplitude, highest concavity time, peak distance, radius at highest concavity, highest concavity deformation amplitude, highest concavity deflection amplitude, highest concavity deflection length, and whole eye movement. In addition, more standard parameters such as corneal radius, IOP and pachymetry are also determined and presented.

Very recently, a new combined Tomography Biomechanical Index (TBI) functionality has been made available for the Corvis. This new analysis has been shown to be highly sensitive and specific for the identification of keratoconus and even forme fruste or sub-clinical keratoconus [65]. Additional studies are needed to confirm the results of this promising capability. Finally, the Corvis is also capable of providing a biomechanically compensated IOP value referred to as bIOP, which was derived using finite element analysis and takes into consideration CCT, age, and dynamic corneal resistance (DCR) parameters. The derivation and clinical interpretation of this measurement is beyond the scope of this chapter.

Corneal Biomechanics in Healthy Human Corneas

A large base of evidence has been established in the literature in the past 15 years since the commercial availability of devices to measure biomechanics in practice. Direct correlation between the available parameters and corneal "rigidity" have not yet been established as it is still unclear what parameters best represent the true corneal modulus of elasticity in vivo. The majority of the publications (nearly 700) have presented findings using the Ocular Response Analyzer due to the fact that it was the first available device. However, there are approximately 175 publications on Corvis already at the time of the writing of this chapter.

In one of the earliest papers on in-vivo corneal biomechanics, Shah et al. reported on Ocular Response Analyzer measurements of CH and CRF, along with CCT in 207 normal eyes of patients with an average age of 62.1 years. They found average CH was 10.7 and CRF was 10.3. CH and CRF were shown to be statistically significantly, but moderately, correlated to CCT. They concluded that CH, CRF, and CCT are related but are not representative of the same physical properties [66]. Numerous subsequent studies on normal subjects have reported similar findings [8, 66–68]. The diurnal variation of CH in normal subjects across a wide range of ages has been studied and reported to be almost constant throughout the day [69, 70]. Three studies to date on normal children and young adults indicate that CH values in children are higher than in adults [71–73]. Three studies on patients with a wide range of ages have shown that CH is weakly negatively correlated with age (decreases) [74, 75]. While there are ex-vivo evidence that the cornea becomes considerably stiffer with age [76, 77] it should be remembered that Corneal Hysteresis is related to viscous damping, not elasticity, and as such it should not be a surprise that it appears to decrease with age.

Corneal Biomechanical Parameters After Cataract Surgery

Cataract surgery requires small corneal incisions, but is typically not considered to have a major biomechanical impact on the cornea, sans the potential for surgically induced astigmatism, which is a minor but semi-frequent undesirable outcome. Studies investigating pre- and post-cataract surgery have shown an initial decrease in CH and CRF with full recovery of these parameters in 1–3 months [78, 79]. These short term biomechanical changes are likely due to corneal edema and the natural post-operative wound healing process. It has also been reported that microincisonal cataract surgery provides a faster biomechanical recovery than a standard phacoemulsification during the first post-operative month [80]. In addition, Denoyer et al. reported that CH was more predictive of post-operative surgically induced astigmatism than incision size [81].

The effects of femtosecond laser-assisted cataract surgery (FLACS) vs phacoemulsification on corneal biomechanics has been studied using the Corvis. Significant differences were found in several parameters between the two groups at 1 week after surgery with FLACS group showing a lesser impact on the corneal biomechanics vs phacoemulsification. Similar to findings with the ORA, these changes in biomechanics were no longer detected at 1 month after surgery indicating the healing of the incision, and the reduction of swelling [82].

Corneal Biomechanical Properties in Fuchs and Corneal Transplants

Corneal pathologies often result in changes in corneal thickness and corneal geometry. Beyond these common and easily measured variables, researchers have long discussed potential alterations of biomechanics in ocular pathology, such as Fuchs' and Keratoconus. Del Buey et al. showed that CH was significantly lower in eyes with Fuchs' (6.9 vs 10.3 in normal controls) even though the central corneal thickness was significantly higher in the Fuchs' eyes (606 vs 538 microns) indicating that CH represents a tissue property, rather than a geometrical aspect of the cornea [83].

Penetrating Keratoplasty (PK) has been studied using biomechanical measurement technologies. Several authors have reported that, compared to normal eyes, post PK eyes have slightly lower CH and CRF [84, 85]. Corvis parameters have been compared between normal and PK eyes as well. Highest concavity time and Corvis radius values showed significant differences. There were no significant relationships between the keratometric data, the size of the donor and recipient, age of the donor and recipient and biomechanical properties obtained by Corvis ST [86].

John et al. demonstrated that CH is significantly lower in eyes following descemetorhexis with endokeratoplasty (DXEK) despite the fact that these corneas are much thicker than (6.94 for DXEK vs 10.51 for normal) [87]. Clemmensen and Hjortdal also reported that Corneal hysteresis and CRF are reduced in Fuchs' endothelial dystrophy as well as after DSAEK [88]. The surprising reduction in CH in post DXEK and DSAEK eyes, despite the substantially greater corneal thickness, may be due to the disruption of the "binding" capability of Dua's layer and Descemet's membrane at the posterior of the cornea.

Corneal Biomechanical Parameters in Refractive Surgery

All refractive surgery procedures that cut, ablate, and/or remove corneal tissue alter the biomechanical properties of the cornea. It is well documented that refractive surgery procedures affect the accuracy of IOP measurements due to the thinner and weaker post-operative cornea, which no longer resists the applied force of a tonometer as an average normal cornea would. When devices to measure corneal biomechanics became available, groups around the world commenced investigations to quantify the biomechanical impact of refractive surgery procedures on the cornea.

Numerous studies have reported a decrease in ORA measures of CH and CRF after myopic and hyperopic LASIK reflecting a weakening of the corneal structure following the procedure [8, 89–91]. For comparable flap thicknesses and ablation depths both CH and CRF decease more in myopic ablation compared to hyperopic ablation. Somewhat surprisingly, it has been shown that postoperative reduction in corneal hysteresis does not correlate strongly with the amount or percentage of corneal tissue removed. This seems to indicate that CH characterizes properties not previously understood and that biomechanical changes induced by refractive surgery may not be predictable based on geometrical changes such as thickness [91]. The time course of biomechanical changes after LASIK have also been studied. It was reported that reductions in CH and CRF were similar at 1 week, 1 month, 3 months and 6 months after surgery [92]. It appears the viscoelastic properties of the cornea do not return toward preoperative levels based on these metrics. Numerous studies using the Corvis have shown significant changes in most Corvis parameters, consistent with what one would expect from biomechanical weakening, including Applanation lengths, velocities, deformation amplitudes, highest concavity and other related parameters [93, 94].

Discerning the biomechanical impact of various methods of flap creation vs the impact of photoablation is a topic of great interest. Gatinel et al. investigated corneal biomechanical changes after only cutting a corneal lamellar flap with no photoablation. The flap was cut on one eye of a patient and CH and CRF were measured before, the day of, and 25 days postoperatively in both eyes. CH and CRF did not change in the control eye, but were significantly reduced in the operated eye. The thickness did not change but it is apparent that flap creation has an independent biomechanical impact [95]. Hamilton et al. investigated changes in corneal biomechanics between mechanical keratome LASIK, Femtosecond flap LASIK, and PRK. While there were no significant differences in ablation depth, delta CH, or delta CRF between the 3 groups, the FS-LASIK group experienced changes in CH and CRF that were more strongly related to the ablation depth, than the change with PRK and LASIK with microkeratome flap creation [96].

More recently studies on small incision lenticule extraction (SMILE) have been conducted and have shown that this procedure also causes significant reduction in biomechanical measurements by ORA and Corvis. ORA Parameters CH and CRF are significantly altered as well as most Corvis parameters. However, it has been shown that SMILE-induced changes are lesser than LASIK [97]. In a study comparing biomechanical differences in corneas treated with SMILE vs femtosecond laser-assisted LASIK (FS-LASIK) almost all Corvis parameters showed significant changes in both groups postoperatively. However, matched pair subgroup analysis of eyes with initially equal CCT, IOP, SE, and difference of pre-to postoperative CCT showed no significant changes in parameters between FS-LASIK and SMILE [98]. This would seem to indicate that FS-LASIK and SMILE induce similar biomechanical changes to the cornea, but more studies are needed to confirm these early results.

Also of interest, the correlation between corneal biomechanics and the corneal short-term response to orthokeratology lens wear has been studied. CH is significantly correlated with changes in steep keratometry and central corneal thickness in patients wearing ortho-k lenses and with changes in steep keratometry during recovery. Overall, higher values of CH result in slower effect and recovery of the ortho-keratologic effect [99].

It is clear, based on the evidence, that refractive surgery has a substantive impact on corneal biomechanical properties. Additional studies using the ORA, Corvis, and other biomechanical assessment tools should help us to increase our understanding of these changes and, ideally, to utilize this knowledge to improve refractive surgery outcomes and to prevent complications.

Corneal Biomechanics in Keratoconus

Keratoconus is a noninflammatory condition of unknown aetiology affecting the central cornea characterized by progressive thinning and steepening of the cornea [100]. Increased distensibility has been reported to be an important factor in the pathogenesis of keratoconus [101]. As such, the desire to understand corneal biomechanical properties in keratoconus eyes is obvious. The hope is that measurements of corneal biomechanical properties could help to predict development of these conditions earlier than conventional diagnostic devices, such as Topography. In addition, identification of eyes with a propensity to develop keratoconus could help eliminate iatrogenic ectasia, a rare but dreaded potential complication from LASIK surgery.

Shah was the first to report ORA parameters of CH and CRF were significantly lower in Keratoconic eyes compared to normal eyes [67]. Since many other studies confirmed this finding [102–106], the severity of keratoconus has been shown to be negatively correlated with CH and CRF [8]. CRF appears to be able to better discriminate between normal and keratoconus eyes, however, using CRF alone to detect KC has a low specificity and sensitivity. Ambrosio et al. identified an optimal CRF cut off value of 9.60 with a sensitivity, specificity and test accuracy of 90.5%, 66% and 77% respectively [107]. Schweitzer et al. evaluated the ability of ORA parameters to distinguish between normal and forme fruste keratoconus (FFKC) eyes. The mean CH and CRF were found to be significantly different between the controls and FFKC eyes with a 9.5 cut-off value providing sensitivity, specificity, and test accuracy similar to previous reports [108].

A case report by Kerautret et al. documented a patient who developed unilateral corneal ectasia after bilateral LASIK. It was observed that the two eyes had similar postoperative CH and CRF values, but that the affected eye produced a very different ORA signal waveform. The waveform applanation peaks were lower amplitude and the area under the peaks, especially the second peak, was greatly reduced compared to the non-ectatic [109]. This was the first published evidence of differences in ORA waveform characteristics in post refractive surgery and ectasia eyes.

Research by Saad, Gatinel, and Luce showed that ORA waveform parameters enable significant separation of normal and forme fruste keratoconus eyes. The waveform parameters far outperformed the CH and CRF parameters [110]. Zarei-Ghanavati et al. investigated the ability of ORA waveform parameters to differentiate between normal post-LASIK eyes and keratoconus eyes. After statistically controlling for the differences in CCT and age, seven parameters were found to be the most useful in distinguishing between the groups. Combining these parameters provided an area under the ROC curve of 0.932. The authors concluded ORA waveform is useful to identify biomechanical conditions [111].

ORA inventor David Luce (1935–2017) utilized these waveform parameters in an analysis of normal and KC data to determine whether the ORA waveform could better differentiate between normal and KC corneas than CH and CRF alone. Signals from 836 normal eyes and nearly 500 clinically identified keratoconus eyes were segregated into subpopulation of severe, moderate, mild, and FFKC were compared mathematically. Of the studied parameters, 12 were combined into the keratoconus match index (KMI), which provides higher sensitivity and specificity in separating normal from KC eyes than CH or CRF [112]. Rocha et al. investigated the ORA KMI in normal, suspect, keratoconus, and asymmetric keratoconus patients who had frank keratoconus in one eye, but topographically normal contralateral eye. The KMI agreed with the topographical identification in the normal, suspect, and keratoconus groups. It also agreed with the topographical indices in the frank keratoconus eye of the asymmetric keratoconus patients. However, in the topographically normal contralateral eyes, the KMI indicated forme fruste keratoconus [113].

While the KMI software appears to be promising in detecting keratoconus, the manufacturer (Reichert Inc) has indicated that the software has not yet been updated to function with newer Generation II and III versions of the Ocular Response Analyzer due to changes in instrumentation hardware, challenges with regulatory approval of the new parameters, and greater company focus on the glaucoma utility of the ORA device.

ORA and Corvis Measurements in Crosslinking (CXL)

Corneal Collagen Crosslinking (CXL) is the world's first medical treatment for keratoconus, intended to halt progression by the formation of chemically bonded crosslinks in the stroma. Numerous authors have studied the effects of CXL on corneal biomechanical measurements using the ORA and Corvis. A variety of publications have shown an absence of significant change in corneal hysteresis and corneal resistance factor by Ocular Response Analyze after CXL [114]. Bak-Nielsen et al. reported on the effects of CXL using the Corvis ST. Patients with both untreated and CXL-treated keratoconus were significantly different from normal patients with respect to the standard Corvis deformation parameters but no significant differences were found between patients with untreated keratoconus and CXL treated keratoconus [115]. These findings are considered by many to be in contrary to anticipated results causing some to question whether the ORA and Corvis are sensitive enough to detect the biomechanical changes induced by crosslinking. Still others have questioned whether or not crosslinking induces measurable biomechanical changes in in-vivo keratoconus patients [116].

Spoerl et al. investigated changes in ORA waveform parameters pre- and post CXL and found that, while the CH and CRF did not change, numerous waveform characteristics were altered by the CXL. The area under peak 2 was noted to be the ORA parameter most able to detect biomechanical changes after CXL. The authors concluded that after CXL keratoconic corneas display altered biomechanical properties, which remain different to those observed in healthy corneas [117].

In more recent investigations certain novel Corvis parameters showed differences between crosslinked corneas and untreated keratoconic corneas. In a small cohort of eyes measured pre- and post CXL (n = 10) Fuchsluger et al. found that Applanation 1 length – Applanation 2 length (A1L – A2L), velocity during second applanation (A2V) and deformation amplitude (DA) were significantly increased in crosslinked keratoconic eyes both compared with untreated keratoconic eyes and with healthy controls. Vinciguerra et al. reported on a series of new DCR (dynamic corneal response) Corvis parameters and found significant increases in SP-A1 and SP-HC and significant decreases in 1/R, DefA, and DA Ratio. It should be noted however that in both studies there were statistically significant changes pre- & post CXL in pachymetry and intraocular pressure and which could influence corneal stiffness parameters [118, 119].

While certain ORA waveform parameters and novel Corvis parameters seem to be promising to distinguish crosslinked from non-treated keratoconus eyes, it is clear that more research is needed in this area.

Corneal Biomechanics and Glaucoma

Glaucoma is an optic neuropathy that involves structural damage to the optic nerve and related vision loss. While these changes occur in the posterior of the eye, there has been ample published evidence over the past 20 years that the cornea provides useful information in the diagnosis of glaucoma. OHTS, the longest running and largest glaucoma trial in history put the cornea on the map in the glaucoma world with its surprise finding that corneal thickness was independently related to the development of glaucoma and more significant in this regard than IOP. Since the publication of OHTS, hundreds of papers have been published investigating corneal biomechanics and their relationship to glaucoma risk.

In the earliest publication to investigate the relevance of the CH measurement in glaucoma, Congdon et al. determined that lower CH, but not CCT, was associated with progressive visual field loss in a series of 230 patients with 5 years of visual field follow up history [120]. Numerous other authors have found that CH is significantly lower in POAG, and is independent from CCT and IOP [121, 122].

Anand et al. investigated CH in patients with asymmetric glaucomatous progression and found that lower CH had the best discriminability for the eye with the worse VF despite there being no difference in CCT or Goldmann IOP values between the two eyes [123]. In a later study by the same group, it was demonstrated that CH was associated with rate of progression in glaucoma. In 153 eyes of 153 patients (mean age 61.3, mean number of VF tests 8.5, and mean follow-up time 5.3 years), progressing eyes had lower CCT and lower CH compared with non-progressing eyes. In the multivariate analysis only peak IOP, age, and CH remained statistically significant [124]. In a prospective longitudinal study by Medeiros, CH was shown to explain a larger proportion of the changes in Visual Field Index than CCT (17.4% vs. 5.2%, respectively) and the effect of IOP on rates of glaucoma progression was dependent on the CH levels [125]. In a similar study it was reported that eyes with lower baseline CH had a higher probability of developing glaucomatous visual field defects in a cohort of pre-perimetric glaucoma suspects followed over 4 years. Each 1-mm Hg lower CH was associated with an increase of 21% in the risk of developing glaucoma [126].

In conclusion, the assessment of corneal biomechanics in vivo is fundamental to predict the corneal behavior to several changes that occur either with age, ocular pathologies or after surgical procedures. Even though a big number of studies have already been published dealing with this issue, mostly utilizing the ORA and Corvis ST, no general reliable conclusions can be drawn as there is a lack of consistency and not enough evidence. Further clinical studies and the implication of new technologies may enable the clinician to foresee the clinical results of various ocular treatments introducing new modalities with higher safety and efficacy.

References

1. Nyquist GW. Rheology of the cornea: experimental techniques and results. Exp Eye Res. 1968;7(2):183–8.
2. Woo SL, Kobayashi AS, Lawrence C, Schlegel WA. Mathematical model of the corneoscleral shell as applied to intraocular pressure-volume relations and applanation tonometry. Ann Biomed Eng. 1972;1(1):87–98.
3. Winkler M, Shoa G, Xie Y, et al. Three-dimensional distribution of transverse collagen fibers in the anterior human corneal stroma. Invest Ophthalmol Vis Sci. 2013;54(12):7293–01.
4. Asejczyk-Widlicka M, Pierscionek BK. Fluctuations in intraocular pressure and the potential effect on aberrations of the eye. Br J Ophthalmol. 2007;91:1054–8.
5. Piñero DP, Nicto JC, Lopez-Miguel A. Characterization of corneal structure in keratoconus. J Cataract Refract Surg. 2012;38:2167–83.
6. Krueger RR, Dupps WJ Jr. Biomechanical effects of femtosecond and microkeratome-based flap creation: prospective contralateral examination of two patients. J Refract Surg. 2007;23:800–7.
7. Kohnen T, Bühren J. Corneal first-surface aberration analysis of the biomechanical effects of astigmatic keratotomy and a microkeratome cut after penetrating keratoplasty. J Cataract Refract Surg. 2005;31:185–9.

8. Ortiz D, Piñero D, Shabayek MH, Arnalich-Montiel F, Alió JL. Corneal biomechanical properties in normal, post-laser in situ keratomileusis, and keratoconic eyes. J Cataract Refract Surg. 2007;33:1371–5.

9. Del Buey MA, Lavilla L, Ascaso FJ, Lanchares E, Huerva V, Cristóbal JA. Assessment of corneal biomechanical properties and intraocular pressure in myopic Spanish healthy population. J Ophthalmol. 2014;905129:2014.

10. Ogbuehi KC, Osuagwu UL. Corneal biomechanical properties: precision and influence on tonometry. Cont Lens Anterior Eye. 2014;37:124–231.

11. Liu J, Roberts CJ. Influence of corneal biomechanical properties on intraocular pressure measurement: quantitative analysis. J Cataract Refract Surg. 2005;31:146–55.

12. Shin J, Kim TW, Park SJ, Yoon M, Lee JW. Changes in biomechanical properties of the cornea and intraocular pressure after myopic laser in situ keratomileusis using a femtosecond laser for flap creation determined using ocular response analyzer and Goldmannn Applanation tonometry. J Glaucoma. 2015 Mar;24(3):195–201.

13. Friedenwald JS. Contribution to the theory and practice of tonometry. Am J Opt. 1937;20:985–1024.

14. Foster CS, Yamamoto GK. Ocular rigidity in keratoconus. Am J Ophthalmol. 1978;86:802–6.

15. Hartstein J, Becker B. Research into the pathogenesis of keratoconus: a new syndrome: low ocular rigidity, contact lenses and keratoconus. Arch Ophthalmol. 1970;84:728–9.

16. Edmund C. Corneal elasticity and ocular rigidity in normal and keratoconic eyes. Acta Ophthalmol (Copenh). 1988;66(2):134–40.

17. Brooks AM, Robertson IF, Mahoney AM. Ocular rigidity and intraocular pressure in keratoconus. Aust J Ophthalmol. 1984;12(4):317–24.

18. Pallikaris IG, Kymionis GD, Ginis HS, Kounis GA, Tsilimbaris MK. Ocular rigidity in living human eyes. Invest Ophthalmol Vis Sci. 2005;46(2):409–14.

19. Kalenak JW, White O. More ocular elasticity? Ophthalmology. 1991;98:411–2.

20. Kymionis GD, Diakonis VF, Kounis G, et al. Ocular rigidity evaluation after photorefractive keratectomy: an experimental study. J Refract Surg. 2008;24(2):173–7.

21. Cronemberger S, Guimaraes CS, Calixto N, et al. Intraocular pressure and ocular rigidity after LASIK. Arq Bras Oftalmol. 2009;72(4):439–43.

22. Lin S-C, Kazemi A, McLaren JW, Moroi SE, Toris CB, Sit AJ. Relationship between ocular rigidity, corneal hysteresis, and corneal resistance factor. Invest Ophthalmol Vis Sci. 2015;56(7):6137.

23. Elsheikh A, Alhasso D, Rama P. Assessment of the epithelium's contribution to corneal biomechanics. Exp Eye Res. 2008;86:445–51.

24. Dawson DG, Grossniklaus HE, Edelhauser HF, McCarey BE. Biomechanical and wound healing characteristics of corneas after excimer laser keratorefractive surgery. J Refract Surg. 2008;24:S90–6.

25. Dua HS, Faraj LA, Said DG, Gray T, Lowe J. Human corneal anatomy redefined: a novel pre-Descemet's layer (Dua's layer). Ophthalmology. 2013;120:1778–85.

26. Yoo L, Reed J, Gimzewski JK, Demer JL. Mechanical interferometry imaging for creep modeling of the cornea. Invest Ophthalmol Vis Sci. 2011;52(11):8420–4.

27. Thomasy SM, Raghunathan VK, Winkler M, et al. Elastic modulus and collagen organization of the rabbit cornea: epithelium to endothelium. Acta Biomater. 2014;10(2):785–91.

28. Torricelli AA, Singh V, Santhiago MR, et al. The corneal epithelial basement membrane: structure, function, and disease. Invest Ophthalmol Vis Sci. 2013;54(9):6390–400.

29. Hogan MJ, Alvarado JA, Weddell E. Histology of the human eye. Philadelphia: WB Saunders; 1971.

30. Krachmer JH, Feder RS, Belin MW. Keratoconus and related noninflammatory corneal thinning disorders. Surv Ophthalmol. 1984;28(4):293–322.

31. Kremer I, Eagle RC, Rapuano CJ, Laibson PR. Histologic evidence of recurrent keratoconus seven years after keratoplasty. Am J Ophthalmol. 1995;119(4):511–2.

32. Seiler T, Matallana M, Sendler S, Bende T. Does Bowman's layer determine the biomechanical properties of the cornea? Refract Corneal Surg. 1992;8(2):139–42.
33. Last JA, Thomasy SM, Croasdale CR, et al. Compliance profile of the human cornea as measured by atomic force microscopy. Micron. 2012;43(12):1293–8.
34. Shih PJ, Wang IJ, Cai WF, Yen JY. Biomechanical simulation of stress concentration and intraocular pressure in corneas subjected to myopic refractive surgical procedures. Sci Rep. 2017;7(1):13906.
35. Aghamohammadzadeh H, Newton RH, Meek KM. X-ray scattering used to map the preferred collagen orientation in the human cornea and limbus. Structure. 2004;12:249–56.
36. Michelacci Y. Collagens and proteoglycans of the corneal extracellular matrix. Braz J Med Biol Res. 2003;36:1037–46.
37. Scott JE. Proteoglycan-fibrillar collagen interactions. Biochem J. 1988;252:313–23.
38. Kao WW-Y, Liu C-Y. Roles of lumican and keratocan on corneal transparency. Glycoconj J. 2002;19:275–85.
39. Funderburgh J, Funderburgh M, Rodrigues M, Krachmer J, Conrad G. Altered antigenicity of keratan sulfate proteoglycan in selected corneal diseases. Invest Ophthalmol Vis Sci. 1990;31:419–28.
40. Praus R, Goldman J. Glycosaminoglycans in human corneal buttons removed at keratoplasty. Ophthalmic Res. 1971;2:223–30.
41. Bueno JM, Gualda EJ, Artal P. Analysis of corneal stroma organization with wavefront optimized nonlinear microscopy. Cornea. 2011;30(6):692–701.
42. Komai Y, Ushiki T. The three-dimensional organization of collagen fibrils in the human cornea and sclera. Invest Ophthalmol Vis Sci. 1991;32(8):2244–58.
43. Winkler M, Chai D, Kriling S, et al. Non-linear optical macroscopic assessment of 3-D corneal collagen organization and axial biomechanics. Invest Ophthalmol Vis Sci. 2011;52(12):8818–27.
44. Dias JM, Ziebarth NM. Anterior and posterior corneal stroma elasticity assessed using nanoindentation. Exp Eye Res. 2013;115:41–6.
45. Labate C, Lombardo M, De Santo MP, et al. Multiscale investigation of the depth-dependent mechanical anisotropy of the human corneal stroma. Invest Ophthalmol Vis Sci. 2015;56(6):4053–60.
46. Mikula ER, Jester JV, Juhasz T. Measurement of an elasticity map in the human cornea. Invest Ophthalmol Vis Sci. 2016;57(7):3282–6.
47. Abass A, Hayes S, White N, Sorensen T, Meek KM. Transverse depth-dependent changes in corneal collagen lamellar orientation and distribution. J R Soc Interface. 2015;12(104):20140717.
48. Chérif HY, Gueudry J, Afriat M, et al. Efficacy and safety of pre-Descemet's membrane sutures for the management of acute corneal hydrops in keratoconus. Br J Ophthalmol. 2015;99(6):773–7.
49. Lombardo M, Parekh M, Serrao S, et al. Two-photon optical microscopy imaging of endothelial keratoplasty grafts. Graefes Arch Clin Exp Ophthalmol. 2017;255(3):575–82.
50. Johnson DH, Bourne WM, Campbell RJ. The ultrastructure of Descemet's membrane. I. Changes with age in normal cornea. Arch Ophthalmol. 1982;100:1942.
51. Danielsen CC. Tensile mechanical and creep properties of Descemet's membrane and lens capsule. Exp Eye Res. 2004;79(3):343–50.
52. Last JA, Liliensiek SJ, Nealey PF, Murphy CJ. Determining the mechanical properties of human corneal basement membranes with atomic force microscopy. J Struct Biol. 2009;167:19–24.
53. Srinivas SP. Dynamic regulation of barrier integrity of the corneal endothelium. Optom Vis Sci. 2010;87:E239–54.
54. Bourne WM, Nelson LR, Hodge DO. Central corneal endothelial cell changes over a ten year period. Invest Ophthalmol Vis Sci. 1997;38:779.

55. Scarcelli G, Pineda R, Yun SH. Brillouin optical microscopy for corneal biomechanics. Invest Ophthalmol Vis Sci. 2012 Jan 20;53(1):185–90. https://doi.org/10.1167/iovs.11-8281.
56. Luce DA. Determining in vivo biomechanical properties of the cornea with an ocular response analyzer. J Cataract Refract Surg. 2005;31(1):156–62.
57. Roberts CJ. Concepts and misconceptions in corneal biomechanics. J Cataract Refract Surg. 2014;40(6):862–9. https://doi.org/10.1016/j.jcrs.2014.04.019.
58. Mikielewicz M, Kotliar K, Barraquer RI, Michael R. Air-pulse corneal applanation signal curve parameters for the characterisation of keratoconus. Br J Ophthalmol. 2011;95(6):793–8.
59. Wolffsohn JS, Safeen S, Shah S, Laiquzzaman M. Changes of corneal biomechanics with keratoconus. Cornea. 2012;31(8):849–54.
60. Hong J, Xu J, Wei A, Deng SX, Cui X, Yu X, Sun X. A new tonometer—the Corvis ST tonometer: clinical comparison with noncontact and Goldmann applanation tonometers. Invest Ophthalmol Vis Sci. 2013;54:659–65.
61. Ambrosio R Jr, Ramos I, Luz A, et al. Dynamic ultra-high speed Scheimpflug imaging for assessing corneal biomechanical properties. Rev Bras Oftalmol. 2013;72
62. Ambrósio R Jr, Ramos I, Luz A, et al. Dynamic ultra high speed Scheimpflug imaging for assessing corneal biomechanical properties. Rev Bras Oftalmol. 2013;72:99–102. https://doi.org/10.1590/S0034-72802013000200005.
63. Ambrósio R Jr, Caiado AL, Guerra FP, Louzada R, Roy AS, Luz A, Dupps WJ, Belin MW. Novel pachymetric parameters based on corneal tomography for diagnosing keratoconus. J Refract Surg. 2011;27(10):753–8. https://doi.org/10.3928/1081597X-20110721-01.
64. Piñero DP, Alcón N. In vivo characterization of corneal biomechanics. J Cataract Refract Surg. 2014;40(6):870–87. https://doi.org/10.1016/j.jcrs.2014.03.021.
65. Ambrósio R Jr, Lopes BT, Faria-Correia F, Salomao MQ, Buhren J, Roberts CJ, Elsheikh A, Vinciguerra R, Vinciguerra P. Integration of Scheimpflug-based corneal tomography and biomechanical assessments for enhancing ectasia detection. J Refract Surg. 2017 Jul 1;33(7):434–43. https://doi.org/10.3928/1081597X-20170426-02.
66. Shah S, Laiquzzaman M, Cunliffe I, et al. The use of the Reichert ocular response analyser to establish the relationship between ocular hysteresis, corneal resistance factor and central corneal thickness in normal eyes. Cont Lens Anterior Eye. 2006;29(5):257–62.
67. Shah S, Laiquzzaman M, Bhojwani R, Mantry S, Cunliffe I. Assessment of the biomechanical properties of the cornea with the ocular response analyzer in normal and keratoconic eyes. Invest Ophthalmol Vis Sci. 2007;48:3026–31.
68. Touboul D, Roberts C, Kerautret J, Garra C, Maurice-Tison S, Saubusse E, Colin J. Correlations between corneal hysteresis, intraocular pressure, and corneal central pachymetry. J Cataract Refract Surg. 2008;34:616–22.
69. Laiquzzaman M, Bhojwani R, Cunliffe I, et al. Diurnal variation of ocular hysteresis in normal subjects: relevance in clinical context. Clin Exp Ophthalmol. 2006;34(2):114–8.
70. Kida T, Liu JH, Weinreb RN. Effect of 24-hour corneal biomechanical changes on intraocular pressure measurement. Invest Ophthalmol Vis Sci. 2006;47(10):4422–6.
71. Kirwan C, O'Keefe M, Lanigan B. Corneal hysteresis and intraocular pressure measurement in children using the Reichert ocular response analyzer. Am J Ophthalmol. 2006;142:990–2.
72. Song Y, Congdon N, Li L, Zhou Z, Choi K, Lam DSC, Pang CP, Xie Z, Liu X, Sharma A, Chen W, Zhang M. Corneal hysteresis and axial length among Chinese secondary school children: the Xichang Pediatric Refractive Error Study (X-PRES) report no. 4. Am J Ophthalmol. 2008;145:819–26.
73. Lim L, Gazzard G, Chan YH, et al. Cornea biomechanical characteristics and their correlates with refractive error in Singaporean children. Invest Ophthalmol Vis Sci. 2008;49(9):3852–7.
74. Kida T, Liu JH, Weinreb RN. Effects of aging on corneal biomechanical properties and their impact on 24-hour measurement of intraocular pressure. Am J Ophthalmol. 2008;146(4):567–72.

75. Kotecha A, Elsheikh A, Roberts CR, et al. Corneal thickness and age-related biomechanical properties of the cornea measured with the ocular response analyzer. Invest Ophthalmol Vis Sci. 2006;47(12):5337–47.
76. Elsheikh A, Wang D, Brown M, Rama P, Campanelli M, Pye D. Assessment of corneal biomechanical properties and their variation with age. Curr Eye Res. 2007;32:11–9.
77. Sherrard ES, Novakovic P, Speedwell L. Age-related changes of the corneal endothelium and stroma as seen in vivo by specular microscopy. Eye. 1987;1:197–203.
78. Kamiya K, Shimizu K, Ohmoto F, Amano R. Evaluation of corneal biomechanical parameters after simultaneous phacoemulsification with intraocular lens implantation and limbal relaxing incisions. J Cataract Refract Surg. 2011 Feb;37(2):265–70. https://doi.org/10.1016/j.jcrs.2010.08.045.
79. Hager A, Loge K, Füllhas MO, Schroeder B, Grossherr M, Wiegand W. Changes in corneal hysteresis after clear corneal cataract surgery. Am J Ophthalmol. 2007;144:341–6.
80. Zhang Z, Yu H, Dong H, Wang L, Jia YD, Zhang SH. Corneal biomechanical properties changes after coaxial 2.2-mm microincision and standard 3.0-mm phacoemulsification. Int J Ophthalmol. 2016;9:230–4. https://doi.org/10.18240/ijo.2016.02.08.
81. Denoyer A, Ricaud X, Van Went C, Labbé A, Baudouin C. Influence of corneal biomechanical properties on surgically induced astigmatism in cataract surgery. J Cataract Refract Surg. 2013 Aug;39(8):1204–10. https://doi.org/10.1016/j.jcrs.2013.02.052.
82. Wei Y, Xu L, Song H. Application of Corvis ST to evaluate the effect of femtosecond laser-assisted cataract surgery on corneal biomechanics. Exp Ther Med. 2017 Aug;14(2):1626–32. https://doi.org/10.3892/etm.2017.4675.
83. del Buey MA, Cristóbal JA, Ascaso FJ, et al. Biomechanical properties of the cornea in Fuchs' corneal dystrophy. Invest Ophthalmol Vis Sci. 2009;50(7):3199–202.
84. Murugesan V, Bypareddy R, Kumar M, Tanuj D, Anita P. Evaluation of corneal biomechanical properties following penetrating keratoplasty using ocular response analyzer. Indian J Ophthalmol. 2014;62:454–60.
85. Fabian ID, Barequet IS, Skaat A, Rechtman E, Goldenfeld M, Roberts CJ, Melamed S. Intraocular pressure measurements and biomechanical properties of the cornea in eyes after penetrating keratoplasty. Am J Ophthalmol. 2011;151:774–81.
86. Modis L Jr, Hassan Z, Szalai E, Flaskó Z, Berta A, Nemeth G. Ocular biomechanical measurements on post-keratoplasty corneas using a Scheimpflug-based noncontact device. Int J Ophthalmol. 2016;9:235–8.
87. John T, Taylor DA, Shimmyo M, et al. Corneal hysteresis following descemetorhexis with endokeratoplasty: early results. Ann Ophthalmol (Skokie). 2007;39:9–14.
88. Clemmensen K, Hjortdal J. Intraocular pressure and corneal biomechanics in Fuchs' endothelial dystrophy and after posterior lamellar keratoplasty. Acta Ophthalmol. 2014 Jun;92(4):350–4.
89. Pepose JS, Feigenbaum SK, Qazi MA, et al. Changes in corneal biomechanics and intraocular pressure following LASIK using static, dynamic, and noncontact tonometry. Am J Ophthalmol. 2007;143:39–47.
90. Chen MC, Lee N, Bourla N, et al. Corneal biomechanical measurements before and after laser in situ keratomileusis. J Cataract Refract Surg. 2008;34:1886–91.
91. Kirwan C, O'Keefe M. Corneal hysteresis using the Reichert ocular response analyser: findings pre- and post-LASIK and LASEK. Acta Ophthalmol. 2008;86:215–8.
92. Kamiya K, Shimizu K, Ohmoto F. Time course of corneal biomechanical parameters after laser in situ keratomileusis. Ophthalmic Res. 2009;42(3):167–71.
93. Pedersen IB, Bak-Nielsen S, Vestergaard AH, Ivarsen A, Hjortdal J. Corneal biomechanical properties after LASIK, ReLEx flex, and ReLEx smile by Scheimpflug-based dynamic tonometry. Graefes Arch Clin Exp Ophthalmol. 2014;252:1329–35.
94. Hassan Z, Modis L Jr, Szalai E, Berta A, Nemeth G. Examination of ocular biomechanics with a new Scheimpflug technology after corneal refractive surgery. Cont Lens Anterior Eye. 2014;37:337–41.

95. Gatinel D, Chaabouni S, Adam PA, Munck J, Puech M, Hoang-Xuan T. Corneal hysteresis, resistance factor, topography, and pachymetry after corneal lamellar flap. J Refract Surg. 2007 Jan;23(1):76–84.

96. Hamilton DR, Johnson RD, Lee N, Bourla N. Differences in the corneal biomechanical effects of surface ablation compared with laser in situ keratomileusis using a microkeratome or femtosecond laser. J Cataract Refract Surg. 2008 Dec;34(12):2049–56. https://doi.org/10.1016/j.jcrs.2008.08.021.

97. Shetty R, Francis M, Shroff R, Pahuja N, Khamar P, Girrish M, Nuijts RMMA, Sinha Roy A. Corneal biomechanical changes and tissue remodeling after SMILE and LASIK. Invest Ophthalmol Vis Sci. 2017 Nov 1;58(13):5703–12. https://doi.org/10.1167/iovs.17-22864.

98. Osman IM, Helaly HA, Abdalla M, Shousha MA. Corneal biomechanical changes in eyes with small incision lenticule extraction and laser assisted in situ keratomileusis. BMC Ophthalmol. 2016 Jul 26;16:123. https://doi.org/10.1186/s12886-016-0304-3.

99. González-Méijome JM, Villa-Collar C, Queirós A, et al. Pilot study on the influence of corneal biomechanical properties over the short-term in response to corneal refractive therapy for myopia. Cornea. 2008;27(4):421–6.

100. Rabinowitz YS. Keratoconus (major review). Surv Ophthalmol. 1998;42:297–319.

101. Edmund C. Assessment of an elastic model in the pathogenesis of keratoconus. Acta Ophthalmol. 1987;65:545–50.

102. Galletti JG, Pförtner T, Bonthoux FF. Improved keratoconus detection by ocular response analyzer testing after consideration of corneal thickness as a confounding factor. J Refract Surg. 2012;28:202–8.

103. Touboul D, Benard A, Mahmoud AM, Gallois A, Colin J, Roberts CJ. Early biomechanical keratoconus pattern measured with an ocular response analyzer: curve analysis. J Cataract Refract Surg. 2011;37:2144–50.

104. Alio JL, Pinero DP, Aleson A, Teus MA, Barraquer RI, Murta J, Maldonado MJ, Castro de Luna G, Gutierrez R, Villa C, Uceda-Montanes A. Keratoconus-integrated characterization considering anterior corneal aberrations, internal astigmatism, and corneal biomechanics. J Cataract Refract Surg. 2011;37:552–68.

105. Fontes BM, Ambrosio R Jr, Velarde GC, Nose W. Corneal biomechanical evaluation in healthy thin corneas compared with matched keratoconus cases. Arq Bras Oftalmol. 2011;74:13–6.

106. Kirwan C, O'Malley D, O'Keefe M. Corneal hysteresis and corneal resistance factor in keratoectasia: findings using the Reichert ocular response analyzer. Ophthalmologica. 2008;222(5):334–7.

107. Fontes BM, Ambrósio R, Jardim D, et al. Corneal biomechanical metrics and anterior segment parameters in mild keratoconus. Ophthalmology. 2010;117(4):673–9.

108. Schweitzer C, Roberts CJ, Mahmoud AM, et al. Screening of forme fruste keratoconus with the ocular response analyzer. Invest Ophthalmol Vis Sci. 2010;51(5):2403–10.

109. Kerautret J, Colin J, Touboul D, et al. Biomechanical characteristics of the ectatic cornea. J Cataract Refract Surg. 2008;34(3):510–3.

110. Luce D, Gatinel D, Saad A. Biomechanical profile of keratoconus suspect eyes. Poster 565, American Academy of ophthalmology annual meeting 2009.

111. Zarei-Ghanavati S, Ramirez-Miranda A, Yu F, Hamilton DR. Corneal deformation signal waveform analysis in keratoconic versus post-femtosecond laser in situ keratomileusis eyes after statistical correction for potentially confounding factors. J Cataract Refract Surg. 2012 Apr;38(4):607–14. https://doi.org/10.1016/j.jcrs.2011.11.033.

112. Labiris G, Giarmoukakis A, Sideroudi H, Song X, Kozobolis V, Seitz B, Gatzioufas Z. Diagnostic capacity of biomechanical indices from a dynamic bidirectional applanation device in pellucid marginal degeneration. J Cataract Refract Surg. 2014 Jun;40(6):1006–12. https://doi.org/10.1016/j.jcrs.2014.03.018.

113. Rocha K. Topographic patterns analysis and ocular response biomechanical keratoconus probability risk score. ASCRS, Boston, 2010. American Society of Cataract and Refractive Surgery, 2010.

114. Goldich Y, Marcovich AL, Barkana Y, et al. Clinical and corneal biomechanical changes after collagen cross-linking with riboflavin and UV irradiation in patients with progressive keratoconus: results after 2 years of follow-up. Cornea. 2012;31:609–14.
115. Bak-Nielsen S, Pedersen IB, Ivarsen A, Hjortdal J. Dynamic Scheimpflug-based assessment of keratoconus and the effects of corneal cross-linking. J Refract Surg. 2014;30:408–14.
116. Gatinel D. The mystery of collagen cross-linking when it comes to in vivo biomechanical measurements. J Refract Surg. 2014 Nov;30(11):727. https://doi.org/10.3928/1081597X-20141021-02.
117. Spoerl E, Terai N, Scholz F, et al. Detection of biomechanical changes after corneal cross-linking using ocular response analyzer software. J Refract Surg. 2011;27(6):452–7.
118. Fuchsluger TA, Brettl S, Geerling G, Kaisers W, ZeitzP F. Biomechanical assessment of healthy and keratoconic corneas (with/without crosslinking) using dynamic ultrahigh-speed Scheimpflug technology and the relevance of the parameter (A1L-A2L). Br J Ophthalmol. 2018 Jun 5;103(4):558–64.
119. Vinciguerra R, Romano V, Arbabi EM, Brunner M, Willoughby CE, Batterbury M, Kaye SB. In vivo early corneal biomechanical changes after corneal cross-linking in patients with progressive keratoconus. J Refract Surg. 2017;33:840–6.
120. Congdon NG, Broman AT, Bandeen-Roche K, et al. Central corneal thickness and corneal hysteresis associated with glaucoma damage. Am J Ophthalmol. 2006;141:868–75.
121. Mangouritsas G, Morphis G, Mourtzoukos S, et al. Association between corneal hysteresis and central corneal thickness in glaucomatous and non-glaucomatous eyes. Acta Ophthalmol. 2009;87(8):901–5.
122. Sullivan-Mee M, Billingsley SC, Patel AD, et al. Ocular response analyzer in subjects with and without glaucoma. Optom Vis Sci. 2008;85:463–70.
123. Anand A, De Moraes CG, Teng CC, et al. Corneal hysteresis and visual field asymmetry in open angle glaucoma. Invest Ophthalmol Vis Sci. 2010;51:6514–8.
124. De Moraes CV, Hill V, Tello C, et al. Lower corneal hysteresis is associated with more rapid glaucomatous visual field progression. J Glaucoma. 2012;21:209–13.
125. Medeiros FA, Meira-Freitas D, Lisboa R, Kuang TM, Zangwill LM, Weinreb RN. Corneal hysteresis as a risk factor for glaucoma progression: a prospective longitudinal study. Ophthalmology. 2013;120:1533–40.
126. Susanna CN, Diniz-Filho A, Daga FB, Susanna BN, Zhu F, Ogata NG, Medeiros FAA. Prospective longitudinal study to investigate corneal hysteresis as a risk factor for predicting development of glaucoma. Am J Ophthalmol. 2018;187:148–52.

Chapter 18
Ocular Rigidity and Glaucoma

Diane N. Sayah and Mark R. Lesk

Introduction: The Relevance of Ocular Rigidity in Glaucoma

Biomechanics is a rapidly developing field, joining physics and biology, and bringing new insights unto physiological and pathophysiological mechanisms. The concept of ocular rigidity (OR), a biomechanical characteristic of the eye or measure of the resistance that the eye exerts against distending forces, was brought forth in 1937 by Jonas S. Friedenwald, a prominent ophthalmologist and scientist, when he proposed the *ocular rigidity function*. This function describes the relationship between the change in ocular volume (V) and intraocular pressure (IOP), when the latter is above 5 mmHg [1]. Friedenwald's ocular rigidity function is:

$$\log \frac{IOP}{IOP_0} = K\left(V - V_0\right)$$

where K is the ocular rigidity coefficient. A greater K value corresponds to a more rigid eye.

While obtained empirically to describe the pressure-volume relationship in the eye, this equation was later demonstrated to be consistent with the mechanical properties of collagen [2, 3]. Alternative and more accurate formulae were developed, however the Friedenwald function remains the most commonly used to calculate the ocular rigidity coefficient clinically [4].

Through his studies on the rigidity of the eye, Friedenwald was seeking to improve the accuracy of tonometry readings and investigate differences between normal and diseased eyes. Indeed, ocular rigidity was clinically relevant due to its influence on the measurement of IOP by indentation tonometry. The conversion

D. N. Sayah · M. R. Lesk (✉)
Department of Ophthalmology, Maisonneuve-Rosemont Hospital Research Center, Université de Montréal, Montreal, QC, Canada

© Springer Nature Switzerland AG 2021
I. Pallikaris et al. (eds.), *Ocular Rigidity, Biomechanics and Hydrodynamics of the Eye*, https://doi.org/10.1007/978-3-030-64422-2_18

table used to estimate IOP from scale readings assumed the same rigidity for all eyes, leading to under- or overestimation of IOP.

While more recent tonometry techniques are less dependent on ocular rigidity, our interest in measuring OR in living human eyes remains. The ability to quantify the structural and material properties of the corneoscleral shell could help elucidate the pathophysiological mechanisms of ocular diseases such as glaucoma, and thus improve their diagnosis and treatment.

Glaucoma is the leading cause of irreversible blindness in the world. An insidious and unpredictable disease, glaucoma causes damage to the retinal ganglion cells (RGC) that form the optic nerve and can remain asymptomatic until major irreversible visual loss has occurred. The clinical hallmark of this disease includes the progressive deformation and excavation of the tissues of the optic nerve head [5], as seen in Fig. 18.1. Once detected, the disease's progression rate cannot be anticipated. Furthermore, the pathogenesis of open-angle glaucoma (OAG), the main form of glaucoma, is poorly understood.

While the development of OAG was traditionally attributed to elevated intraocular pressure (IOP), the susceptibility of individual eyes to glaucomatous damage is variable. Nearly half of OAG patients have IOP within the normal range [6], going up to almost 90% of patients in some populations [7]. In contrast, most patients with elevated IOP do not develop glaucoma [8]. This suggests that factors other than IOP must also underlie the susceptibility of the optic nerve head (ONH) to glaucomatous injury.

The realization that a given IOP can result in very different stresses and strains at the ONH in different eyes led to an entire field of research known as ocular

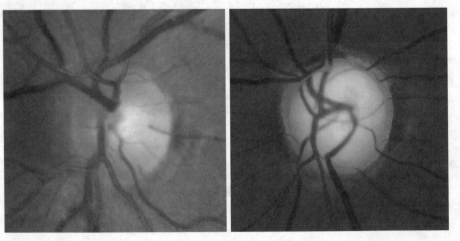

Normal Optic Nerve   Glaucomatous Optic Nerve

Fig. 18.1 Glaucomatous optic neuropathy is characterized by the progressive deformation and excavation of tissues at the optic nerve head. Thinning of the neuroretinal rim due to axonal loss, increased cupping and bowing of the lamina cribrosa are clinical hallmarks of this disease (Drs Sayah and Lesk)

biomechanics. Central to this theory is the fact that the retinal axons that unite at the ONH to form the optic nerve leave the eye through the lamina cribrosa. The lamina is the major load-bearing tissue of the ONH and is accepted as both a site of discontinuity and weakness in the corneo-scleral shell of the eye and as the most likely site of damage to ONH axons [9–13]. The *mechanical theory* postulates that elevated mechanical stresses lead to axonal damage and loss of retinal ganglion cells [14].

There is mounting evidence that the stiffness of the sclera and the lamina cribrosa are important risk factors in the development and progression of glaucomatous optic neuropathy, perhaps more so than IOP [15]. This chapter will review the most prominent findings pertaining to this topic, and will present the evidence on the link between OR and OAG. It will focus on OR and other relevant biomechanical metrics and their alteration in glaucoma, and is meant to be complementary to the other chapters in this textbook.

The Main Findings of Ocular Rigidity in Glaucoma

The following sections will present the main findings pertaining to the biomechanical properties of the eye in glaucoma, from the most anterior to the most posterior structures. The outer coat of the eye is formed by the cornea and the sclera, two tough connective tissues that make up the corneoscleral shell. Posteriorly, the corneoscleral shell is pierced by the scleral canal through which the retinal ganglion cells' (RGC) axons exit the eye on their way to the brain. The lamina cribrosa (LC), a specialized region of the sclera, spans the scleral canal. It is clear that remodeling of these tissues occurs in glaucoma, thus altering the mechanical environment of the optic nerve head. The properties of these structures will be briefly reviewed with an emphasis on their relevance in glaucoma. The trabecular meshwork, region of interest for the aqueous outflow and IOP regulation in glaucoma, will also be presented.

For additional information on the biomechanical properties of each of these structures, please refer to the corresponding chapters in this textbook.

The Cornea

The cornea is the anterior extension of the sclera, and its viscoelastic properties and thickness contribute to the overall rigidity of the eye. The main biomechanical properties of the cornea which can be currently measured and studied in glaucoma are the central corneal thickness (CCT), corneal hysteresis (CH), corneal resistance factor (CRF), and many others that have been studied less extensively.

Corneal Thickness

CCT is most frequently measured using ultrasound pachymetry, optical pachymetry, Scheimpflug imaging or anterior segment optical coherence tomography [16]. Initially, CCT was used in the clinical management of glaucoma to correct IOP readings [17]. This correction was later shown to be inadequate due to the absence of algorithm to accurately predict the true IOP corrected for CCT [18]. The Ocular Hypertension Treatment Study (OHTS) was the first to demonstrate the importance of CCT as a predictor for the development of OAG [8]. In this study, a CCT of 555 μm or less was associated with a threefold increased risk of developing OAG. Further investigation has confirmed CCT to be an independent predictor for the development of primary open-angle glaucoma (POAG) [8, 19] as well as a risk factor for the development of visual field (VF) loss in glaucoma patients [20].

Several experiments were carried out to better understand the link between CCT and posterior structures of the eye in glaucoma. While this association remains unclear, due to the absence of correlation between CCT and laminar and scleral thicknesses [21, 22], a thinner cornea was suggested to be associated with a more compliant lamina cribrosa due to larger displacement of the LC with IOP reduction in eyes with lower CCT [23]. Furthermore, an inverse relationship was found between CCT and optic disc size or area, perhaps indicating larger and more deformable optic discs with lower CCT [24]. In a study involving non-invasive measurement of OR, a positive albeit weak correlation was also found between OR and CCT, indicating that subjects with a thinner cornea may have a more compliant sclera [25]. In a similar clinical study, no relationship between OR and CCT was found, arguably due to low statistical power [26].

In subjects with no corneal pathology, CCT remains relatively stable. CCT was reportedly lower in subjects from African descent (AD) and Hispanics compared to Caucasians [27–30], although this difference was later shown to be dependent upon CH [31]. While CCT also decreases with age, and can be altered with some topical treatments [32–34], it is not known to change over time in glaucoma patients as their disease advances [35].

Corneal Viscoelastic Properties

CH and CRF can be measured in vivo using the Ocular Response Analyzer (ORA; Reichert Ophthalmic Instruments, Inc., Buffalo, NY, USA), a non-contact tonometer that measures the biomechanical response of the eye to a rapid air jet-induced deformation at the cornea [36]. The Corneal Visualization Scheimpflug Technology tonometer (Corvis ST: CST; Oculus, Wetzlar, Germany), a more recent device, visualizes and measures corneal deformation also in response to an air impulse using a high-speed Scheimpflug camera [37]. It measures numerous parameters, many of which have been shown to be correlated with CH and CRF [38].

CH and CRF are considered to be analogous to the viscous and elastic properties of the cornea respectively. Both parameters have been shown to be relevant in glaucoma. Typically, average CH and CRF values in non-diseased eyes are around 10.5 mmHg [39, 40]. CH was found to be significantly lower in POAG [41–44] compared to controls, while both CH and CRF were found to be highest in OHT eyes [45]. Numerous studies also associated a lower CH with an increased risk of glaucoma progression [46–49]. Furthermore, in a study investigating CH in asymmetric glaucoma progression, worse eyes had significantly lower CH than the less damaged eyes (8.2 ± 1.9 vs. 8.9 ± 1.9 mmHg; $p < 0.001$), while CCT and IOP did not significantly differ between eyes. CH was thus the most discriminative index for predicting the eye with worse VF in asymmetric OAG [50]. Moreover, when comparing corneal biomechanical factors, reported findings showed lower CH values to be predictive of glaucoma progression, more so than CCT [46, 47].

How these corneal properties are linked to optic nerve susceptibility and glaucomatous damage remains unclear, although no correlation was found between these parameters and OR [51]. Some speculate that the viscoelasticity of the corneal extracellular matrix (ECM) could be related to the properties of the ECM in the LC and peripapillary sclera (PPS). This would mean that an eye with a more deformable cornea (low CH) may also be more vulnerable to IOP-induced ONH damage. Some studies on the relationship between CH and ONH morphology have found lower CH to be associated with larger cup-to-disc ratio [52, 53], deeper cup in untreated POAG [52] and small rim area [53]. However, another study did not find such correlations in a large, non-glaucomatous cohort [54]. When subjected to an acute but transient IOP elevation, glaucomatous eyes have shown a correlation between CH and optic nerve surface displacement, whereas controls did not [42]. When IOP was reduced in POAG subjects, greater change in ONH cup area occurred in POAG eyes with lower CH when controlling for baseline IOP and IOP change, but this was not significant when all factors were included in the multivariate model [55]. Similarly, no significant association was found between CH and RNFL thickness in glaucomatous subjects when multivariate analyses were carried out [56, 57].

CH is a dynamic property. While it has been shown to decrease only slightly with age [58], it has been shown to have a mild inverse relationship with IOP [59, 60]. Consequently, CH can be altered following IOP-lowering therapies such as with topical prostaglandin analogues (PGA) [33]. Other surgical IOP-lowering strategies also showed increased CH post-operatively [60, 61], while maintaining a lower CH in the treated eye compared to the contralateral healthy eye in some cases [60]. Furthermore, low-baseline CH, but not CCT, can be predictive of a greater magnitude of IOP reduction following treatments such as PGA (29 vs. 7.6% IOP reduction with mean CH 7.0 mmHg vs. 11.9 mmHg respectively, $p = 0.006$) [62] and selective laser trabeculoplasty (SLT) [63]. Ethnic differences point to lower CH in subjects of African Descent (AD) [31], in both healthy and glaucomatous eyes [64]. Whether this could be linked to the higher predilection of AD subjects of developing glaucoma remains unknown.

In summary, CH may be more relevant in glaucoma than CCT by its stronger association with disease severity, risk of progression, and effectiveness of glaucoma treatments [65]. How these findings can be related to ONH biomechanics remains to be elucidated.

The Sclera

The sclera is the fibrous envelope of the eye. Since the sclera is responsible for the majority of the ocular globe's rigidity, it is not surprising that the Friedenwald equation can be derived from the mechanical properties (stress-strain relationship) of its primary constituent, collagen [2, 3]. In his original study, Friedenwald derived the ocular rigidity function empirically from experiments on enucleated eyes. Most OR measurements since then were performed in cadaver eyes [14, 66–68] or in vivo by means of Schiotz tonometry, either paired readings or differential tonometry using both indentation and applanation tonometry, or by laser interferometry and ocular pulse amplitude measurements [1, 23, 69]. More recently, numerical modeling has provided insight into the profound effect of biomechanical properties of the corneoscleral shell on the level of stress exerted on the ONH [15, 70–72]. These models have shown that forces at the ONH are considerably higher than the IOP [73]. Furthermore, finite element modeling suggested that scleral stiffness could be the most important biomechanical factor in determining stress and strain at the ONH [15].

Until now, reported outcomes on the association between OR and glaucoma remain mitigated. Inflation studies in cadaver eyes, and in vivo studies using indirect measurements showed higher OR in eyes with established glaucoma [69, 74–76]. More recent studies reported an inverse correlation between glaucomatous neuroretinal damage and OR [51], low OR in OAG [25, 77], and highest OR in ocular hypertensives (OHT) with no glaucomatous damage [25]. Finally, using intraoperative cannulation, one experiment showed no difference between diseased and healthy eyes [78]. How can these results be reconciled? The idea that perhaps OR is altered during the course of the disease is an interesting one, although this has not been assessed yet. As early as 1960, Drance postulated that while OR seems to be increased in long-standing glaucoma, decreased OR in untreated glaucoma patients was possible [76]. Discrepancies may also be due to confounding factors which can influence OR values. Some of these factors include:

1. *Post-mortem changes*: Experiments using enucleated eyes often yield higher values of OR when compared to in vivo measurements. This is thought to result from the influence of the vasculature and extraocular muscles in living eyes, and of edema in postmortem eyes [26, 79–81]. While comparison of glaucomatous and non-glaucomatous eyes remains possible, limited knowledge as to the prior state of the eyes and the history of the disease is available when using human cadaver eyes. Furthermore, dynamic behavior cannot be easily assessed using cadaver eyes.

2. *Glaucoma stage or severity*: In most studies, glaucomatous patients are chosen following diagnostic criteria including signs of axonal and VF damage [69, 75]. Since VF defects are detected only after a substantial proportion, 30–50% of RGCs are lost [82, 83], these subjects have established glaucoma. Therefore, OR is not often measured near the initiation of glaucoma, and changes may have occurred that modify the initial OR. As well, these cross-sectional experiments

do not permit the assessment of how OR changes during the course of glaucoma. Perhaps longitudinal studies will help establish whether OR could be low in early stages and increases with advanced disease, as proposed by Drance [76].

3. *IOP and IOP-lowering therapy*: In several studies investigating OR in glaucoma, recruited patients are on IOP-lowering therapy. Due to the dependence of OR on IOP, results thus need to be interpreted with caution [4]. Furthermore, commonly used IOP-lowering medications may have an effect on OR possibly through alterations of the sclera's composition [1, 77, 84].

4. *Ocular volume*: The relationship between OR and the diameter or volume of the eye is well known. OR is thought to be lower in longer eyes, such as in axial myopia [25, 85]. Myopia is also a known risk factor for glaucoma, with a two- to threefold increased risk of glaucoma compared with non-myopes [86, 87]. Theoretically, this would be due to greater IOP-induced strain in larger eyes [88], and needs to be controlled for in clinical studies investigating OR.

5. *Age*: There is evidence for the association between aging and increased OR [1, 26, 89]. Induced crosslinking from the accumulation of advanced glycation end products in tissues with aging could be at fault [90, 91]. These age-related changes in the composition and thickness of the sclera and ONH would increase LC and PPS stiffness [92, 93]. Since aging is also a risk factor for glaucoma, a high OR would then be thought to be associated with glaucoma. However, this may not be the case as demonstrated by more recent clinical and computational studies [15, 25] and needs to be further investigated.

6. *Ethnic differences in OR*: Through inflation studies and ONH reconstructions from cadaver eyes, ethnic differences were observed between eyes from African descent (AD) and those from European descent (ED). PPS stiffness was reported to be higher in aging AD eyes compared to ED eyes [94]. Similarly, AD eyes showed an increase in scleral thickness and LC depth with age, whereas ED eyes did not [93].

7. *Measurement techniques*: Different approaches, both invasive and non-invasive, to measure OR have been used and are described in more detail in another chapter. Each has advantages and limitations, which renders results pertaining to OR in glaucoma to be interpreted with caution. Historically, OR was measured in living human eyes using differential tonometry. This technique consisted of comparing Schiötz and Goldmann tonometry results, but was later considered inaccurate primarily due to the dependence of both indentation and applanation tonometry on the biomechanical properties of the eye [95–98]. The most significant source of this variability in OR coefficients originates from the use of weights in Schiötz tonometry, which compress the ocular wall and displace a significant amount of intraocular fluid [95, 98], but also through the erroneous assumption that the OR of all eyes is standard in the applicability of the conversion table which provides the IOP reading in mmHg [95, 99, 100].

Other non-invasive methods were developed to measure OR based on Friedenwald's equation. The first method estimated the ocular volume change (ΔV) by measuring the movement between the cornea and inner retina in response to the cardiac pulse, also known as the fundus pulse amplitude (FPA)

[69]. Another group measured the change in axial length (AL) following pharmacological IOP reduction to estimate OR [75]. Both methods consisted of measuring the anterior to posterior expansion of the corneoscleral shell, which is itself dependent on the ocular rigidity [101]. Instead of measuring the response of ocular coats to an increase in volume, choroidal laser Doppler flowmetry was used to estimate the amount of blood injected in the eye with each cardiac pulse as an indicator of ΔV to estimate OR. However this gave only relative values because choroidal blood flow was measured in arbitrary units [25].

Due to the difficulties of quantifying ΔV with other methods, anterior chamber manometry remained the main technique to directly calculate OR in vivo [26, 79, 102, 103]. This technique is used at the outset of surgery and involves injecting small increments of fluid into the anterior chamber while measuring the resultant change in IOP. It could be considered the "gold standard" for clinical OR measurements, however its invasive nature limited its applicability in clinical use. Instead of injecting known volumes of fluid in the eye and measuring resulting IOP changes to estimate OR, our group has recently developed a non-invasive, clinical method to directly measure OR in living human eyes [104]. The approach is based on video-rate Spectral Domain optical coherence tomography (OCT) and Pascal Dynamic Contour Tonometry (DCT) to measure ΔV and the pulsatile IOP change respectively. It acquires a time-series at least 8 mm wide of the submacular choroid with OCT images captured at 8 Hz, and through automated segmentation of choroidal boundaries, measures the pulsatile choroidal thickness change. The change in choroidal thickness during the cardiac cycle is then extrapolated to ΔV using a mathematical model of the eye [105]. OR measurements obtained using this method have been shown to be strongly correlated ($r = 0.853$, $p < 0.001$) with those obtained invasively in the same eyes, confirming the validity of the method [105]. The repeatability of OR coefficients was also confirmed [105]. In addition, OR differences between non-myopic and myopic eyes were found using this technique, showing lower OR in axial myopia. While the development of an accurate and non-invasive instrument to measure OR in a clinical setting had limited the study of OR on a large scale, recent studies revealed that lower OR was significantly associated with greater RNFL and ganglion cell damage across the spectrum of glaucoma [51].

The mechanism by which the sclera is altered in glaucoma has not been established, and in vivo studies indicating OR alterations in glaucoma remain sparse. Changes in the content and composition of collagen fibers in glaucomatous eyes and in suspected glaucomatous eyes were found [106]. However, while increased OR in established glaucoma may be related to stiffness or thickness of the sclera, no relationship was found between OR and scleral thickness [107]. This reinforces that to better understand the fundamental biomechanical paradigm and the forces that lead to ONH damage, it is perhaps necessary to evaluate OR in conjunction with other factors such as the biomechanical properties of the PPS and the LC, which make major contributions to the stresses and strains in the ONH.

The Lamina Cribrosa/Optic Nerve Head

An extension of the sclera, the LC is a porous disc at the base of the optic nerve head through which the axons composing the optic nerve leave the eye. It features a complex three-dimensional structure composed of a network of flexible beams of connective tissue. As it spans the scleral canal, this fenestrated and vascularized tissue provides mechanical as well as metabolic support to the retinal ganglion cells' axons as they leave the eye [108].

Biomechanically, the LC is a structure of great interest and is thought to be the principal site of axonal damage in glaucoma [9, 12, 109]. The LC is significantly more compliant and thinner compared to the surrounding sclera. It corresponds to about one-tenth of the sclera's stiffness and one-third of the PPS thickness [108]. It is thus considered a 'weak spot' in the corneoscleral shell [73]. Its vulnerability is further exacerbated by its surroundings. On one side the intraocular space and on the other the retrobulbar space represent high (IOP) and low (cerebrospinal fluid pressure, or CSFP) pressure environments respectively, creating a translaminar pressure gradient (TLPG) across this barrier [110]. The TLPG, estimated as the difference between IOP and CSFP divided by the laminar thickness [111, 112], would generally produce an outward bowing of the LC. IOP-induced circumferential stress can also act on the ONH via the corneoscleral shell and PPS to expand the scleral canal. Both these elements can give rise to considerable stress and strain which in turn can induce morphological changes within these structures, but also disrupt axoplasmic flow within the RGC axons at the LC level [109, 113–116] and impinge on the delicate ONH vasculature [117]. LC deformation is thus mediated by IOP, CSFP, as well as the geometrical and material properties of the sclera and LC of the individual eye [108]. Eye-specific characteristics thus mediate the susceptibility to glaucoma in individuals at any given IOP.

Chronic IOP elevation and transient IOP elevations were found to produce tissue remodeling in the ONH through various pathways, including through the activation of astrocytes and LC cells [118–121]. Stretching induces remodeling of the extracellular matrix in the LC [122–124]. This remodeling can influence the stiffness of the LC and in turn, play a role in the development of OAG. Laminar stiffness is shown to increase with age [68, 90, 125], more so in patients of African origin [93, 126, 127]. A plethora of studies have investigated LC mobility in ex vivo [14, 66–68, 128] and histological studies [14, 129–132] as well as in monkey eyes [129, 133, 134] and living human eyes [135–139], and more recently through engineering modeling [15, 70, 140]. Some have suggested an initial hypercompliance in early glaucoma [129, 134] and most have documented increased rigidity later in the course of the disease [14, 66–68, 128, 129, 133, 135, 141]. Morphologically, glaucomatous changes to the laminar structure have been shown to manifest as posteriorizing of the LC insertion into the sclera, increased cupping and focal laminar defects [108]. Focal defects such as laminar holes and disinsertions were found to be linked with disk hemorrhages [142–145] and RNFL defects [146, 147]. Enlargement of the laminar pores were also found, particularly in the superior and inferior quadrants where early glaucomatous RNFL defects and VF loss are most common [130]. Laminar posteriorizing was greater in glaucomatous eyes compared to controls [148], and greater LC depth was found in high-tension glaucoma compared to NTG [149]. Posteriorizing of the LC insertion and peripheral LC were shown in OAG eyes compared with age-matched controls, the latter being more displaced in the vertical meridian [150]. This was consistent with the findings in asymmetric glaucoma where prelaminar tissue was thinner and the LC was more posterior in the eye with VF loss compared to the contralateral eye with no VF defect [151].

In experiments involving significant IOP reduction or elevation, LC displacement was shown to bend in either direction (i.e. inward or outward) [152, 153]. This can be dependent on its initial position and the stiffness of the surrounding tissue. When OAG subjects were divided in three groups according to disease severity, and anterior LC depth (ALD) was imaged using OCT prior to and after significant IOP reduction, the results showed posterior displacement of the LC in the group with lesser VF damage, anterior displacement in the group with moderate damage and close to no displacement in subjects with greater glaucoma damage [152]. Perhaps these results suggest that the LC is stiffer in advanced glaucoma, and that the group with less VF damage has a more compliant sclera. In other words, while a compliant PPS would expand with high IOP, producing a taut pulling of the lamina and an expansion of the scleral canal, IOP reduction would reverse this expansion. The LC would hence move outward, back to its original position as the IOP is reduced, as illustrated in Fig. 18.2. However, this remains to be verified.

As more imaging tools are developed to study the biomechanical behavior of the LC, a small and relatively inaccessible structure of the eye, it will become possible to assess glaucomatous changes over time through longitudinal studies. However, confounding factors including age-related changes in stiffness of the laminar tissues and ethnic differences will continue to challenge our understanding of the disease process.

The Trabecular Meshwork

IOP is maintained through careful equilibrium between aqueous humor production by the ciliary processes and evacuation mainly through the trabecular or uveoscleral pathway. The trabecular, or conventional, pathway is responsible for 85% of aqueous humor outflow from the eye. Its primary constituent is the trabecular meshwork (TM). Involved in IOP regulation and IOP elevation in glaucoma, it is a region of great interest in glaucoma research. This is particularly true when considering that increased resistance of aqueous outflow through the TM is a known risk factor for glaucoma and can cause ocular hypertension [8, 100].

From a biomechanical perspective, the stiffness of the TM is relevant in the development of glaucoma. Since the TM cells are contractile [154], this may cause

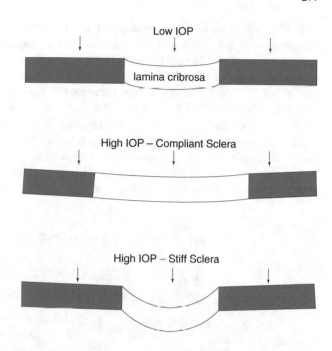

Fig. 18.2 Behavior of the lamina cribrosa when subjected to low or high IOP. When the sclera is compliant, increased IOP pulls the LC taut due to the expansion of the sclera and scleral canal. When the sclera is rigid, minimal scleral deformation occurs. Instead, the LC deforms posteriorly under the effect of IOP. (Reprinted from Sigal et al. [164] with permission from Elsevier)

an increased outflow resistance [155]. On the other hand, this can also lead to tissue remodeling [156], and subsequent TM stiffness alteration. Some evidence points to increased TM stiffness in glaucoma [157, 158]. The mechanism through which this occurs remains unknown.

The measurement of TM stiffness can be challenging in living human eyes. More importantly, interpreting both ex vivo and in vivo measurements can be problematic as many agents, including topical glaucoma medications can alter TM function and potentially TM stiffness [159]. Much like other tissues of the eye, additional confounding factors include age and ethnic differences. Aging was found to increase TM stiffness by a factor of two [160] and TM structural differences, mainly a tendency for shorter TM height, were found in patients of African origin compared to Asians and Caucasians [161].

The exact significance of TM stiffness, how it is affected by IOP and how it is linked to outflow resistance remains unclear and needs to be further investigated to better understand the pathogenesis of glaucoma [158, 159, 162, 163].

Discussion on Competing Hypotheses

The biomechanical paradigm of glaucoma (see Fig. 18.3) stipulates that IOP produces stress and strain within ocular tissues which ultimately lead to RGC damage [71]. The ONH's response to these biomechanical stimuli has been found to depend on eye-specific geometrical and material properties. This is thought to determine an individual's predisposition to develop OAG. Interestingly, in finite element models the stiffness of the sclera was the most influential property on the biomechanical response of the ONH to IOP. Over the last 80 years, the role of ocular rigidity in the pathophysiology of this blinding disease has been studied. Despite the numerous studies on this topic, the association between OR and glaucoma remains unclear, and competing hypotheses are highly debated. On one side, OR is thought to be higher in glaucomatous eyes, producing higher IOP fluctuations due to rigid ocular walls, and hence more deformation at the ONH. On the other side, OR is thought to be lower in early glaucoma, engendering axonal stretching and damage. According to this theory, increased OR would occur at later stages of the disease. Challenges that researchers face when studying OR range from a plethora of confounding

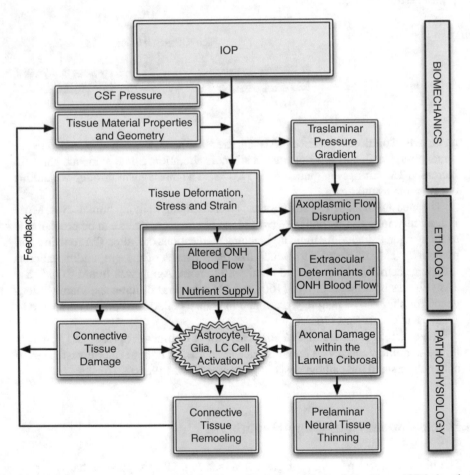

Fig. 18.3 Representation scheme of the biomechanical paradigm of glaucoma. IOP-induced deformation, stress and strain produce alterations in physiological processes which ultimately lead to axonal loss and glaucomatous damage. (Reprinted from Sigal et al. [164] with permission from Elsevier.)

factors, both ocular and systemic, including ocular volume and shape, scleral thickness, choroidal blood volume, age and ethnicity, which can have an effect on OR [4]. The difficulty in diagnosing glaucoma at the earliest phase of the disease is another obstacle. The lack of longitudinal studies to show whether OR contributes primarily to glaucoma or is altered due to the disease hinders our knowledge of this parameter.

Until recently, there was no reliable, non-invasive clinical method to measure OR directly in living human eyes. Hence, interpretation of results with non-invasive techniques had to be done carefully, and invasive methods were not suitable for large scale testing. Ongoing studies using our novel OCT-based method to measure OR will provide insight into the link between OR and glaucoma [104, 105, 165] through assessment of OR differences across the glaucoma spectrum [51] and through longitudinal assessment of OR throughout the progression of the disease. To provide a complete picture of the optic nerve's biomechanical responses in glaucoma, LC compliance also needs to be assessed in vivo. Most attempts to study LC compliance measure laminar displacement with IOP change [23, 135, 136, 138, 139, 152, 153, 166] or pulsatility [167–169]. While early studies used scanning laser ophthalmoscopy to measure mean cup depth, IOP-induced deformation of the prelaminar neural tissue was not found to be a good surrogate for the deformation of the LC [70]. Improved imaging methods such as OCT are now used for the direct visualization of the LC deeper in the ONH tissue [170]. While this remains a challenge, coupling the laminar biomechanical properties with OR measurements in a same eye would be ideal to understand how RGC axonal damage is mediated by scleral and laminar interactions. We think that perhaps glaucoma predisposition occurs from a mismatch between scleral and laminar stiffness. However, this hypothesis remains to be fully assessed.

A newly considered biomechanical risk factor for glaucoma pertains to ocular motility or extraocular muscles and their impact on ONH deformation. It would seem that adduction, or the movement of the eye towards the nose, imposes strain on the ONH and peripapillary structures [171]. It is hypothesized that repetitive movement of the eye over a long period might lead to the development of glaucomatous optic neuropathy in vulnerable eyes, independently from IOP. This is corroborated by finite element modeling which suggests that greater mechanical stress and strain are exerted in the ONH region during adduction, more so than would elevated IOP [172]. According to these findings, it might be beneficial to limit adduction in certain individuals as therapy to prevent optic nerve sheath tethering [173], but much more research is required.

Clinicians and researchers must remember competing hypotheses when studying OR in glaucoma. For example, in addition to the more evident clinical data such as age, ethnicity, IOP history, systemic cardiovascular status, and migraine, alterations to less clinically accessible factors such as ocular blood flow, vasospasticity, CSF pressure, glial cell function, and axonal susceptibility between individuals must be considered among many other factors. Some of these factors can be assessed through clinical measurements and others will become accessible through genetic testing.

Currently, the only evidence-based treatment to prevent the progression of OAG is to lower IOP, regardless of baseline IOP [174–177]. This supports the importance of biomechanics in OAG. IOP reduction can be carried out using pharmaceuticals, laser trabeculoplasty, surgical procedures, or a combination of these methods. However, current therapeutic options to lower IOP may also bring forth changes in the biomechanical properties of the corneoscleral shell, as discussed previously [1, 32, 77]. Commonly used hypotensive drugs may thus have an impact on OR measurements. On the other hand, while studies unequivocally show the benefit of IOP-lowering therapy in slowing structural and functional loss in glaucoma, this does not always halt the progression of the disease. Hence, the prevention and treatment of glaucoma remain an unsolved problem. This has fueled the development of neuroprotective treatments which do not rely on IOP reduction. Several experiments have shown some promise in protecting RGC following injury [178–184]. One of them demonstrated that human recombinant insulin administered as eye drops could regenerate RGCs in glaucoma [185].

Given that the biomechanical properties of the sclera and LC are involved in axonal damage in glaucoma, altering these properties may also protect against the disease. Attempts to alter the stiffness of these ocular tissues to prevent initial RGC injury have been carried out [186]. Therapeutic approaches could include targeting the matrix metallo-proteinases which modify collagen stiffness, or UV-crosslinking of collagen as is currently performed for corneal ectasias [187] and has been attempted in the sclera [188–190]. Of course, a central question to this treatment option remains: is a stiffer or a more compliant sclera protective against IOP-induced stress and strain? Experimental studies in models systems have started to approach this question [186, 191].

Conclusion

Despite the tremendous progress that has been achieved in understanding how biomechanical properties of the eye are critical in glaucoma, the pathophysiological mechanisms leading to axonal degeneration in this blinding disease remain unclear. We believe that the interplay between scleral and laminar stiffness must be evaluated to provide a complete picture of how glaucoma develops. Reliable, non-invasive ocular rigidity measurement methods will help us to better understand whether having a low or high OR suggests a predisposition for POAG or whether it simply reflects a change caused by the condition. Perhaps measurement of OR would also help predict the progression of OAG in patients, hence giving clinicians the ability to identify which patients will require more aggressive treatment. The study of ocular rigidity could also lead to new avenues of therapy for glaucoma to ultimately prevent vision loss.

References

1. Friedenwald JS. Contribution to the theory and practice of tonometry. Am J Ophthalmol. 1937;20:985–1024.
2. Ethier CR, Johnson M, Ruberti J. Ocular biomechanics and biotransport. Annu Rev Biomed Eng. 2004;6:249–73.
3. Greene PR. Closed-form ametropic pressure-volume and ocular rigidity solutions. Am J Optom Physiol Optic. 1985;62(12):870–8.
4. Pallikaris IG, Dastiridou AI, Tsilimbaris MK, Karyotakis NG, Ginis HS. Ocular rigidity. Expert Rev Ophthalmol. 2010;5(3):343–51.
5. Foster PJ, Buhrmann R, Quigley HA, Johnson GJ. The definition and classification of glaucoma in prevalence surveys. Br J Ophthalmol. 2002;86(2):238–42.
6. Sommer A, Tielsch JM, Katz J, Quigley HA, Gottsch JD, Javitt J, et al. Relationship between intraocular pressure and primary open angle glaucoma among white and black Americans. The Baltimore Eye Survey. Arch Ophthalmol. 1991;109(8):1090–5.
7. Suzuki Y, Iwase A, Araie M, Yamamoto T, Abe H, Shirato S, et al. Risk factors for open-angle glaucoma in a Japanese population: the Tajimi Study. Ophthalmology. 2006;113(9):1613–7.
8. Gordon MO, Beiser JA, Brandt JD, Heuer DK, Higginbotham EJ, Johnson CA, et al. The Ocular Hypertension Treatment Study: baseline factors that predict the onset of primary open-angle glaucoma. Arch Ophthalmol. 2002;120(6):714–20. discussion 829–30
9. Quigley H, Anderson DR. The dynamics and location of axonal transport blockade by acute intraocular pressure elevation in primate optic nerve. Investig Ophthalmol. 1976;15(8):606–16.
10. Quigley HA, Anderson DR. Distribution of axonal transport blockade by acute intraocular pressure elevation in the primate optic nerve head. Invest Ophthalmol Vis Sci. 1977;16(7):640–4.
11. Quigley HA, Flower RW, Addicks EM, McLeod DS. The mechanism of optic nerve damage in experimental acute intraocular pressure elevation. Invest Ophthalmol Vis Sci. 1980;19(5):505–17.
12. Quigley HA, Addicks EM, Green WR, Maumenee AE. Optic nerve damage in human glaucoma. II. The site of injury and susceptibility to damage. Arch Ophthalmol. 1981;99(4):635–49.
13. Quigley HA, Addicks EM, Green WR. Optic nerve damage in human glaucoma. III. Quantitative correlation of nerve fiber loss and visual field defect in glaucoma, ischemic neuropathy, papilledema, and toxic neuropathy. Arch Ophthalmol. 1982;100(1):135–46.
14. Yan DB, Coloma FM, Metheetrairut A, Trope GE, Heathcote JG, Ethier CR. Deformation of the lamina cribrosa by elevated intraocular pressure. Br J Ophthalmol. 1994;78(8):643–8.
15. Sigal IA, Flanagan JG, Ethier CR. Factors influencing optic nerve head biomechanics. Invest Ophthalmol Vis Sci. 2005;46(11):4189–99.
16. Wolffsohn JS, Davies LN. Advances in anterior segment imaging. Curr Opin Ophthalmol. 2007;18(1):32–8.
17. Copt RP, Thomas R, Mermoud A. Corneal thickness in ocular hypertension, primary open-angle glaucoma, and normal tension glaucoma. Arch Ophthalmol. 1999;117(1):14–6.
18. Herndon LW. Measuring intraocular pressure-adjustments for corneal thickness and new technologies. Curr Opin Ophthalmol. 2006;17(2):115–9.
19. Medeiros FA, Weinreb RN, Sample PA, Gomi CF, Bowd C, Crowston JG, et al. Validation of a predictive model to estimate the risk of conversion from ocular hypertension to glaucoma. Arch Ophthalmol. 2005;123(10):1351–60.
20. Medeiros FA, Sample PA, Zangwill LM, Bowd C, Aihara M, Weinreb RN. Corneal thickness as a risk factor for visual field loss in patients with preperimetric glaucomatous optic neuropathy. Am J Ophthalmol. 2003;136(5):805–13.

21. Jonas JB, Holbach L. Central corneal thickness and thickness of the lamina cribrosa in human eyes. Invest Ophthalmol Vis Sci. 2005;46(4):1275–9.
22. Oliveira C, Tello C, Liebmann J, Ritch R. Central corneal thickness is not related to anterior scleral thickness or axial length. J Glaucoma. 2006;15(3):190–4.
23. Lesk MR, Hafez AS, Descovich D. Relationship between central corneal thickness and changes of optic nerve head topography and blood flow after intraocular pressure reduction in open-angle glaucoma and ocular hypertension. Arch Ophthalmol. 2006;124(11):1568–72.
24. Pakravan M, Parsa A, Sanagou M, Parsa CF. Central corneal thickness and correlation to optic disc size: a potential link for susceptibility to glaucoma. Br J Ophthalmol. 2007;91(1):26–8.
25. Wang J, Freeman EE, Descovich D, Harasymowycz PJ, Kamdeu Fansi A, Li G, et al. Estimation of ocular rigidity in glaucoma using ocular pulse amplitude and pulsatile choroidal blood flow. Invest Ophthalmol Vis Sci. 2013;54(3):1706–11.
26. Pallikaris IG, Kymionis GD, Ginis HS, Kounis GA, Tsilimbaris MK. Ocular rigidity in living human eyes. Invest Ophthalmol Vis Sci. 2005;46(2):409–14.
27. Brandt JD, Beiser JA, Kass MA, Gordon MO. Central corneal thickness in the Ocular Hypertension Treatment Study (OHTS). Ophthalmology. 2001;108(10):1779–88.
28. Hahn S, Azen S, Ying-Lai M, Varma R, Los Angeles Latino Eye Study Group. Central corneal thickness in Latinos. Invest Ophthalmol Vis Sci. 2003;44(4):1508–12.
29. Nemesure B, Wu SY, Hennis A, Leske MC, Barbados Eye Study Group. Corneal thickness and intraocular pressure in the Barbados eye studies. Arch Ophthalmol. 2003;121(2):240–4.
30. Shimmyo M, Ross AJ, Moy A, Mostafavi R. Intraocular pressure, Goldmann applanation tension, corneal thickness, and corneal curvature in Caucasians, Asians, Hispanics, and African Americans. Am J Ophthalmol. 2003;136(4):603–13.
31. Haseltine SJ, Pae J, Ehrlich JR, Shammas M, Radcliffe NM. Variation in corneal hysteresis and central corneal thickness among black, hispanic and white subjects. Acta Ophthalmol. 2012;90(8):e626–31.
32. Meda R, Wang Q, Paoloni D, Harasymowycz P, Brunette I. The impact of chronic use of prostaglandin analogues on the biomechanical properties of the cornea in patients with primary open-angle glaucoma. Br J Ophthalmol. 2017;101(2):120–5.
33. Tsikripis P, Papaconstantinou D, Koutsandrea C, Apostolopoulos M, Georgalas I. The effect of prostaglandin analogs on the biomechanical properties and central thickness of the cornea of patients with open-angle glaucoma: a 3-year study on 108 eyes. Drug Des Devel Ther. 2013;7:1149–56.
34. Brandt JD, Gordon MO, Beiser JA, Lin SC, Alexander MY, Kass MA, et al. Changes in central corneal thickness over time: the ocular hypertension treatment study. Ophthalmology. 2008;115(9):1550–6, 1556.e1.
35. Chauhan BC, Hutchison DM, LeBlanc RP, Artes PH, Nicolela MT. Central corneal thickness and progression of the visual field and optic disc in glaucoma. Br J Ophthalmol. 2005;89(8):1008–12.
36. Luce DA. Determining in vivo biomechanical properties of the cornea with an ocular response analyzer. J Cataract Refract Surg. 2005;31(1):156–62.
37. Hong J, Xu J, Wei A, Deng SX, Cui X, Yu X, et al. A new tonometerDOUBLEHYPHEN-the Corvis ST tonometer: clinical comparison with noncontact and Goldmann applanation tonometers. Invest Ophthalmol Vis Sci. 2013;54(1):659–65.
38. Matsuura M, Hirasawa K, Murata H, Yanagisawa M, Nakao Y, Nakakura S, et al. The relationship between corvis ST tonometry and ocular response analyzer measurements in eyes with glaucoma. PLoS One. 2016;11(8):e0161742.
39. Shah S, Laiquzzaman M, Bhojwani R, Mantry S, Cunliffe I. Assessment of the biomechanical properties of the cornea with the ocular response analyzer in normal and keratoconic eyes. Invest Ophthalmol Vis Sci. 2007;48(7):3026–31.
40. Carbonaro F, Andrew T, Mackey DA, Spector TD, Hammond CJ. The heritability of corneal hysteresis and ocular pulse amplitude: a twin study. Ophthalmology. 2008;115(9):1545–9.

41. Mangouritsas G, Morphis G, Mourtzoukos S, Feretis E. Association between corneal hysteresis and central corneal thickness in glaucomatous and non-glaucomatous eyes. Acta Ophthalmol. 2009;87(8):901–5.
42. Wells AP, Garway-Heath DF, Poostchi A, Wong T, Chan KC, Sachdev N. Corneal hysteresis but not corneal thickness correlates with optic nerve surface compliance in glaucoma patients. Invest Ophthalmol Vis Sci. 2008;49(8):3262–8.
43. Abitbol O, Bouden J, Doan S, Hoang-Xuan T, Gatinel D. Corneal hysteresis measured with the Ocular Response Analyzer in normal and glaucomatous eyes. Acta Ophthalmol. 2010;88(1):116–9.
44. Sullivan-Mee M, Katiyar S, Pensyl D, Halverson KD, Qualls C. Relative importance of factors affecting corneal hysteresis measurement. Optom Vis Sci. 2012;89(5):E803–11.
45. Shah S, Laiquzzaman M, Mantry S, Cunliffe I. Ocular response analyser to assess hysteresis and corneal resistance factor in low tension, open angle glaucoma and ocular hypertension. Clin Exp Ophthalmol. 2008;36(6):508–13.
46. Medeiros FA, Meira-Freitas D, Lisboa R, Kuang TM, Zangwill LM, Weinreb RN. Corneal hysteresis as a risk factor for glaucoma progression: a prospective longitudinal study. Ophthalmology. 2013;120(8):1533–40.
47. Congdon NG, Broman AT, Bandeen-Roche K, Grover D, Quigley HA. Central corneal thickness and corneal hysteresis associated with glaucoma damage. Am J Ophthalmol. 2006;141(5):868–75.
48. De Moraes CV, Hill V, Tello C, Liebmann JM, Ritch R. Lower corneal hysteresis is associated with more rapid glaucomatous visual field progression. J Glaucoma. 2012;21(4):209–13.
49. Zhang C, Tatham AJ, Abe RY, Diniz-Filho A, Zangwill LM, Weinreb RN, et al. Corneal hysteresis and progressive retinal nerve fiber layer loss in glaucoma. Am J Ophthalmol. 2016;166:29–36.
50. Anand A, De Moraes CG, Teng CC, Tello C, Liebmann JM, Ritch R. Corneal hysteresis and visual field asymmetry in open angle glaucoma. Invest Ophthalmol Vis Sci. 2010;51(12):6514–8.
51. Sayah DN, Mazzaferri J, Descovich D, Costantino S, Lesk MR. The association between ocular rigidity and neuroretinal damage in glaucoma. Invest Ophthalmol Vis Sci. 2020;61(13):11.
52. Prata TS, Lima VC, Guedes LM, Biteli LG, Teixeira SH, de Moraes CG, et al. Association between corneal biomechanical properties and optic nerve head morphology in newly diagnosed glaucoma patients. Clin Exp Ophthalmol. 2012;40(7):682–8.
53. Khawaja AP, Chan MP, Broadway DC, Garway-Heath DF, Luben R, Yip JL, et al. Corneal biomechanical properties and glaucoma-related quantitative traits in the EPIC-Norfolk Eye Study. Invest Ophthalmol Vis Sci. 2014;55(1):117–24.
54. Carbonaro F, Hysi PG, Fahy SJ, Nag A, Hammond CJ. Optic disc planimetry, corneal hysteresis, central corneal thickness, and intraocular pressure as risk factors for glaucoma. Am J Ophthalmol. 2014;157(2):441–6.
55. Prata TS, Lima VC, de Moraes CG, Guedes LM, Magalhaes FP, Teixeira SH, et al. Factors associated with topographic changes of the optic nerve head induced by acute intraocular pressure reduction in glaucoma patients. Eye (Lond). 2011;25(2):201–7.
56. Mansouri K, Leite MT, Weinreb RN, Tafreshi A, Zangwill LM, Medeiros FA. Association between corneal biomechanical properties and glaucoma severity. Am J Ophthalmol. 2012;153(3):419–27. e1
57. Vu DM, Silva FQ, Haseltine SJ, Ehrlich JR, Radcliffe NM. Relationship between corneal hysteresis and optic nerve parameters measured with spectral domain optical coherence tomography. Graefes Arch Clin Exp Ophthalmol. 2013;251(7):1777–83.
58. Fontes BM, Ambrosio R Jr, Alonso RS, Jardim D, Velarde GC, Nose W. Corneal biomechanical metrics in eyes with refraction of -19.00 to +9.00 D in healthy Brazilian patients. J Refract Surg. 2008;24(9):941–5.
59. Ang GS, Bochmann F, Townend J, Azuara-Blanco A. Corneal biomechanical properties in primary open angle glaucoma and normal tension glaucoma. J Glaucoma. 2008;17(4):259–62.

60. Sun L, Shen M, Wang J, Fang A, Xu A, Fang H, et al. Recovery of corneal hysteresis after reduction of intraocular pressure in chronic primary angle-closure glaucoma. Am J Ophthalmol. 2009;147(6):1061–6, 1061.e1–2.

61. Pakravan M, Afroozifar M, Yazdani S. Corneal biomechanical changes following trabeculectomy, phaco-trabeculectomy, ahmed glaucoma valve implantation and phacoemulsification. J Ophthalmic Vis Res. 2014;9(1):7–13.

62. Agarwal DR, Ehrlich JR, Shimmyo M, Radcliffe NM. The relationship between corneal hysteresis and the magnitude of intraocular pressure reduction with topical prostaglandin therapy. Br J Ophthalmol. 2012;96(2):254–7.

63. Hirneiss C, Sekura K, Brandlhuber U, Kampik A, Kernt M. Corneal biomechanics predict the outcome of selective laser trabeculoplasty in medically uncontrolled glaucoma. Graefes Arch Clin Exp Ophthalmol. 2013;251(10):2383–8.

64. Detry-Morel M, Jamart J, Hautenauven F, Pourjavan S. Comparison of the corneal biomechanical properties with the Ocular Response Analyzer(R) (ORA) in African and Caucasian normal subjects and patients with glaucoma. Acta Ophthalmol. 2012;90(2):e118–24.

65. Deol M, Taylor DA, Radcliffe NM. Corneal hysteresis and its relevance to glaucoma. Curr Opin Ophthalmol. 2015;26(2):96–102.

66. Levy NS, Crapps EE. Displacement of optic nerve head in response to short-term intraocular pressure elevation in human eyes. Arch Ophthalmol. 1984;102(5):782–6.

67. Yan DB, Flanagan JG, Farra T, Trope GE, Ethier CR. Study of regional deformation of the optic nerve head using scanning laser tomography. Curr Eye Res. 1998;17(9):903–16.

68. Albon J, Purslow PP, Karwatowski WS, Easty DL. Age related compliance of the lamina cribrosa in human eyes. Br J Ophthalmol. 2000;84(3):318–23.

69. Hommer A, Fuchsjager-Mayrl G, Resch H, Vass C, Garhofer G, Schmetterer L. Estimation of ocular rigidity based on measurement of pulse amplitude using pneumotonometry and fundus pulse using laser interferometry in glaucoma. Invest Ophthalmol Vis Sci. 2008;49(9):4046–50.

70. Sigal IA, Flanagan JG, Tertinegg I, Ethier CR. Finite element modeling of optic nerve head biomechanics. Invest Ophthalmol Vis Sci. 2004;45(12):4378–87.

71. Sigal IA, Ethier CR. Biomechanics of the optic nerve head. Exp Eye Res. 2009;88(4):799–807.

72. Burgoyne CF, Downs JC, Bellezza AJ, Suh JK, Hart RT. The optic nerve head as a biomechanical structure: a new paradigm for understanding the role of IOP-related stress and strain in the pathophysiology of glaucomatous optic nerve head damage. Prog Retin Eye Res. 2005;24(1):39–73.

73. Bellezza AJ, Hart RT, Burgoyne CF. The optic nerve head as a biomechanical structure: initial finite element modeling. Invest Ophthalmol Vis Sci. 2000;41(10):2991–3000.

74. Coudrillier B, Tian J, Alexander S, Myers KM, Quigley HA, Nguyen TD. Biomechanics of the human posterior sclera: age- and glaucoma-related changes measured using inflation testing. Invest Ophthalmol Vis Sci. 2012;53(4):1714–28.

75. Ebneter A, Wagels B, Zinkernagel MS. Non-invasive biometric assessment of ocular rigidity in glaucoma patients and controls. Eye (Lond). 2009;23(3):606–11.

76. Drance SM. The coefficient of scleral rigidity in normal and glaucomatous eyes. Arch Ophthalmol. 1960;63:668–74.

77. Agrawal KK, Sharma DP, Bhargava G, Sanadhya DK. Scleral rigidity in glaucoma, before and during topical antiglaucoma drug therapy. Indian J Ophthalmol. 1991;39(3):85–6.

78. Dastiridou AI, Tsironi EE, Tsilimbaris MK, Ginis H, Karyotakis N, Cholevas P, et al. Ocular rigidity, outflow facility, ocular pulse amplitude, and pulsatile ocular blood flow in open-angle glaucoma: a manometric study. Invest Ophthalmol Vis Sci. 2013;54(7):4571–7.

79. Eisenlohr JE, Langham ME, Maumenee AE. Manometric studies of the pressure-volume relationship in living and enucleated eyes of individual human subjects. Br J Ophthalmol. 1962;46(9):536–48.

80. Eisenlohr JE, Langham ME. The relationship between pressure and volume changes in living and dead rabbit eyes. Investig Ophthalmol. 1962;1:63–77.

81. Ytteborg J. The role of intraocular blood volume in rigidity measurements on human eyes. Acta Ophthalmol. 1960;38:410–36.
82. Kerrigan-Baumrind LA, Quigley HA, Pease ME, Kerrigan DF, Mitchell RS. Number of ganglion cells in glaucoma eyes compared with threshold visual field tests in the same persons. Invest Ophthalmol Vis Sci. 2000;41(3):741–8.
83. Harwerth RS, Carter-Dawson L, Shen F, Smith EL 3rd, Crawford ML. Ganglion cell losses underlying visual field defects from experimental glaucoma. Invest Ophthalmol Vis Sci. 1999;40(10):2242–50.
84. Trier K, Ribel-Madsen SM. Latanoprost eye drops increase concentration of glycosaminoglycans in posterior rabbit sclera. J Ocul Pharmacol Ther. 2004;20(3):185–8.
85. Dastiridou AI, Ginis H, Tsilimbaris M, Karyotakis N, Detorakis E, Siganos C, et al. Ocular rigidity, ocular pulse amplitude, and pulsatile ocular blood flow: the effect of axial length. Invest Ophthalmol Vis Sci. 2013;54(3):2087–92.
86. Boland MV, Quigley HA. Risk factors and open-angle glaucoma: classification and application. J Glaucoma. 2007;16(4):406–18.
87. Mitchell P, Hourihan F, Sandbach J, Wang JJ. The relationship between glaucoma and myopia: the Blue Mountains Eye Study. Ophthalmology. 1999;106(10):2010–5.
88. Quigley HA. The contribution of the sclera and lamina cribrosa to the pathogenesis of glaucoma: diagnostic and treatment implications. Prog Brain Res. 2015;220:59–86.
89. Friberg TR, Lace JW. A comparison of the elastic properties of human choroid and sclera. Exp Eye Res. 1988;47(3):429–36.
90. Tezel G, Luo C, Yang X. Accelerated aging in glaucoma: immunohistochemical assessment of advanced glycation end products in the human retina and optic nerve head. Invest Ophthalmol Vis Sci. 2007;48(3):1201–11.
91. Malik NS, Moss SJ, Ahmed N, Furth AJ, Wall RS, Meek KM. Ageing of the human corneal stroma: structural and biochemical changes. Biochim Biophys Acta. 1992;1138(3):222–8.
92. Fazio MA, Grytz R, Morris JS, Bruno L, Gardiner SK, Girkin CA, et al. Age-related changes in human peripapillary scleral strain. Biomech Model Mechanobiol. 2014;13(3):551–63.
93. Girkin CA, Fazio MA, Yang H, Reynaud J, Burgoyne CF, Smith B, et al. Variation in the three-dimensional histomorphometry of the normal human optic nerve head with age and race: lamina cribrosa and peripapillary scleral thickness and position. Invest Ophthalmol Vis Sci. 2017;58(9):3759–69.
94. Fazio MA, Grytz R, Morris JS, Bruno L, Girkin CA, Downs JC. Human scleral structural stiffness increases more rapidly with age in donors of African descent compared to donors of European descent. Invest Ophthalmol Vis Sci. 2014;55(11):7189–98.
95. Jackson CR. Schiotz tonometers. An assessment of their usefulness. Br J Ophthalmol. 1965;49(9):478–84.
96. Gloster J, Perkins ES. Ocular rigidity and tonometry. Proc R Soc Med. 1957;50(9):667–74.
97. Perkins ES, Gloster J. Further studies on the distensibility of the eye. Br J Ophthalmol. 1957;41(8):475–86.
98. Moses RA, Grodzki WJ. Ocular rigidity in tonography. Doc Ophthalmol. 1969;26:118–29.
99. Friedenwald JS. Tonometer calibration; an attempt to remove discrepancies found in the 1954 calibration scale for Schiotz tonometers. Trans Am Acad Ophthalmol Otolaryngol. 1957;61(1):108–22.
100. Grant WM. Clinical measurements of aqueous outflow. AMA Arch Ophthalmol. 1951;46(2):113–31.
101. Silver DM, Farrell RA, Langham ME, O'Brien V, Schilder P. Estimation of pulsatile ocular blood flow from intraocular pressure. Acta Ophthalmol Suppl. 1989;191:25–9.
102. Ytteborg J. The effect of intraocular pressure on rigidity coefficient in the human eye. Acta Ophthalmol. 1960;38:548–61.
103. Ytteborg J. Further investigations of factors influencing size of rigidity coefficient. Acta Ophthalmol. 1960;38:643–57.

104. Beaton L, Mazzaferri J, Lalonde F, Hidalgo-Aguirre M, Descovich D, Lesk MR, et al. Non-invasive measurement of choroidal volume change and ocular rigidity through automated segmentation of high-speed OCT imaging. Biomed Opt Express. 2015;6(5):1694–706.

105. Sayah DN, Mazzaferri J, Ghesquière P, Duval R, Rezende F, Costantino S, et al. Non-invasive in vivo measurement of ocular rigidity: clinical validation and method improvement. Exp Eye Res. 2019;190:107831.

106. Tengroth B, Ammitzboll T. Changes in the content and composition of collagen in the glaucomatous eyeDOUBLEHYPHENbasis for a new hypothesis for the genesis of chronic open angle glaucomaDOUBLEHYPHENa preliminary report. Acta Ophthalmol. 1984;62(6):999–1008.

107. Perkins ES. Ocular volume and ocular rigidity. Exp Eye Res. 1981;33(2):141–5.

108. Downs JC, Girkin CA. Lamina cribrosa in glaucoma. Curr Opin Ophthalmol. 2017;28(2):113–9.

109. Anderson DR, Hendrickson A. Effect of intraocular pressure on rapid axoplasmic transport in monkey optic nerve. Investig Ophthalmol. 1974;13(10):771–83.

110. Jonas JB, Ritch R, Panda-Jonas S. Cerebrospinal fluid pressure in the pathogenesis of glaucoma. Prog Brain Res. 2015;221:33–47.

111. Lee DS, Lee EJ, Kim TW, Park YH, Kim J, Lee JW, et al. Influence of translaminar pressure dynamics on the position of the anterior lamina cribrosa surface. Invest Ophthalmol Vis Sci. 2015;56(5):2833–41.

112. Morgan WH, Yu DY, Alder VA, Cringle SJ, Cooper RL, House PH, et al. The correlation between cerebrospinal fluid pressure and retrolaminar tissue pressure. Invest Ophthalmol Vis Sci. 1998;39(8):1419–28.

113. Gaasterland D, Tanishima T, Kuwabara T. Axoplasmic flow during chronic experimental glaucoma. 1. Light and electron microscopic studies of the monkey optic nervehead during development of glaucomatous cupping. Invest Ophthalmol Vis Sci. 1978;17(9):838–46.

114. Quigley HA, Addicks EM. Chronic experimental glaucoma in primates. II. Effect of extended intraocular pressure elevation on optic nerve head and axonal transport. Invest Ophthalmol Vis Sci. 1980;19(2):137–52.

115. Quigley HA, Guy J, Anderson DR. Blockade of rapid axonal transport. Effect of intraocular pressure elevation in primate optic nerve. Arch Ophthalmol. 1979;97(3):525–31.

116. Minckler DS, Bunt AH, Johanson GW. Orthograde and retrograde axoplasmic transport during acute ocular hypertension in the monkey. Invest Ophthalmol Vis Sci. 1977;16(5):426–41.

117. Zhao DY, Cioffi GA. Anterior optic nerve microvascular changes in human glaucomatous optic neuropathy. Eye (Lond). 2000;14(Pt 3B):445–9.

118. Qu J, Chen H, Zhu L, Ambalavanan N, Girkin CA, Murphy-Ullrich JE, et al. High-magnitude and/or high-frequency mechanical strain promotes peripapillary scleral myofibroblast differentiation. Invest Ophthalmol Vis Sci. 2015;56(13):7821–30.

119. Schneider M, Fuchshofer R. The role of astrocytes in optic nerve head fibrosis in glaucoma. Exp Eye Res. 2016;142:49–55.

120. Wallace DM, O'Brien CJ. The role of lamina cribrosa cells in optic nerve head fibrosis in glaucoma. Exp Eye Res. 2016;142:102–9.

121. Hernandez MR. The optic nerve head in glaucoma: role of astrocytes in tissue remodeling. Prog Retin Eye Res. 2000;19(3):297–321.

122. Quigley HA, Brown A, Dorman-Pease ME. Alterations in elastin of the optic nerve head in human and experimental glaucoma. Br J Ophthalmol. 1991;75(9):552–7.

123. Morrison JC, Dorman-Pease ME, Dunkelberger GR, Quigley HA. Optic nerve head extracellular matrix in primary optic atrophy and experimental glaucoma. Arch Ophthalmol. 1990;108(7):1020–4.

124. Pena JD, Netland PA, Vidal I, Dorr DA, Rasky A, Hernandez MR. Elastosis of the lamina cribrosa in glaucomatous optic neuropathy. Exp Eye Res. 1998;67(5):517–24.

125. Albon J, Karwatowski WS, Avery N, Easty DL, Duance VC. Changes in the collagenous matrix of the aging human lamina cribrosa. Br J Ophthalmol. 1995;79(4):368–75.

126. Luo H, Yang H, Gardiner SK, Hardin C, Sharpe GP, Caprioli J, et al. Factors influencing central lamina cribrosa depth: a multicenter study. Invest Ophthalmol Vis Sci. 2018;59(6):2357–70.
127. Behkam R, Kollech HG, Jana A, Hill A, Danford F, Howerton S, et al. Racioethnic differences in the biomechanical response of the lamina cribrosa. Acta Biomater. 2019;88:131–40.
128. Zeimer RC, Ogura Y. The relation between glaucomatous damage and optic nerve head mechanical compliance. Arch Ophthalmol. 1989;107(8):1232–4.
129. Bellezza AJ, Rintalan CJ, Thompson HW, Downs JC, Hart RT, Burgoyne CF. Deformation of the lamina cribrosa and anterior scleral canal wall in early experimental glaucoma. Invest Ophthalmol Vis Sci. 2003;44(2):623–37.
130. Quigley HA, Addicks EM. Regional differences in the structure of the lamina cribrosa and their relation to glaucomatous optic nerve damage. Arch Ophthalmol. 1981;99(1):137–43.
131. Quigley HA, Hohman RM, Addicks EM, Massof RW, Green WR. Morphologic changes in the lamina cribrosa correlated with neural loss in open-angle glaucoma. Am J Ophthalmol. 1983;95(5):673–91.
132. Jonas JB, Berenshtein E, Holbach L. Anatomic relationship between lamina cribrosa, intraocular space, and cerebrospinal fluid space. Invest Ophthalmol Vis Sci. 2003;44(12):5189–95.
133. Burgoyne CF, Quigley HA, Thompson HW, Vitale S, Varma R. Early changes in optic disc compliance and surface position in experimental glaucoma. Ophthalmology. 1995;102(12):1800–9.
134. Heickell AG, Bellezza AJ, Thompson HW, Burgoyne CF. Optic disc surface compliance testing using confocal scanning laser tomography in the normal monkey eye. J Glaucoma. 2001;10(5):369–82.
135. Azuara-Blanco A, Harris A, Cantor LB, Abreu MM, Weinland M. Effects of short term increase of intraocular pressure on optic disc cupping. Br J Ophthalmol. 1998;82(8):880–3.
136. Lesk MR, Spaeth GL, Azuara-Blanco A, Araujo SV, Katz LJ, Terebuh AK, et al. Reversal of optic disc cupping after glaucoma surgery analyzed with a scanning laser tomograph. Ophthalmology. 1999;106(5):1013–8.
137. Bowd C, Weinreb RN, Lee B, Emdadi A, Zangwill LM. Optic disk topography after medical treatment to reduce intraocular pressure. Am J Ophthalmol. 2000;130(3):280–6.
138. Irak I, Zangwill L, Garden V, Shakiba S, Weinreb RN. Change in optic disk topography after trabeculectomy. Am J Ophthalmol. 1996;122(5):690–5.
139. Raitta C, Tomita G, Vesti E, Harju M, Nakao H. Optic disc topography before and after trabeculectomy in advanced glaucoma. Ophthalmic Surg Lasers. 1996;27(5):349–54.
140. Sigal IA, Flanagan JG, Tertinegg I, Ethier CR. Reconstruction of human optic nerve heads for finite element modeling. Technol Health Care. 2005;13(4):313–29.
141. Levy NS, Crapps EE, Bonney RC. Displacement of the optic nerve head. Response to acute intraocular pressure elevation in primate eyes. Arch Ophthalmol. 1981;99(12):2166–74.
142. Sharpe GP, Danthurebandara VM, Vianna JR, Alotaibi N, Hutchison DM, Belliveau AC, et al. Optic disc hemorrhages and laminar disinsertions in glaucoma. Ophthalmology. 2016;123(9):1949–56.
143. Lee EJ, Kim TW, Kim M, Girard MJ, Mari JM, Weinreb RN. Recent structural alteration of the peripheral lamina cribrosa near the location of disc hemorrhage in glaucoma. Invest Ophthalmol Vis Sci. 2014;55(4):2805–15.
144. Kim YK, Jeoung JW, Park KH. Effect of focal lamina cribrosa defect on disc hemorrhage area in glaucoma. Invest Ophthalmol Vis Sci. 2016;57(3):899–907.
145. Park SC, Hsu AT, Su D, Simonson JL, Al-Jumayli M, Liu Y, et al. Factors associated with focal lamina cribrosa defects in glaucoma. Invest Ophthalmol Vis Sci. 2013;54(13):8401–7.
146. Kim YK, Park KH. Lamina cribrosa defects in eyes with glaucomatous disc haemorrhage. Acta Ophthalmol. 2016;94(6):e468–73.
147. You JY, Park SC, Su D, Teng CC, Liebmann JM, Ritch R. Focal lamina cribrosa defects associated with glaucomatous rim thinning and acquired pits. JAMA Ophthalmol. 2013;131(3):314–20.

148. Kim YW, Jeoung JW, Kim DW, Girard MJ, Mari JM, Park KH, et al. Clinical assessment of lamina cribrosa curvature in eyes with primary open-angle glaucoma. PLoS One. 2016;11(3):e0150260.
149. Li L, Bian A, Cheng G, Zhou Q. Posterior displacement of the lamina cribrosa in normal-tension and high-tension glaucoma. Acta Ophthalmol. 2016;94(6):e492–500.
150. Kim YW, Kim DW, Jeoung JW, Kim DM, Park KH. Peripheral lamina cribrosa depth in primary open-angle glaucoma: a swept-source optical coherence tomography study of lamina cribrosa. Eye (Lond). 2015;29(10):1368–74.
151. Kim DW, Jeoung JW, Kim YW, Girard MJ, Mari JM, Kim YK, et al. Prelamina and lamina cribrosa in glaucoma patients with unilateral visual field loss. Invest Ophthalmol Vis Sci. 2016;57(4):1662–70.
152. Quigley H, Arora K, Idrees S, Solano F, Bedrood S, Lee C, et al. Biomechanical responses of lamina cribrosa to intraocular pressure change assessed by optical coherence tomography in glaucoma eyes. Invest Ophthalmol Vis Sci. 2017;58(5):2566–77.
153. Agoumi Y, Sharpe GP, Hutchison DM, Nicolela MT, Artes PH, Chauhan BC. Laminar and prelaminar tissue displacement during intraocular pressure elevation in glaucoma patients and healthy controls. Ophthalmology. 2011;118(1):52–9.
154. Sigal IA, Roberts MD, Girard MJA, Burgoyne CF, Downs JC. Chapter 20: biomechanical changes of the optic disc. In: Levin LA, Albert DM, editors. Ocular disease: mechanisms and management. London: Elsevier; 2010. p. 153–64.
155. Lepple-Wienhues A, Stahl F, Wiederholt M. Differential smooth muscle-like contractile properties of trabecular meshwork and ciliary muscle. Exp Eye Res. 1991;53(1):33–8.
156. Wiederholt M, Thieme H, Stumpff F. The regulation of trabecular meshwork and ciliary muscle contractility. Prog Retin Eye Res. 2000;19(3):271–95.
157. Fuchshofer R, Tamm ER. The role of TGF-beta in the pathogenesis of primary open-angle glaucoma. Cell Tissue Res. 2012;347(1):279–90.
158. Last JA, Pan T, Ding Y, Reilly CM, Keller K, Acott TS, et al. Elastic modulus determination of normal and glaucomatous human trabecular meshwork. Invest Ophthalmol Vis Sci. 2011;52(5):2147–52.
159. Wang K, Johnstone MA, Xin C, Song S, Padilla S, Vranka JA, et al. Estimating human trabecular meshwork stiffness by numerical modeling and advanced oct imaging. Invest Ophthalmol Vis Sci. 2017;58(11):4809–17.
160. Wang K, Read AT, Sulchek T, Ethier CR. Trabecular meshwork stiffness in glaucoma. Exp Eye Res. 2017;158:3–12.
161. Morgan JT, Raghunathan VK, Chang YR, Murphy CJ, Russell P. The intrinsic stiffness of human trabecular meshwork cells increases with senescence. Oncotarget. 2015;6(17):15362–74.
162. Chen RI, Barbosa DT, Hsu CH, Porco TC, Lin SC. Ethnic differences in trabecular meshwork height by optical coherence tomography. JAMA Ophthalmol. 2015;133(4):437–41.
163. Xin C, Johnstone M, Wang N, Wang RK. OCT study of mechanical properties associated with trabecular meshwork and collector channel motion in human eyes. PLoS One. 2016;11(9):e0162048.
164. Xin C, Song S, Johnstone M, Wang N, Wang RK. Quantification of pulse-dependent trabecular meshwork motion in normal humans using phase-sensitive OCT. Invest Ophthalmol Vis Sci. 2018;59(8):3675–81.
165. Sayah DN, Szigiato AA, Mazzaferri J, Descovich D, Duval R, Rezende FA, Costantino S, Lesk MR. Correlation of ocular rigidity with intraocular pressure spike after intravitreal injection of bevacizumab in exudative retinal disease. Br J Ophthalmol. 2021;105(3):392–6.
166. Kadziauskiene A, Jasinskiene E, Asoklis R, Lesinskas E, Rekasius T, Chua J, et al. Long-term shape, curvature, and depth changes of the lamina cribrosa after trabeculectomy. Ophthalmology. 2018;125(11):1729–40.
167. Hidalgo-Aguirre M, Gitelman J, Lesk MR, Costantino S. Automatic segmentation of the optic nerve head for deformation measurements in video rate optical coherence tomography. J Biomed Opt. 2015;20(11):116008.

168. Hidalgo-Aguirre M, Costantino S, Lesk MR. Pilot study of the pulsatile neuro-peripapillary retinal deformation in glaucoma and its relationship with glaucoma risk factors. Curr Eye Res. 2017;42(12):1620–7.
169. Singh K, Dion C, Godin AG, Lorghaba F, Descovich D, Wajszilber M, et al. Pulsatile movement of the optic nerve head and the peripapillary retina in normal subjects and in glaucoma. Invest Ophthalmol Vis Sci. 2012;53(12):7819–24.
170. Lee EJ, Kim TW, Weinreb RN, Park KH, Kim SH, Kim DM. Visualization of the lamina cribrosa using enhanced depth imaging spectral-domain optical coherence tomography. Am J Ophthalmol. 2011;152(1):87–95.e1.
171. Chang MY, Shin A, Park J, Nagiel A, Lalane RA, Schwartz SD, et al. Deformation of optic nerve head and peripapillary tissues by horizontal duction. Am J Ophthalmol. 2017;174:85–94.
172. Shin A, Yoo L, Park J, Demer JL. Finite element biomechanics of optic nerve sheath traction in adduction. J Biomech Eng. 2017;139(10):1010101–10101010.
173. Suh SY, Clark RA, Demer JL. Optic nerve sheath tethering in adduction occurs in esotropia and hypertropia, but not in exotropia. Invest Ophthalmol Vis Sci. 2018;59(7):2899–904.
174. Morrison JC, Nylander KB, Lauer AK, Cepurna WO, Johnson E. Glaucoma drops control intraocular pressure and protect optic nerves in a rat model of glaucoma. Invest Ophthalmol Vis Sci. 1998;39(3):526–31.
175. Heijl A, Leske MC, Bengtsson B, Hyman L, Bengtsson B, Hussein M, et al. Reduction of intraocular pressure and glaucoma progression: results from the Early Manifest Glaucoma Trial. Arch Ophthalmol. 2002;120(10):1268–79.
176. Kass MA, Heuer DK, Higginbotham EJ, Johnson CA, Keltner JL, Miller JP, et al. The Ocular Hypertension Treatment Study: a randomized trial determines that topical ocular hypotensive medication delays or prevents the onset of primary open-angle glaucoma. Arch Ophthalmol. 2002;120(6):701–13. discussion 829-30
177. Garway-Heath DF, Crabb DP, Bunce C, Lascaratos G, Amalfitano F, Anand N, et al. Latanoprost for open-angle glaucoma (UKGTS): a randomised, multicentre, placebo-controlled trial. Lancet. 2015;385(9975):1295–304.
178. Huang W, Fileta JB, Dobberfuhl A, Filippopolous T, Guo Y, Kwon G, et al. Calcineurin cleavage is triggered by elevated intraocular pressure, and calcineurin inhibition blocks retinal ganglion cell death in experimental glaucoma. Proc Natl Acad Sci U S A. 2005;102(34):12242–7.
179. Ji JZ, Elyaman W, Yip HK, Lee VW, Yick LW, Hugon J, et al. CNTF promotes survival of retinal ganglion cells after induction of ocular hypertension in rats: the possible involvement of STAT3 pathway. Eur J Neurosci. 2004;19(2):265–72.
180. Martin KR, Quigley HA, Zack DJ, Levkovitch-Verbin H, Kielczewski J, Valenta D, et al. Gene therapy with brain-derived neurotrophic factor as a protection: retinal ganglion cells in a rat glaucoma model. Invest Ophthalmol Vis Sci. 2003;44(10):4357–65.
181. McKinnon SJ, Lehman DM, Tahzib NG, Ransom NL, Reitsamer HA, Liston P, et al. Baculoviral IAP repeat-containing-4 protects optic nerve axons in a rat glaucoma model. Mol Ther. 2002;5(6):780–7.
182. Nakazawa T, Nakazawa C, Matsubara A, Noda K, Hisatomi T, She H, et al. Tumor necrosis factor-alpha mediates oligodendrocyte death and delayed retinal ganglion cell loss in a mouse model of glaucoma. J Neurosci. 2006;26(49):12633–41.
183. Neufeld AH, Das S, Vora S, Gachie E, Kawai S, Manning PT, et al. A prodrug of a selective inhibitor of inducible nitric oxide synthase is neuroprotective in the rat model of glaucoma. J Glaucoma. 2002;11(3):221–5.
184. Schwartz M. Neurodegeneration and neuroprotection in glaucoma: development of a therapeutic neuroprotective vaccine: the Friedenwald lecture. Invest Ophthalmol Vis Sci. 2003;44(4):1407–11.
185. Agostinone J, Alarcon-Martinez L, Gamlin C, Yu WQ, Wong ROL, Di Polo A. Insulin signalling promotes dendrite and synapse regeneration and restores circuit function after axonal injury. Brain. 2018;141(7):1963–80.

186. Steinhart MR, Cone FE, Nguyen C, Nguyen TD, Pease ME, Puk O, et al. Mice with an induced mutation in collagen 8A2 develop larger eyes and are resistant to retinal ganglion cell damage in an experimental glaucoma model. Mol Vis. 2012;18:1093–106.
187. Mohammadpour M, Masoumi A, Mirghorbani M, Shahraki K, Hashemi H. Updates on corneal collagen cross-linking: indications, techniques and clinical outcomes. J Curr Ophthalmol. 2017;29(4):235–47.
188. Strouthidis NG, Girard MJ. Altering the way the optic nerve head responds to intraocular pressure—a potential approach to glaucoma therapy. Curr Opin Pharmacol. 2013;13(1):83–9.
189. Wollensak G, Spoerl E. Collagen crosslinking of human and porcine sclera. J Cataract Refract Surg. 2004;30(3):689–95.
190. Spoerl E, Boehm AG, Pillunat LE. The influence of various substances on the biomechanical behavior of lamina cribrosa and peripapillary sclera. Invest Ophthalmol Vis Sci. 2005;46(4):1286–90.
191. Girard MJ, Suh JK, Bottlang M, Burgoyne CF, Downs JC. Biomechanical changes in the sclera of monkey eyes exposed to chronic IOP elevations. Invest Ophthalmol Vis Sci. 2011;52(8):5656–69.

Chapter 19
Ocular Rigidity and Age Related Macular Degeneration

Miltiadis K. Tsilimbaris

Theoretical Correlation: The Vascular Theory of AMD

As early as 1937 Friedenwald [1] stressed the role of elevated scleral rigidity in the aging eye and in the same year Verhoeff [2] attributed the pathogenesis of AMD to impairment of choroidal blood flow. But it was Ephraim Friedman that first proposed a possible direct correlation between scleral rigidity and age related macular degeneration as part of his hypothesis on a vascular pathogenesis of AMD [3]. According to this theory, the sclera, becoming increasingly "rigid" and noncompliant, because of age or other causes, limits the filling of the vortex veins, and thereby increases the resistance to venous outflow. This relative obstruction ultimately leads to dilatation and decompensation of the choroidal venous system at the posterior pole, compromising Bruch's membrane, the choriocapillaris, and the retinal pigment epithelium of the macular area. Friedman's vascular model underwent several revisions becoming gradually more elaborated and attempting to incorporate the role of atherosclerosis and blood pressure in the pathophysiology of AMD [4, 5]. However, in all versions the hemodynamic consequence of stiffening of the eye's scleral cell remained central for the hypothesis. The lipoid infiltration of the sclera, Bruch membrane, and the walls of blood vessels is considered one of the main etiologic factors that result in decreased compliance of the sclera, Bruch membrane, and the choroidal vessels. Scleral rigidity, in turn, plays a central role interfering with choroidal venous drainage of retinal lipoproteins which are considered a major pathogenic factor for the retinal damage seen in AMD [6].

M. K. Tsilimbaris (✉)
University of Crete Medical School, Heraklion, Crete, Greece
e-mail: tsilimb@med.uoc.gr

© Springer Nature Switzerland AG 2021
I. Pallikaris et al. (eds.), *Ocular Rigidity, Biomechanics and Hydrodynamics of the Eye*, https://doi.org/10.1007/978-3-030-64422-2_19

Existing Evidence: Scleral Rigidity Measurements in AMD

In their 1989 paper Friedman et al measured the coefficient of scleral rigidity (CSR) of the eyes of 29 patients with age-related macular degeneration [7]. CSR of the right and left eyes of the 29 ARMD patients was 0.023 (0.006) and 0.024 (0.004), respectively. The mean CSR (standard deviation) of the right and left eyes of the 25 controls was 0.018 (0.005) and 0.020 (0.007), respectively. The differences in CSR between cases and controls were statistically significant for both the right eye ($P = 0.0003$) and the left eye ($P = 0.009$). The coefficient was found to be significantly higher than that of 25 control patients, frequency matched for age. Age and axial length did not seem to affect this correlation. Authors concluded that their data suggested that an increased scleral rigidity may be a significant risk factor for the development of the disorder. The data produced by this work was the first direct indication that a correlation may exist between scleral rigidity and AMD.

The failure to distinguish between dry and wet AMD cases as well as the relative inaccurate rigidity measurement using Perkins and Schiotz tonometers can be considered as weaknesses of this work.

Our group repeated the measurement of ocular rigidity in patients with AMD using the direct manometric system described in Chap. 2. Thirty-two patients with AMD (16 with neovascular and 16 with non-neovascular AMD) and 44 age-matched control patients (control group) were measured prior to a scheduled cataract operation [8]. No statistically significant difference in ocular rigidity measurements between patients with AMD and control subjects was found (AMD group: 0.0142 [0.0077] vs. control group: 0.0125 [0.0049]; $P = 0.255$), and this was in accordance with our previous study of scleral rigidity measurement in living eyes [9]. However, when we examined separately the two subgroups of patients with AMD (neovascular and nonneovascular AMD), the average ocular rigidity measurements were higher in patients with neovascular AMD vs. both control subjects and patients with non-neovascular AMD (neovascular AMD group: 0.0186 [0.0078] vs. control group: 0.0125 [0.0048] $P = 0.014$ vs. non-neovascular AMD group: 0.0104 [0.0053] $P = 0.004$) (Fig. 19.1). Thus, this was the second study to find a possible correlation between scleral rigidity and age related macular degeneration. The different measurement method as well as possible difference in composition of the study groups may be the reason for the differences compared to Friedman's et al. study.

Interpretation and Future Directions

Although both studies have significant limitations (small sample sizes, limited phenotypic grouping of AMD) and they contain some contradictory findings, they provide a considerable indication of a possible correlation between ocular rigidity and AMD.

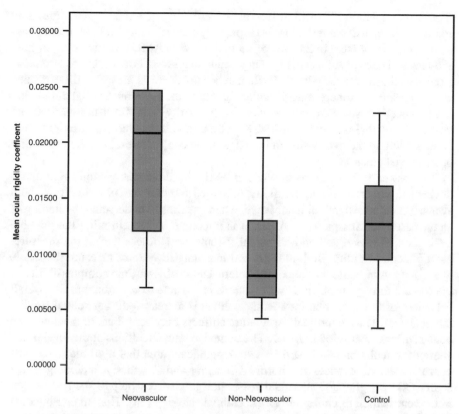

Fig. 19.1 Mean ocular rigidity coefficient in patients with neovascular (n = 16) and non-neovascular age-related macular degeneration (n = 16) and in control subjects (n = 44). (From Pallikaris et al. [8])

According to Friedman this correlation is etiopathogenic. Ocular haemodynamic abnormalities observed in AMD are considered the result of an increasingly rigid sclera that acts to encapsulate the ocular vasculature in a more incompressible compartment, leading to a success of events that end up with the phenotype of AMD. However, based on the existing data, this is hard to prove. There is always the possibility that increased scleral rigidity is an epiphenomenon of AMD and not an etiologic factor [10]. Clarification of this correlation can have obvious advantages. Ocular rigidity can be modified with appropriate intervention. We have described such an intervention that is based on the intraocular implantation of a compressible miniature airbag [11]. The presence of the intraocular air reservoir can augment the capacity of intraocular volume increase with minimal pressure raise. This can modify the hemodynamic balance of the globe, and optimally reverse the effects of increased ocular stiffness.

Other investigators, while agreeing with Friedman's starting point about AMD sharing both risk factors and pathogenetic mechanisms with atherosclerosis, have focused their research in the possible role of local hemodynamic alterations of the choroidal circulation [12] and in the role of stiffening of retinal vasculature. Sato and co-workers, using a retinal laser Doppler system, measured retinal arterial haemodynamic parameters in 25 eyes of 25 patients with AMD and nine eyes of nine age-matched control subjects [13]. They found that blood flow in retinal arteries is more pulsatile in patients with AMD than in healthy controls. Based on these results, they suggest that an increasing vascular rigidity in the systemic arterial circulation can be directly associated with an increasing severity of AMD. Authors postulate that it is likely that patients with AMD have a stiffer, less compliant arterial vasculature leading to the eye, although here again one could not exclude the possibility of an epiphenomenon.

The answer to the question of whether AMD-related haemodynamic abnormalities are due to increased scleral rigidity, increased systemic vascular rigidity, or both awaits further investigation. In any case, when one tries to understand the finding of an increased ocular rigidity in AMD, it is important to keep in mind the possible interaction of scleral cell and choroidal vasculature stiffness during the measurement of ocular rigidity. Both indirect and manometric systems measure the whole eye rigidity. And while the role of the scleral cell is obvious, the compressibility of the choroid through backwards venous flow, is possible to contribute in the overall behaviour of the eye when intraocular volume is increased during scleral rigidity measurement. Thus, choroidal vasculature stiffness may contribute to the increased ocular stiffness measured in AMD. The hemodynamic alterations at the level of the choroidal circulation in AMD represent a significant area that until today remains obscure. Recent advances in choroidal imaging and flowmetry, including swept source OCT imaging and choroidal vessel flowgraphy may help to shed more light in the contribution of choroid in AMD pathophysiology [14]. This, in combination with the development of accurate, non-invasive technology for the measurement of ocular rigidity [15] may permit the design of clinical studies of adequate power to clarify the possible role of sclera and choroidal vasculature in AMD and their interplay in ocular rigidity measurement.

In conclusion, the available data indicate the existence of possible correlation between ocular rigidity and age related macular degeneration, but the pathogenic nature of this correlation is uncertain. Advancements in imaging, ocular hemodynamic evaluation and non-invasive rigidity recording, may facilitate the clarification of the etiologic correlation between ocular rigidity and AMD, opening the way for new therapeutic interventions.

References

1. Friedenwald JS. Contribution to the theory and practice of tonometry. Am J Ophthalmol. 1937;20:985–1024.
2. Verhoeff FH, Grossman HP. Pathogenesis of disciform degeneration of the macula. Arch Ophthalmol. 1937;18:561–85.
3. Friedman E. Scleral rigidity, venous obstruction, and age-related macular degeneration: a working hypothesis. In: BenEzra D, Ryan SJ, Glaser BM, et al., editors. Ocular circulation

and neovascularization, Documenta Ophthalmologica Proceedings Series, vol. 50. Dordrecht: NijhoffjJunk; 1987. p. 197–204.

4. Friedman E. A hemodynamic model of the pathogenesis of age-related macular degeneration. Am J Ophthalmol. 1997;124(5):677–82.
5. Friedman E. Update of the vascular model of AMD. Br J Ophthalmol. 2004;88(2):161–3.
6. Friedman E. The pathogenesis of age-related macular degeneration. Am J Ophthalmol. 2008;146(3):348–9.
7. Friedman E, Ivry M, Ebert E, Glynn R, Gragoudas E, Seddon J. Increased scleral rigidity and age-related macular degeneration. Ophthalmology. 1989;96(1):104–8.
8. Pallikaris IG, Kymionis GD, Ginis HS, Kounis GA, Christodoulakis E, Tsilimbaris MK. Ocular rigidity in patients with age-related macular degeneration. Am J Ophthalmol. 2006;141(4):611–5.
9. Pallikaris IG, Kymionis GD, Ginis HS, Kounis GA, Tsilimbaris MK. Ocular rigidity in living human eyes. Invest Ophthalmol Vis Sci. 2005;46(2):409–14.
10. Pulido J. Scleral rigidity and macular degeneration: pathophysiologic or epiphenomenon? Am J Ophthalmol. 2006;141(4):731–2.
11. Pallikaris I, Tsilibaris MK, Kounis G, Kymionis G, Harilaos G. Device and method for the increase of ocular elasticity and prevention of macular degeneration. https://patents.google.com/patent/US20020026240
12. Gelfand BD, Ambati JA. Revised hemodynamic theory of age-related macular degeneration. Trends Mol Med. 2016;22(8):656–70.
13. Sato E, Feke GT, Menke MN, Wallace McMeel J. Retinal haemodynamics in patients with age-related macular degeneration. Eye (Lond). 2006;20(6):697–702.
14. Wei X, Balne PK, Meissner KE, Barathi VA, Schmetterer L, Agrawal R. Assessment of flow dynamics in retinal and choroidal microcirculation. Surv Ophthalmol. 2018;63(5):646–64.
15. Pallikaris I, Ginis HS, De Brouwere D, Tsilimbaris MK. A novel instrument for the non-invasive measurement of intraocular pressure and ocular rigidity. Invest Ophthalmol Vis Sci. 2006;47:2268.

Chapter 20
Ocular Rigidity and Diabetes

Athanassios Giarmoukakis and Theonitsa Panagiotoglou

Introduction

Diabetes mellitus is a group of metabolic diseases characterized by significant heterogeneity [1]. According to the International Diabetes Federation (IDF), the global prevalence of diabetes in adults was 8.3% (382 million people) in 2013, being expected to rise up to 10.1% (beyond 592 million people) by 2035 [2]. In addition, the development of diabetic complications represent a major cause of morbidity and mortality, as well as a substantial worldwide public health burden [2]. Diabetic retinopathy (DR) is one of the most common diabetic complications that can lead to severe vision-loss if left undiagnosed and untreated [3]. In fact, DR is the leading cause of visual impairment in adults [4].

The main feature of diabetes is the dysfunction in the metabolism of carbohydrates, fats and proteins, due to compromised secretion and action of insulin [1, 2]. This dysfunction results in high levels of blood glucose (hyperglycemia), which in turn trigger certain biochemical pathways that are considered key factors for the pathogenesis of the disease and its complications [5]. Moreover, these metabolic and biochemical changes in diabetes are known to exert a significant impact on physical properties of different human tissues [6–8], including ocular tissues [6, 7], that could potentially suggest a possible relationship between the disease and ocular biomechanics, as well.

A. Giarmoukakis (✉)
Department of Ophthalmology, Medical School, University of Crete,
Heraklion, Crete, Greece

University Hospital of Heraklion, Heraklion, Crete, Greece

T. Panagiotoglou
Department of Ophthalmology, Medical School, University of Crete,
Heraklion, Crete, Greece

The Effect of Diabetes on Tissue Biochemical and Biomechanical Properties

A number of interconnecting and up-regulated biochemical pathways have been proposed as potential links between hyperglycemia and diabetic retinopathy. These include increased polyol pathway flux, activation of protein kinase C (PKC) pathway, increased expression of growth factors such as vascular endothelial growth factor (VEGF) and insulin-like growth factor-1 (IGF-1) and increased oxidative stress [5]. This up-regulation is the hallmark of the pathogenesis of the disease's complications [5]. Moreover, the increased protein glycation and the formulation of its products, such as the advanced glycation end products (AGEs), constitute fundamental factors for the manifestation of vascular diabetic complications, including diabetic retinopathy [5, 7–9]. In addition, AGEs promote an increase in thickness and stiffness of basement membranes (BMs), which has been specifically noticed in BMs of the retinal vasculature [7, 10], affecting their morphological and biomechanical properties [7]. BM thickening may also result in a loss of vascular elasticity, therefore changing vascular biomechanical properties, that is considered a contributing factor to elevated blood pressure, as well [11, 12]. BMs are extracellular matrix components that are important for the structural integrity of different tissues [13]. Major BM proteins include among others different types of collagen (type IV and XVIII), laminin and a series of proteoglycans [13]. It is considered that AGEs can lead to changes in the physical properties of tissues either by excessive intermolecular cross-linking, altering the biochemical profile of BMs and collagen molecule, thus modifying the intermolecular and cell-collagen interactions or by connecting to cellular receptors modifying their role [7–9]. Therefore, based on the high distribution of collagen and proteoglycans in the human cornea and sclera [14, 15] and the increased levels of AGEs found in different ocular tissues of diabetic patients [16–18], it has been hypothesized that diabetes may promote changes in the biomechanical properties of the eye and hence in OR, as well [19].

Ocular Rigidity as Measured in Diabetes

Despite the well-documented and thoroughly studied ocular complications of diabetes mellitus [20], as well as the well-established knowledge concerning the possible pathophysiologic mechanisms that may suggest alterations of ocular tissue physical properties in diabetes, as discussed in the previous section, little is known up to date with regard to the actual effect of the disease on OR.

As already mentioned within the context of the present book, OR measurements in human eyes have been obtained mainly by either paired Schiotz tonometry, based on the Friedenwald's equation [21], or by invasive manometry-based devises [19, 22], which are considered to provide direct and more precise measurements [22]. Implementing the Friedenwald's equation, Arora and Prasad were the first to report on OR measurements in patients with different stages of DR [23]. They concluded that no differences in scleral rigidity between individuals with and without DR could be documented [23]. In another study, Pallikaris et al. reported on OR measurements on a large sample of living human eyes that were obtained by a direct manometric measurement device at different intraocular pressures (IOPs) [22]. In addition, they attempted to explore any possible relationship between OR and different demographic, ocular and systemic factors, including diabetes mellitus [22]. According to their results, no significant correlation was detected between the OR coefficient and the presence of diabetes mellitus [22]. Nevertheless, it should be noted that this study did not check the actual presence of diabetic retinopathy among study participants but it was based only on personal history data with regard to diabetes mellitus and other systemic disease. Towards this direction, in a more recent study of the same research team, Panagiotoglou et al. assessed OR in patients with diagnosed non-proliferative DR (NPDR) [19], using a similar measurement setting with Pallikaris et al. [22]. Study participants were further divided into two subgroups according to NPDR severity (mild NPDR group, moderate and severe NPDR group), while OR measurements were compared to those of an age-matched control group with no signs of diabetic retinopathy or history of diabetes. Despite the fact that no significant differences were recorded in OR coefficient between the control and NPDR groups, as well as between the two NPDR sub-groups, authors described a tendency towards higher OR values with increasing disease severity [19].

Conclusions and Future Perspectives

It has been suggested that changes in OR may have significant clinical implications by affecting other ocular parameters such as IOP and ocular blood flow [22], while possibly playing an important role in the pathogenesis and clinical course of different ocular conditions, including glaucoma and age-related macular degeneration (AMD) [24, 25]. Nevertheless, the invasive nature of its most precise measurement technique (i.e. manometry-based systems) remains the most significant factor that limits its wide implementation.

Regarding OR in diabetes, there has been supporting evidence that diabetes induces physical changes in different ocular tissues that may constitute contributing factors for possible alterations of ocular biomechanics [6, 7, 16–18]. On the other hand, up to date, there are only a few studies that have attempted an assessment of their relationship in clinical settings, with their results failing to support any changes of OR in diabetic patients [19, 22, 23]. Nevertheless, significant limitations of these studies, such as the relative small number of patients and the lack of uniformity in the applied measurement technique [19, 23], suggest the need for further investigation. Therefore, future studies with larger cohorts are considered necessary, in order to elucidate the relationship between OR and diabetic retinopathy, as well as to further evaluate any possible impact of the disease severity and stage on OR and ocular biomechanics.

References

1. Kharroubi AT, Darwish HM. Diabetes mellitus: the epidemic of the century. World J Diabetes. 2015;6(6):850–67.
2. International Diabetes Federation. IDF diabetes atlas. 6th ed. Brussels: International Diabetes Federation; 2013. https://www.idf.org/e-library/epidemiology-research/diabetes-atlas/19-atlas-6th-edition.html
3. Lee R, Wong TY, Sabanayagam C. Epidemiology of diabetic retinopathy, diabetic macular edema and related vision loss. Eye Vis (Lond). 2015;2:17.
4. Cheung N, Mitchell P, Wong TY. Diabetic retinopathy. Lancet. 2010;376(9735):124–36.
5. Brownlee M. Biochemistry and molecular cell biology of diabetic complications. Nature. 2001;414(6865):813–20.
6. Scheler A, Spoerl E, Boehm AG. Effect of diabetes mellitus on corneal biomechanics and measurement of intraocular pressure. Acta Ophthalmol. 2012;90(6):e447–51.
7. To M, Goz A, Camenzind L, et al. Diabetes-induced morphological, biomechanical, and compositional changes in ocular basement membranes. Exp Eye Res. 2013;116:298–307.
8. Gautieri A, Redaelli A, Buehler MJ, Vesentini S. Age- and diabetes-related nonenzymatic crosslinks in collagen fibrils: candidate amino acids involved in Advanced Glycation End-products. Matrix Biol. 2014;34:89–95.
9. Paul RG, Bailey AJ. Glycation of collagen: the basis of its central role in the late complications of ageing and diabetes. Int J Biochem Cell Biol. 1996;28(12):1297–310.
10. Tsilibary EC. Microvascular basement membranes in diabetes mellitus. J Pathol. 2003;200(4):537–46.
11. Durham JT, Herman IM. Microvascular modifications in diabetic retinopathy. Curr Diabetes Rep. 2011;11(4):253–64.
12. Zatz R, Brenner BM. Pathogenesis of diabetic microangiopathy. The hemodynamic view. Am J Med. 1986;80(3):443–53.
13. Halfter W, Candiello J, Hu H, et al. Protein composition and biomechanical properties of in vivo-derived basement membranes. Cell Adh Migr. 2013;7(1):64–71.
14. Massoudi D, Malecaze F, Galiacy SD. Collagens and proteoglycans of the cornea: importance in transparency and visual disorders. Cell Tissue Res. 2016;363(2):337–49.
15. Watson PG, Young RD. Scleral structure, organisation and disease. A review. Exp Eye Res. 2004;78(3):609–23.
16. Kase S, Ishida S, Rao NA. Immunolocalization of advanced glycation end products in human diabetic eyes: an immunohistochemical study. J Diabetes Mellitus. 2011;1:57–62.
17. Sato E, Mori F, Igarashi S, Abiko T, Takeda M, Ishiko S, Yoshida A. Corneal advanced glycation end products increase in patients with proliferative diabetic retinopathy. Diabetes Care. 2001;24(3):479–82.
18. Hadley JC, Meek KM, Malik NS. The effect of glycation on charge distribution and swelling behaviour of corneal and scleral collagen. Invest Ophthalmol Vis Sci. 1996;37:4636.
19. Panagiotoglou T, Tsilimbaris M, Ginis H, et al. Ocular rigidity and outflow facility in nonproliferative diabetic retinopathy. J Diabetes Res. 2015;2015:141598.
20. Poh S, Mohamed Abdul RB, Lamoureux EL, et al. Metabolic syndrome and eye diseases. Diabetes Res Clin Pract. 2016;113:86–100.
21. Friedenwald JS. Contribution to the theory and practice of tonometry. Am J Ophthalmol. 1937;20:985–1024.
22. Pallikaris IG, Kymionis GD, Ginis HS, Kounis GA, Tsilimbaris MK. Ocular rigidity in living human eyes. Invest Ophthalmol Vis Sci. 2005;46(2):409–14.
23. Arora VK, Prasad VN. The intraocular pressure and diabetes—a correlative study. Indian J Ophthalmol. 1989;37(1):10–2.
24. Detorakis ET, Pallikaris IG. Ocular rigidity: biomechanical role, in vivo measurements and clinical significance. Clin Exp Ophthalmol. 2013;41(1):73–81.
25. Pallikaris IG, Kymionis GD, Ginis HS, Kounis GA, Christodoulakis E, Tsilimbaris MK. Ocular rigidity in patients with age-related macular degeneration. Am J Ophthalmol. 2006;141(4):611–5.

Chapter 21
Ocular Rigidity and High Myopia

Georgios Bontzos

Myopia Epidemiology and Structural Changes

Myopia is creating an advancing global epidemic; its current prevalence is estimated to be around 27%, affecting 1.45 billion people [1]. The incidence of myopia has increased dramatically over the last decades, reaching 70–80% in many Eastern Asia countries [2] and 30–40% in Western countries [3]. It is predicted that almost 50% of the world population will be myopic by 2050 [4]. A younger onset of myopia is particularly worrying since younger eyes experience faster progression of myopia.

The myopic eye is elongated and its altered architecture is accompanied with structural changes of the choroid and the sclera [5]. Several ocular complications, like earlier cataract development [6], glaucoma and retinal degenerations are associated with high myopia. Common retinal disorders in high myopia include myopic choroidal neovascularization, chorioretinal atrophy, myopic traction maculopathy, posterior staphyloma and retinal detachment [7]. Although the ocular mechanisms leading to myopia are not completely understood, it is likely to be driven from a complex interaction of environmental factors and the effects of multiple genes during the emmetropization process. Current approaches suggest that the sclera plays a key role with changes in biomechanical properties and biomechanical environment occurring the process of eye elongation controlled by both cellular and extracellular matrix factors [8].

G. Bontzos (✉)
University Hospital of Heraklion, Heraklion, Crete, Greece
e-mail: gbontzos@hotmail.gr

© Springer Nature Switzerland AG 2021
I. Pallikaris et al. (eds.), *Ocular Rigidity, Biomechanics and Hydrodynamics of the Eye*, https://doi.org/10.1007/978-3-030-64422-2_21

Ocular Rigidity and Globe Expansion

Since its implementation *ocular rigidity* has been associated with eye dimensions. It is generally considered as a surrogate parameter related to the biomechanical properties of the whole globe. The ocular volume is tended with a confined structure of the outer coats of cornea and sclera which protect the eye from external trauma. These structures are of fundamental importance in understanding the mechanical and material properties of the eye [9]. It is notable that, sclera is more prone to distortion than the cornea from intraocular and extraocular muscle forces. Greene [10] showed that an incremental increase in intraocular pressure does not change the corneal curvature, while scleral curvature increases linearly with pressure. Thus, it is commonly accepted that ocular rigidity is related to the elasticity of the sclera.

The sclera is a dynamic tissue which provides a strong framework that support the visual apparatus of the inner eye. With its significant malleability, it can adapt to extraocular forces by altering its properties, as data suggest from ex-vivo analyses [8]. In-vivo human studies also support this theory, although data is more limited [11, 12]. Moreover, in high myopia, the sclera is significantly thinner than the emmetropic eye and gradually expands under the force of intraocular pressure. Studies from cadaver human eyes showed that collagen fiber bundles are thinned and their size is decreased in myopia [13, 14] (Fig. 21.1). Gottlieb [15] investigated

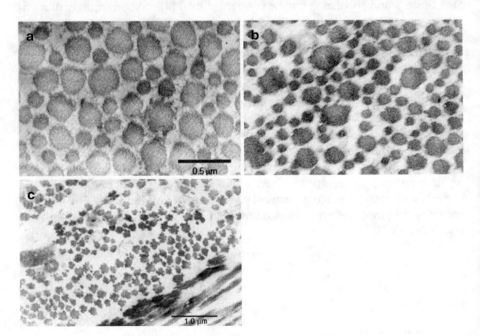

Fig. 21.1 Collagen fibrils of the sclera in emmetropic and myopic human eyes. The highly myopic human sclera shows greater variability in collagen fibril diameters and contains an increased number of smaller diameter collagen fibrils (**a, b**). Additionally, an increase in unusual star-shaped fibrils is observed on cross section (**c**). (Adapted from: Curtin et al. [14])

the biomechanics of the weakened sclera during myopia development and high-lighted the role of cellular and matrix factors as well as the reduced myofibroblasts in the process of eye elongation. The mechanical stress forces on the sclera during near work have been hypothesized to contribute in myopia development [10]. Greene [10], calculated the distribution of forces on the sclera during accommodation and proposed that the effect of extraocular muscles during convergence has a significant effect on the progression of myopia. Nevertheless, more studies are needed on the elasticity and rigidity of the eye to evaluate how mechanical factors affect the eye, and help in understanding how the eye responds to such environmental stimuli and how it expands in myopia.

Ocular Rigidity as Measured in Myopia

The degree of expansion of the outer coat of the eye with increase in volume, is affected by the elastic properties of the cornea and sclera. When in 1937, Friedenwald [16], introduced the theory of ocular rigidity, he described a measure of resistance that the eye exerts to distending forces. He proposed a coefficient of ocular rigidity (K), based on a logarithmic pressure-volume relationship, as derived from experimental data on enucleated eyes. This parameter describes the elasticity of the ocular shell, especially the sclera, cornea and the compressibility of the choroid, assuming that the other ocular compartments are practically incompressible. In his mathematic formula, Friedenwald's coefficient K had an average value of 0.025. Coefficient K is inversely proportional to ocular volume, resulting in a high correlation between ocular rigidity and axial length. It has been postulated that this due to the larger volume of such eyes both by Phillips [17] and Perkins [18]. The latter calculated a coefficient of rigidity that included the volume of each myopic eye and suggested that myopic eyes do not exhibit apparent changes in scleral distensibility [18].

In his original study, Friedenwald [16], demonstrated that scleral rigidity is lower in myopic eyes of one to five diopters than emmetropic controls. Interestingly however, he found that in myopic eyes of more than five diopters rigidity gradually reached normal levels. In extreme myopia, ocular rigidity actually displayed higher values then normative data. His results were also confirmed by later studies. Honmura has shown a significant negative correlation between rigidity and axial length [19]. Ocular volume was an important parameter, in the pressure-volume relationship, in the rigidity equation as described in a later study by Silver and Geyer [20]. Moreover, Castrén and Pohjola [21] suggested that scleral rigidity was lower in myopes than non-myopes, and since scleral rigidity was lower at adolescence than adulthood, lower scleral rigidity could be a contributing factor of myopia progression at this age group [22]. In her recent studies, Dastiridou [23] also reported a significant negative correlation between ocular rigidity coefficient and axial length in an in-vivo manometric study of human eyes (Fig. 21.2). In contrast, ocular rigidity is believed to be increased in hyperopic eyes [24]. Despite the

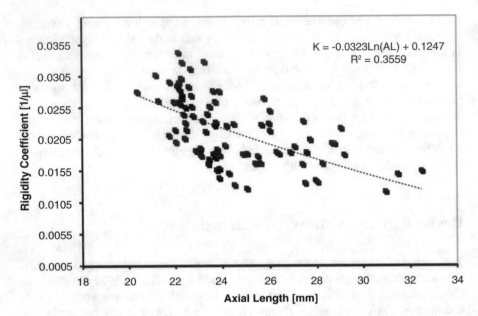

Fig. 21.2 Scatterplot of the relationship between ocular rigidity coefficient and axial length as measured by Dastiridou et al. [23]

growing data that support the hypothesis of lower ocular rigidity in myopic eyes, there are studies which do not verify this statement. For instance, Wong and Yap [25] found poor correlation between refractive error and ocular rigidity, in Chinese population, a group predisposed to myopia. In addition, Schmid [26] did not found significant difference in ocular rigidity between a myopic group of children (−3.43D) and an emmetropic one.

Measurement Techniques and Limitations

When calculating the ocular rigidity in many mathematical formulations, the ocular volume is a key parameter. The relationship between ocular volume and rigidity can be observed in clinical practice by the fact that pressure spikes after an intravitreal injection differ among axial lengths [27]. The ocular volume itself, depends on the shape of the eye. When in 1966, Friedman [28] worked on a spherical model of the eye, by applying Laplace's Law, he pointed out that the stress experienced by the walls of the eye is directly related to intraocular pressure and volume and inversely related to the thickness of the walls. However, the shape of the eye is not a perfect sphere; in fact, in high myopic and hyperopic eyes the lateral and vertical diameters can display significant discrepancies. Generally, it has been measured that, myopic eyes are elongated relative to emmetropic eyes, more in length than in height [29, 30] (Fig. 21.3). This fact can partially explain why results are not consistent, among

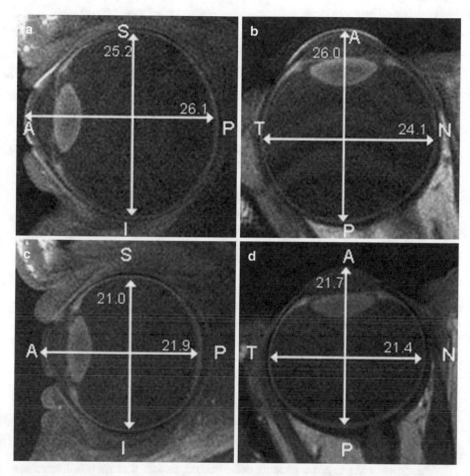

Fig. 21.3 Sagittal and axial MRI figures of emmetropic and myopic human eyes. Top panels (**a**, **b**) show an elongated myopic eye with increased measured dimensions. Lower panels (**c, d**) show an emmetropic eye. We can observe how the myopic eye is longer towards the anteroposterior axis (26.1 mm) compared to its width (24.1 mm) and height (25.2 mm). emmetropic eye (Reprint from Atchison et al. [29])

different studies, in the relation between axial length and ocular rigidity. Moreover, in cases of posterior staphylomas the eyeball shape can be further distorted as presented by Ohno-Matsui [31]. The regional inconsistency of curvature and the deformation of the sclera result in variability of the applied forces by intra- or extraocular stresses on the outer coats of the eye. The effect of a distorted eye on the rigidity measurements is also supported by the study of Friberg and Fourman [32] who studied eyes previously undergone scleral buckling. They found significantly reduced ocular rigidity which was attributed to the changes in eye shape and stress distribution. It should be noted here that, the buckling material is also important when evaluating ocular rigidity. In a later study [33], it was found the silicone buckling resulted in significantly lower ocular rigidity than metal, as observed in postmortem enucleated eyes.

Up to this day, Friedenwald's equation [16] is considered the gold-standard for calculating ocular rigidity. However, his methodology has received criticism for two main reasons [34]. Firstly, the data that were used for calculations were taken from enucleated eyes, neglecting the effect of extraocular muscles and the environment of the orbital cavity. Secondly, one should take under consideration the post-mortem changes such as the edema and the consequent thickening tissues. The intact living eye is also affected by the active blood flow and the vascular rigidity [35–37]. Considering these drawbacks, several measurement techniques have been described to estimate the ocular rigidity. The first method to evaluate in-vivo the pressure-volume relationship were performed in human eyes schedules for enucleation [34]. A manometric system was used and the eye was injected with known volume of saline after intraocular cannulation [34, 38, 39]. Later, Pallikaris [12] presented a methodology of direct manometric measurements performed before cataract surgery in human eyes under retrobulbar anesthesia. However, the invasive nature of this technique restricts its clinical utility. Attempts have been made to estimate ocular rigidity with non-invasive techniques. Ebneter [40] proposed a method based on measurement of axial length changes after oral administration of acetazolamide. The measured axial length decrease per mmHg of intraocular reduction can be used to estimate ocular rigidity. Recently, Detorakis [41] proposed an non-invasive technique based on the comparative measurements of Goldmann applanation tonometry which deforms the corneal apex and displaces aqueous humor and Dynamic Contour Tonometry which respects the globe geometry. The differences between pressure and volume can then be applied in Friedenwald's mathematic formula [16]. It is doubtful though, if simple non-invasive techniques can be used in large myopic eyes, since the constant K has to be reconsidered in these cases. The only study until today, to measure the ocular rigidity in a large number of living human eyes has been reported by Dastiridou [23] who suggested that axial length could comprise an independent factor of differences in ocular rigidity measurements.

When measuring myopic patients concomitant factors that may influence the integrity of rigidity measurements have to be considered. Increased axial length might be associated with keratoconus, glaucoma and retinal degenerations. For example, the reduction of ocular rigidity in keratoconus, is attributed to the reduced corneal rigidity rather than higher axial length [42]. Ocular rigidity in myopic patients should also be classified in different age groups. Aging, is related to structural alteration of the ocular walls and increase rigidity [43–45]. The increased scleral resistance allows less blood flow through the choroidal vessels [46].

Clinical Role and Future Perspective

Ocular rigidity is a macroscopic parameter that depends on the architecture and material properties of the globe. Its role in the pathogenesis of various ophthalmic conditions has been recognised. Unfortunately, the clinical use of ocular rigidity is limited due to its invasive technique. So far, a negative association has been reported between axial length and rigidity (Fig. 21.2). It has been hypothesized that, in myopia, the degeneration of the outer coats of the eye and especially the sclera is the key factor behind these reduced values. It remains to be elucidated whether extreme myopia is correlated with ocular rigidity and which measurement technique yields the most accurate and reliable results. Therefore ocular rigidity calculations need to be verified within a wide range of axial lengths using different methodologies. Ocular rigidity measurements can also expand our understanding towards the pathogenesis of myopia. For future studies, ocular rigidity should also be measured in young patients who can be re-examined in a later stage of their life, to evaluate whether differences in ocular rigidity are correlated with possible changes in axial length.

References

1. Holden BA, Wilson DA, Jong M, Sankaridurg P, Fricke TR, Smith EL III, et al. Myopia: a growing global problem with sight-threatening complications. Community Eye Health. 2015;28(90):35.
2. Sun J, Zhou J, Zhao P, Lian J, Zhu H, Zhou Y, et al. High prevalence of myopia and high myopia in 5060 Chinese university students in Shanghai. Invest Ophthalmol Vis Sci. 2012;53(12):7504–9.
3. Kempen JH, Mitchell P, Lee KE, Tielsch JM, Broman AT, Taylor HR, et al. The prevalence of refractive errors among adults in the United States, Western Europe, and Australia. Arch Ophthalmol. 2004;122(4):495–505.
4. Holden BA, Fricke TR, Wilson DA, Jong M, Naidoo KS, Sankaridurg P, et al. Global prevalence of myopia and high myopia and temporal trends from 2000 through 2050. Ophthalmology. 2016;123(5):1036–42.
5. Curtin BJ, Karlin DB. Axial length measurements and fundus changes of the myopic eye. Am J Ophthalmol. 1971;71(1 Pt 1):42–53.
6. Tuft SJ, Bunce C. Axial length and age at cataract surgery. J Cataract Refract Surg. 2004;30(5):1045–8.
7. Vongphanit J, Mitchell P, Wang JJ. Prevalence and progression of myopic retinopathy in an older population. Ophthalmology. 2002;109(4):704–11.
8. McBrien NA, Jobling AI, Gentle A. Biomechanics of the sclera in myopia: extracellular and cellular factors. Optom Vis Sci. 2009;86(1):E23–30.
9. Asejczyk-Widlicka M, Pierscionek BK. Fluctuations in intraocular pressure and the potential effect on aberrations of the eye. Br J Ophthalmol. 2007;91(8):1054–8.
10. Greene PR. Mechanical considerations in myopia: relative effects of accommodation, convergence, intraocular pressure, and the extraocular muscles. Am J Optom Physiol Optic. 1980;57(12):902–14.
11. Dastiridou AI, Ginis HS, De Brouwere D, Tsilimbaris MK, Pallikaris IG. Ocular rigidity, ocular pulse amplitude, and pulsatile ocular blood flow: the effect of intraocular pressure. Invest Ophthalmol Vis Sci. 2009;50(12):5718–22.
12. Pallikaris IG, Kymionis GD, Ginis HS, Kounis GA, Tsilimbaris MK. Ocular rigidity in living human eyes. Invest Ophthalmol Vis Sci. 2005;46(2):409–14.
13. Curtin BJ, Teng CC. Scleral changes in pathological myopia. Trans Am Acad Ophthalmol Otolaryngol. 1958;62(6):777–88. discussion 88–90
14. Curtin BJ, Iwamoto T, Renaldo DP. Normal and staphylomatous sclera of high myopia. An electron microscopic study. Arch Ophthalmol. 1979;97(5):912–5.

15. Gottlieb MD, Joshi HB, Nickla DL. Scleral changes in chicks with form-deprivation myopia. Curr Eye Res. 1990;9(12):1157–65.
16. Friedenwald JS. Contribution to the theory and practice of tonometry. Am J Ophthalmol. 1937;20(10):985–1024.
17. Phillips CI, Storey JK. Glaucoma geometry. Exp Eye Res. 1971;11(1):140–1.
18. Perkins ES. Ocular volume and ocular rigidity. Exp Eye Res. 1981;33(2):141–5.
19. Honmura S. Studies on the relationship between ocular tension and myopia. I. Later refractive changes of rabbits' eyes after peripheral iridectomy. Nippon Ganka Gakkai Zasshi. 1968;72(6):671–87.
20. Silver DM, Geyer O. Pressure-volume relation for the living human eye. Curr Eye Res. 2000;20(2):115–20.
21. Castren JA, Pohjola S. Refraction and scleral rigidity. Acta Ophthalmol. 1961;39:1011–4.
22. Castren J, Pohjola S. Scleral rigidity at puberty. Acta Ophthalmol. 1961;39:1015–9.
23. Dastiridou AI, Ginis H, Tsilimbaris M, Karyotakis N, Detorakis E, Siganos C, et al. Ocular rigidity, ocular pulse amplitude, and pulsatile ocular blood flow: the effect of axial length. Invest Ophthalmol Vis Sci. 2013;54(3):2087–92.
24. Goldmann H, Schmidt T. [Friedenwald's rigidity coefficient]. Ophthalmologica. 1957;133(4–5):330–5; discussion, 5–6.
25. Wong E, Yap MKH. Factors affecting ocular rigidity in the Chinese. Clin Exp Optom. 1991;74(5):156–9.
26. Schmid KL, Li RW, Edwards MH, Lew JK. The expandability of the eye in childhood myopia. Curr Eye Res. 2003;26(2):65–71.
27. Kotliar K, Maier M, Bauer S, Feucht N, Lohmann C, Lanzl I. Effect of intravitreal injections and volume changes on intraocular pressure: clinical results and biomechanical model. Acta Ophthalmol Scand. 2007;85(7):777–81.
28. Friedman B. Stress upon the ocular coats: effects of scleral curvature scleral thickness, and intra-ocular pressure. Eye Ear Nose Throat Mon. 1966;45(9):59–66.
29. Atchison DA, Jones CE, Schmid KL, Pritchard N, Pope JM, Strugnell WE, et al. Eye shape in emmetropia and myopia. Invest Ophthalmol Vis Sci. 2004;45(10):3380–6.
30. Tabernero J, Schaeffel F. More irregular eye shape in low myopia than in emmetropia. Invest Ophthalmol Vis Sci. 2009;50(9):4516–22.
31. Ohno-Matsui K. Proposed classification of posterior staphylomas based on analyses of eye shape by three-dimensional magnetic resonance imaging and wide-field fundus imaging. Ophthalmology. 2014;121(9):1798–809.
32. Friberg TR, Fourman SB. Scleral buckling and ocular rigidity. Clinical ramifications. Arch Ophthalmol. 1990;108(11):1622–7.
33. Whitacre MM, Emig MD, Hassanein K. Effect of buckling material on ocular rigidity. Ophthalmology. 1992;99(4):498–502.
34. Eisenlohr JE, Langham ME, Maumenee AE. Manometric studies of the pressure-volume relationship in living and enucleated eyes of individual human subjects. Br J Ophthalmol. 1962;46(9):536–48.
35. McEwen WK, St Helen R. Rheology of the human sclera. Unifying formulation of ocular rigidity. Ophthalmologica. 1965;150(5):321–46.
36. Ytteborg J. The role of intraocular blood volume in rigidity measurements on human eyes. Acta Ophthalmol. 1960;38:410–36.
37. Lam AK, Chan ST, Chan H, Chan B. The effect of age on ocular blood supply determined by pulsatile ocular blood flow and color Doppler ultrasonography. Optom Vis Sci. 2003;80(4):305–11.
38. Prijot E, Weekers R. [Contribution to the study of the rigidity of the normal human eye]. Ophthalmologica 1959;138:1–9.
39. Ytteborg J. Influence of bulbar compression on rigidity coefficient of human eyes, in vivo and encleated. Acta Ophthalmol. 1960;38:562–77.

40. Ebneter A, Wagels B, Zinkernagel MS. Non-invasive biometric assessment of ocular rigidity in glaucoma patients and controls. Eye (Lond). 2009;23(3):606–11.
41. Detorakis ET, Tsaglioti E, Kymionis G. Non-invasive ocular rigidity measurement: a differential tonometry approach. Acta Med (Hradec Kralove). 2015;58(3):92–7.
42. Shah S, Laiquzzaman M, Bhojwani R, Mantry S, Cunliffe I. Assessment of the biomechanical properties of the cornea with the ocular response analyzer in normal and keratoconic eyes. Invest Ophthalmol Vis Sci. 2007;48(7):3026–31.
43. Ravalico G, Toffoli G, Pastori G, Croce M, Calderini S. Age-related ocular blood flow changes. Invest Ophthalmol Vis Sci. 1996;37(13):2645–50.
44. Gaasterland D, Kupfer C, Milton R, Ross K, McCain L, MacLellan H. Studies of aqueous humour dynamics in man. VI. Effect of age upon parameters of intraocular pressure in normal human eyes. Exp Eye Res. 1978;26(6):651–6.
45. Friedman E, Ivry M, Ebert E, Glynn R, Gragoudas E, Seddon J. Increased scleral rigidity and age-related macular degeneration. Ophthalmology. 1989;96(1):104–8.
46. Friedman E. Update of the vascular model of AMD. Br J Ophthalmol. 2004;88(2):161–3.

Chapter 22
Ocular Rigidity and Uveitis

Anna I. Dastiridou, Nikolaos Ziakas, and Sofia Androudi

Introduction

The term uveitis refers to inflammation of the uveal tissues in the eye. The uvea includes the iris, the ciliary body and the choroid. Infectious causes and autoimmune diseases can cause certain types of uveitis, while idiopathic forms are not uncommon. Specific findings can in some cases guide the diagnosis and treatment, together with ancillary testing.

It is understood that the biomechanical properties of ocular tissues and also, intraocular pressure, with the mechanical load that it exerts, can change considerably during the course of a uveitic attack. In fact, uveitis can cause a wide range of clinical manifestations from the anterior and/or posterior segment. Remodeling of extracellular matrix and changes in collagen content in ocular tissues may lead to changes in the elastic and viscous properties of the ocular tissues, especially those of the choroid, cornea and sclera.

A. I. Dastiridou (✉)
2nd Ophthalmology Department, Aristotle University of Thessaloniki, Thessaloniki, Greece

School of Medicine, University of Thessalia, Larissa, Greece

N. Ziakas
2nd Department of Ophthalmology, Papageorgiou Hospital, Aristotle University of Thessaloniki, Thessaloniki, Greece

S. Androudi
Ophthalmology Clinic, University Hospital of Larissa, University of Thessalia, Volos, Greece
e-mail: androudi@otenet.gr

© Springer Nature Switzerland AG 2021
I. Pallikaris et al. (eds.), *Ocular Rigidity, Biomechanics and Hydrodynamics of the Eye*, https://doi.org/10.1007/978-3-030-64422-2_22

Evidence from Studies on Ocular Rigidity

The first report of ocular rigidity (OR) measurements in uveitis comes from Friedenwald, who tested 18 eyes with this diagnosis [1]. In those eyes, the OR was elevated and this finding was consistent, irrespective of the status of the intraocular pressure or the presence of secondary glaucoma. The mean ocular rigidity in this group measured 0.034. In eyes with uveitis, the presence of ocular inflammation, the release of prostaglandins and the vascular congestion might have led one to expect a lower OR. In the course of a uveitic attack, there are also changes in the outflow routes, with studies pointing to an increase in the uveoscleral pathway, and often a decrease in the conventional route of outflow. Inflammation may in fact alter the scleral elasticity and also choroidal blood flow. Furthermore, the intraocular pressure in uveitis can be normal, decreased, for instance due to ciliary body shut down, or even elevated, due to secondary ocular hypertension or glaucoma. This could also affect the measured OR. Our current knowledge on the inflammatory cascade that takes place in a uveitic attack suggests that cytokines play an important role [2].

The results of his study, led Friedenwald hypothesize that certain inflammation mediators or byproducts may have a stiffening effect on the sclera [1]. Due to inherent difficulties of measuring tissue elasticity in the eye, it is unknown if this hypothesis holds true. Furthermore, most studies in the biomechanics of the uveitic eye as presented in the following section are probably pointing to the opposite direction.

Cornea Biomechanics in Uveitis

Interestingly, recent studies have looked at the effects of uveitis on the corneal hysteresis (CH) and cornea resistance factor (CRF) that are measured with the Ocular Response Analyser (ORA, Reichert Ophthalmic Instruments, Buffalo, NY, USA) [3]. The ORA has the ability to provide quantitative parameters that characterize the viscous (CH) and elastic (CRF) properties of the cornea, based on the cornea response to a jet of air [4]. In addition, the Corvis ST can measure several biomechanical properties of the eye and provide estimates of the stiffness of the cornea and extracorneal tissues [5].

In a study analyzing measurements with the ORA from 85 eyes with inactive recurrent anterior uveitis of diverse etiology, the authors reported lower CH and lower CRF in patients, compared to controls, whereas no difference was found in CCT between the groups [6]. Patients enrolled in that study had been diagnosed with idiopathic anterior uveitis, multiple sclerosis-related uveitis, sarcoidosis-associated uveitis, Behcet uveitis and HLA B27-associated anterior uveitis. This study also searched for associations with disease duration or frequency of the attacks and found no correlation.

Studies have since provided specific evidence on ORA changes in different disease groups. In a study comparing IOP and cornea biomechanics with ORA in patients with systemic lupus erythematosus and controls, the authors found that CH and CRF were both lower in patients compared to controls, whereas there was no difference in central corneal thickness [7]. In fact, Goldmann-related IOP also measured lower, while corneal-compensated IOP was the same between patients and controls, suggesting that altered cornea properties in patients with SLE may lead to a falsely low IOP reading in these patients.

Cornea biomechanical properties were also studied in patients suffering from rheumatoid arthritis. Cornea hysteresis has been reported to be lower in both studies available in the literature, using ORA [8, 9]. In the study by Tas et al., the authors also found decreased cornea resistance factor in rheumatoid arthritis patients [9].

It has also been reported that Fuchs' uveitis patients demonstrate decreased CRF and CH [10]. In that study, patients with unilateral Fuchs uveitis were tested and compared to age matched controls. CH and CFR were significantly lower in the uveitic eyes, compared to contralateral eyes and eyes from healthy controls [11].

Contrary to findings in rheumatoid arthritis and lupus, ORA measurements in scleroderma patients showed that CRF and IOPg (Goldmann-correlated intraocular pressure) were higher, compared to controls, while no difference was found in CH or corneal thickness [12]. Systemic sclerosis is a disease of autoimmune origin, characterized by deposition of excessive amounts of collagen and fibrosis in various organs. ORA measurements helped to demonstrate that there are changes in the biomechanical properties of the cornea that are associated with this condition. Therefore, IOP may be overestimated in these patients on routine testing.

Finally, the properties of the cornea were also assessed in a series of pediatric noninfectious uveitis patients [13]. Again, in those patients, with a mean age of 10 years old, CRF measured lower compared to the control group, while corneal hysteresis and central cornea thickness did not differ between the groups.

Finally, there is also evidence in the literature that uveitis patients have altered biomechanical properties as measured using the Corvis ST (Oculus). The authors in this cross-sectional study enrolled 76 patients with systemic autoimmune disease, including mostly patients with rheumatoid arthritis and HLA-B27 related uveitis, but also other diagnosis, such as Adamantiadis-Behcet's uveitis, systemic lupus erythematosus, sarcoidosis, seronegative arthritis and granulomatosis with polyangiitis, and compared them to controls [14]. Parameters, namely corneal stiffness, extracorneal tissue stiffness and extracorneal tissue viscosity were estimated based on a biomechanical model) [15]. They found that corneal stiffness and extracorneal tissue viscosity were lower in the uveitic group. Although this cross-sectional includes eyes with very diverse history and manifestations of disease, it provides initial evidence that the biomechanics of the uveitic eye are altered. Further follow up studies may clarify the series of events in the pathophysiology of each disease phenotype.

References

1. Friedenwald JS. Contribution to the theory and practice of tonometry. Am J Opthalmology. 1937;20:985.
2. Weinstein JE, Pepple KL. Cytokines in uveitis. Curr Opin Ophthalmol. 2018;29:267–74.
3. Lau W, Pye D. A clinical description of Ocular Response Analyzer measurements. Invest Ophthalmol Vis Sci. 2011;52:2911–6.
4. Luce DA. Determining in vivo biomechanical properties of the cornea with an oeular response analyzer. Cataract Refract Surg. 2005;31:156–62.
5. Matalia J, Francis M, Tejwani S, Dudeja G, Rajappa N, Sinha Roy A. Role of age and myopia in simultaneous assessment of corneal and extracorneal tissue stiffness by air-puff applanation. J Refract Surg. 2016;32:486–93.
6. Turan-Vural E, Torun Acar B, Sevim MS, Buttanri IB, Acar S. Corneal biomechanical properties in patients with recurrent anterior uveitis. Ocul Immunol Inflamm. 2012;20:349–53.
7. Yazici AT, Kara N, Yuksel K, et al. The biomechanical properties of the cornea in patients with systemic lupus erythematosus. Eye. 2011;25:1005–9.
8. Prata TS, Sousa AK, Garcia Filho CA, Lm D, Paranhos A Jr. Assessment of corneal biomechanical properties and intraocular pressure in patients with rheumatoid arthritis. Can J Ophthalmol. 2009;44:602.
9. Taş M, Öner V, Özkaya E, Durmuş M. Evaluation of corneal biomechanical properties in patients with rheumatoid arthritis: a study by ocular response analyzer. Ocul Immunol Inflamm. 2014;22:224–7.
10. Inal M, Tan S, Demirkan S, Burulday V, Gündüz Ö, Örnek K. Evaluation of optic nerve with strain and shear wave elastography in patients with Behçet's disease and healthy subjects. Ultrasound Med Biol. 2017;43(7):1348–54.
11. Sen E, Ozdal P, Balikoglu-Yilmaz M, Nalcacioglu Yuksekkaya P, Elgin U, Tirhiş MH, Ozturk F. Are there any changes in corneal biomechanics and central corneal thickness in Fuchs' uveitis? Ocul Immunol Inflamm. 2016;24(5):561–7.
12. Emre S, Kaykçoglu Ö, Ates H, et al. Corneal hysteresis, corneal resistance factor, and intraocular pressure measurement in patients with scleroderma using the reichert ocular response analyzer. Cornea. 2010;29(6):628–31.
13. Sen E, Balikoglu-Yilmaz M, Ozdal P. Corneal biomechanical properties and central corneal thickness in pediatric noninfectious uveitis: a controlled study. Eye Contact Lens. 2018;44(Suppl 2):S60–4.
14. Mahendradas P, Francis M, Vala R, Gowda PB, Kawali A, Shetty R, Sinha Roy A. Quantification of ocular biomechanics in ocular manifestations of systemic autoimmune diseases. Ocul Immunol Inflamm. 2019;27(7):1127–37.
15. Sinha Roy A, Kurian M, Matalia H, Shetty R. Air-puff associated quantification of nonlinear biomechanical properties of the human cornea in vivo. J Mech Behav Biomed Mater. 2015;48:173–82.

Chapter 23
Biomechanics of Scleral Buckling and Effects on Eye Geometry

Benjamin W. Botsford, Asad F. Durrani, Raed Aldhafeeri, Patrick Smolinski, and Thomas R. Friberg

Introduction

Scleral buckling has been in use since 1949 for treatment of retinal detachments. Indentation of the sclera facilitates apposition of the retinal pigment epithelium to the neurosensory retina by decreasing vitreous tractional forces. Buckling may vary widely, and surgeons choose among different types and shapes of buckle elements, different degrees of indentation (buckle height), buckle locations, and extent of the circumference of the globe being buckled. Buckles can be implants or exoplants, the latter of which is typically performed due to the difficulty in creating partial thickness scleral flaps required for scleral implants. The mechanical nature of the buckling process places stresses on the ocular structures, affecting the biomechanics and overall geometry of the eye. This chapter seeks to delineate the geometric and biomechanical effects of scleral buckling on the human eye.

B. W. Botsford · A. F. Durrani
Department of Ophthalmology, University of Pittsburgh School of Medicine, Pittsburgh, PA, USA
e-mail: beb2579@med.cornell.edu; afd20@pitt.edu

T. R. Friberg (✉)
Department of Ophthalmology, University of Pittsburgh School of Medicine, Pittsburgh, PA, USA

Department of Bioengineering, University of Pittsburgh Swanson School of Engineering, Pittsburgh, PA, USA
e-mail: friberg@pitt.edu

R. Aldhafeeri · P. Smolinski
Department of Mechanical Engineering and Materials Science, Swanson School of Engineering, University of Pittsburgh, Pittsburgh, PA, USA
e-mail: rba10@pit.edu; patsmol@pitt.edu

© Springer Nature Switzerland AG 2021
I. Pallikaris et al. (eds.), *Ocular Rigidity, Biomechanics and Hydrodynamics of the Eye*, https://doi.org/10.1007/978-3-030-64422-2_23

Axial Length Changes with Scleral Buckling

As scleral buckling induces conformational changes in the eye, the refractive properties of the eye often change after surgery. Most eyes will have a myopic shift post
scleral-buckling due to an increase in axial length (elongation effect). However, this
change in axial length is dependent upon several factors, including the type of
buckle used, the shape of the element, the height of the buckle, buckle material, the
location of the buckle, and the placement of the sutures holding the buckle in place.

With solid silicone encircling buckles, axial length is generally increased, as
circumferential shortening of the eye by the buckle increases the anteroposterior
dimension of the globe. As the eye adopts a more prolate shape, the axial length
increases, inducing myopia. Several studies have shown variable changes in axial
length after buckling due to heterogeneity of technique and buckle type, with
authors reporting axial lengthening of 0.47, 0.99, 0.58, 1.28, and 0.81 mm [1–5].
One study showed similar changes in axial length across different age groups, suggesting that age-related changes in eye tissue has little impact upon the final axial
length [6]. Authors differed in their use of segmental elements, buckle width, and
shape. Additionally, factors like buckle height and position behind the limbus are
often not described.

An encircling buckle of significant height (indentation), however, may cause the
axial length of the eye to actually decrease [1]. Rubin showed that for a 2 mm wide
encircling band element, a high buckle induced a reduction in axial length of
0.35 mm, while low and moderate degrees of indentation increased the axial length
by 0.44 and 1.09 mm [7]. The decrease in axial length with buckling is attributed to
the eye adopting a dumbbell shape with high buckles, as well as invagination of the

a   b

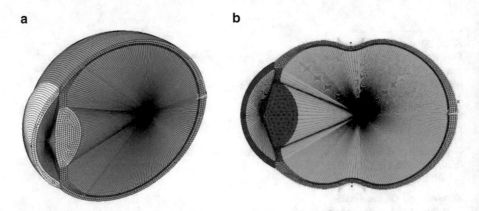

Fig. 23.1 Finite element model of the eye before and after axial lengthening induced by scleral
buckling. (**a**) Whole eye finite element model (**b**) Whole eye finite element model after equatorial
encircling buckle

sclera anterior and posterior to the buckle along the mattress sutures, especially with round or oval and thicker buckle elements [8]. Scleral invagination and anteroposterior lengthening through circumferential indentation are balanced against each other, and remain in flux after surgery, as tension of the sutures and tightness of the buckle element may vary. An example of encircling buckle can be seen in Fig. 23.1, in a finite element model created by Aldhafeeri [9].

The change in axial length after buckling is an important consideration for patients subsequently undergoing cataract removal and intraocular lens (IOL) placement after retinal detachment surgery. Fluctuations in biometrics affect IOL calculations, and therefore stability in eye geometry should be established before an IOL is chosen. One study looked at a large series of patients who underwent scleral buckling and noted that axial length stabilized at 3 months [3]. Other authors showed an increase of 0.77 mm in axial length at 1 month, which decreased to 0.57 mm at 1 year after treatment [10]. Part of this change over time has been attributed to the repetitive stretching of the encircling buckle element, causing stress relaxation over time [11]. This is unlikely as the buckle material is not the primary determinant of ocular rigidity and in our opinion such a change is more likely due to the creep of the sclera over time [12].

For segmental buckles, hyperopic as well as myopic shifts have been described. Variable outcomes have been reported, which depend upon the location of the segmental buckle on the globe, the concurrent use of an encircling element, the circumferential extent of the segmental buckle, buckle height, buckle material, and the shape of the buckle. Some clinical studies have reported that the axial length increased by the amount of 0.98, 0.6, 0.77 and 0.48 mm and the extent of the buckle had no effect [1, 10, 13, 14]. Other studies have demonstrated hyperopic shifts with segmental buckling [5, 15]. No significant change has also been reported in one study that used implants placed on the sclera under partial thickness scleral flaps [16].

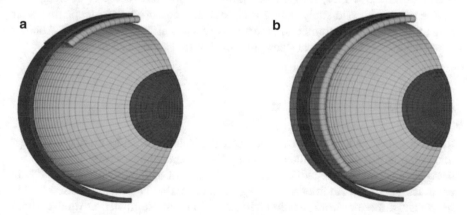

a   b

Fig. 23.2 Finite element models of the eye with (**a**) 90° buckle extant and (**b**) 270° buckle extant

To better understand the effect of buckling on the globe, Aldhafeeri created a detailed finite element analysis model of the eye. He simulated the effect of scleral buckling on eye geometry and biomechanics. In this model, the axial length was increased in both encircling and segmental buckles, an effect driven predominantly by indentation, with width, extent, and thickness of the buckle elements having smaller roles. Segmental buckle models are seen in Fig. 23.2.

Effects of Scleral Buckling on the Biomechanics of the Cornea

Scleral buckling can affect the cornea in numerous ways, including corneal steepness, astigmatism, corneal hysteresis (CH) and corneal resistance factor (CRF). As the sclera is not particularly elastic, buckle forces can be transmitted to the viscoelastic cornea, affecting these properties depending on the nature of the buckle. It is important to consider that corneal changes may also be caused by suturing techniques, buckle height selection, and other manipulations during surgery.

Corneal Power

The cornea provides two-thirds of the eye's refractive power and buckle forces can alter corneal power. Change in corneal power following buckle surgery is highly variable, and measurements differ between studies largely due to variation in buckling technique. Encircling buckle-induced changes in corneal power have been shown to be +0.01, −1.7, +1.8, 1.58 and 0 diopters (D) [15, 17–20]. This change with encircling buckles may be due to central corneal steepening with peripheral corneal flattening post-operatively [15]. For segmental buckles, change in cornea power for segmental buckles has been shown to be −2.2, −0.23, −0.22, 0.5, −1.1, 0.2, and −0.07 D [10, 14, 15, 17, 19–21]. Some authors have noted these changes to be transient, with one study noting a significant central corneal steepening after surgery of 1.8 D that returned to preoperative values after 6 months [18]. Another study reported central corneal steepening lasting for as long as 3 months [20].

Astigmatism

Regarding astigmatic optical errors induced after scleral buckling, regular and irregular astigmatism are more likely to arise from segmental or radial buckles. One study noted that 46% of radial buckles had >2 D of astigmatism vs. only 8% in encircled eyes [22]. Additionally, in segmental or radial buckles, increased buckle height and a more anterior location will result in more astigmatism. Another study demonstrated astigmatism of 0.31 D for segmental and 2.75 D for encircled eyes [2], while others showed mean central corneal astigmatism at 1 week, 1 month, and

3 months was 4.3 ± 2.0 D, 3.3 ± 1.6 D, and 3.1 ± 1.0 D, respectively for encircled eyes [21]. Ornek noted a significant increase in total (1.6 D) and irregular astigmatism (0.28 D) in the first month that was transient in eyes with encircling buckles, returning to normal after around 6 months [18]. Topographic changes in the cornea noted in the first week after surgery have also been reported to return to preoperative values at 1 month [23].

Kinoshita et al. performed a vector analysis of corneal astigmatism and noted that segmental buckles spanning 1–2 quadrants produced 1.65 D of astigmatism while those spanning only one or >2 quadrants displayed 1.09 D, suggesting that buckle extent is an important determinant for the amount of astigmatism induced [17]. Okada demonstrated that the direction of the astigmatism vector is in the direction of the center of the buckle and displayed greater astigmatism with more anterior buckles [1]. Okamoto noted that scleral buckling surgery significantly increased higher order aberrations at 2 weeks, 1 month, and 3 months postoperatively, with greater and more prolonged changes seen with segmental over encircling buckling [24]. They also noted coma was negative in cases of upper segment buckling.

Effects of Buckling in Thinned Corneas

Little data exists for the effects of scleral buckling in eyes with corneal thinning. One series describes two patients that had previous encircling buckles who underwent LASIK and developed significant corneal ectasia with corneal steepening (16 D and 8 D), though the stromal thicknesses under the flap were <250 microns [25]. The first case showed flattening of 3D after buckle removal [25]. A response to this article reported good success of LASIK post buckling in one patient [26].

In Aldhafeeri's model, increased indentation and corneal thinning had large effects on increasing cornea power post-buckling. For example, a 5 mm buckle with a 180° extent at a 1 mm indentation, the change in cornea power was 0.12, 0.16 and

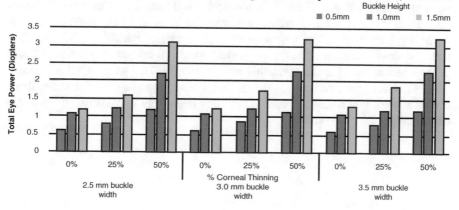

Fig. 23.3 Changes in total eye power with equatorial encircling band in eyes with corneal thinning at different buckle width and height. Adapted from Aldhafeeri [9]

1.21 D for 0, 25 and 50% cornea thinning, respectively [9]. In an eye with 50% corneal thinning, a 5 mm buckle with 90°, 180° and 270° buckle extent at a 1 mm indentation the change in cornea power was 1.45, 1.21 and 0.85 D, respectively [9]. For 0% thinned cornea, the results from Aldhafeeri's model are close to the reported power change by previous clinical studies. Results for equatorial encircling bands for different buckle widths and heights at 0, 25, and 50% corneal thinning are shown in Fig. 23.3 [9].

Astigmatism was induced by indentation and thinning where higher steepening occurred at the meridian parallel to center of the buckle for all models. A 5 mm buckle with a 180° extent at 1 mm indentation had astigmatism error of about 0.09, 0.22 and 1.35 D for 0, 25 and 50% cornea thinning, respectively. Tilting of the cornea was noticed away from buckling location. For corneas with normal thickness, corneal tilt decreased with increasing buckle extent in the model with 1.69, 1.15 and 0.24 degrees of tilt for 90°, 180° and 270° buckle extent, respectively.

Corneal Hysteresis and Corneal Resistance Factor

The inherent viscoelastic nature of the cornea allows it to absorb and dissipate energy when stress is applied such as with applanation. Measurement of this viscous damping property is defined as corneal hysteresis (CH). Only a few studies have looked at the effect of scleral buckling on CH. In a study of 56 eyes, 27 of which underwent encircling buckle and 29 of which underwent segmental buckling, a statistically significant decrease in CH was found in the segmental buckle group whereas no difference was found in the encircling buckle group [27]. The direct consequences of decreased corneal hysteresis have yet to be established, however, decreased hysteresis has been noted in many disorders of the eye such as Fuchs' dystrophy, keratoconus, and glaucoma [28].

Whereas corneal hysteresis is a measure of the viscous damping of the cornea, corneal resistance factor (CRF) is a biomechanical measure of the cornea that is dominated by its elastic properties. In a study of 56 eyes, 27 of which underwent encircling buckle and 29 of which underwent segmental buckling, CRF, like CH, was significantly decreased in the segmental buckle group and again no significant difference was found in the encircling buckle group [27]. Again, the direct consequences of decreased corneal resistance factor have yet to be established but these results suggest that segmental scleral buckling negatively impacts the viscous and elastic properties of the cornea.

Effects of Scleral Buckling on Anterior Chamber Depth

Scleral buckling may also affect the geometry of the anterior chamber and drainage angle. Information on how buckling affects such structures is important for both refractive specialists as well as the general ophthalmologist, as glaucoma develops in 1–5% of patients post buckling surgery [29]. Scleral buckling has been demonstrated to decrease anterior chamber depth. The reduction in anterior chamber depth is thought to be due to ciliary body edema from reduced uveal or choroidal circulation, which occurs in the early post-operative period and may peak around post-operative day 3 [30, 31]. This edema can be accompanied by both supraciliary effusion, ciliary rotation, and may also increase lens thickness. All these sequelae may raise intraocular pressure, as well as increase the refractive power of the eye through forward displacement of the lens-iris diaphragm [4].

The degree to which anterior chamber depth is shallowed varies between studies. Huang et al. demonstrated that AC depth went from 3.20 to 3.01 mm at 6 months (~6% decrease), and then slightly increased to 3.03 mm at 12 months [4]. Kawahara et al. noted shallowing of the anterior chamber in all eyes that underwent encircling buckles and 60% of eyes that underwent segmental buckles [32]. While most studies showed anterior chamber depth shallowing persisted, Goezinne et al. demonstrated shallowing of anterior chamber at 9 months with return to normal depth at 1 year in a series of 38 eyes treated with encircling element and radial or segmental buckle [33]. Wong et al. showed anterior chamber depth decreased 3.84–3.32 at 12 months in eyes treated with encircling buckle, with stabilization of values at week 1 [3]. Two other studies noted anterior chamber shallowing of 0.204 and 0.20 mm [21, 34].

Regarding angle structure changes with encircling bands, anterior segment optical coherence tomography studies have demonstrated trabecular iris angle, angle opening distance, and trabecular iris space area were all significantly decreased at 1 month of follow-up, without an accompanying change in intraocular pressure [35]. Similarly, using ultrasound biomicroscopy, Pavlin et al. demonstrated a greater than 5° decrease in angle opening in 73% of patients who went scleral buckling 1 week after surgery with the ciliary body and iris root rotated anteriorly [36]. Furthermore, the ciliary body and iris root were rotated anteriorly in all patients in this study.

Aldhafeeri, in his finite element model, demonstrated that anterior chamber depth did decrease about 1% with scleral buckling, but noted that in eyes with 50% corneal thinning, anterior chamber depth was slightly increased by buckling [9]. This does not account for all the changes in anterior chamber depth seen with buckling in clinical studies, and this model does not account for ciliary body edema and rotation that occur in vivo. However, the effect of scleral buckling on anterior chamber depth in eyes with thinned corneas has yet to be established in the current literature.

Volume Changes Induced by Scleral Buckling

As a sphere contains the largest amount of volume for the least amount of surface area, indentation from scleral buckling surgery will cause a reduction in volume by creating a more oblong shape, displacing fluid from the vitreous cavity. Volume change after scleral buckling surgery has been evaluated by Thompson et al. in a study on cadaver eyes in which a 5 mm radial buckle displaced 5% of volume, a 2.5-mm silicone encircling band displaced up to 12% of the vitreous volume, and a 7-mm hard silicone band displaced 33–43% depending on the height [37]. Shi et al. demonstrated through MRI of the eye that volume after encircling buckle decreased by an average of 1.72 mL [38]. The volume displaced can be determined from the following formula: $V = c \frac{\pi}{360} \left(2r * h * h^2 \right) \left(w1 + w2 \right)$, where V is the volume displaced in mm³, c is the circumference of the buckle in degrees, r is the radius of the eye in mm, h is the height of the buckle in mm, w1 is the width of the buckle anterior to the equator in mm, and w2 is the width of the buckle posterior to the equator in mm [39].

In Aldhafeeri's model, volume decreased with buckle indentation. They noted a 0.65, 1.82 and 3.17% reduction of the original volume, respectively, for 1/3, 2/3 and 1 mm of indentation with a 5 mm buckle and 180° extent [9]. The buckling parameters he used for his study were selected by a vitreoretinal surgeon [12] as were some of the scleral and choroidal elasticity constants [40].

Effects of Scleral Buckling on Ocular Rigidity

Ocular rigidity is a measure of an eyes elasticity and is the change in intraocular pressure for a given change in volume. This can be influenced by myopia, intraocular gas, and buckling surgery [12]. Ocular rigidity can be estimated as the slope of the line generated by plotting the log of pressure against change in volume [41]. This formula assumes rigidity to be constant for an eye regardless of intraocular pressure. Various additional formulas have been developed, including pressure/volume curves using the van der Werff formula: $\Delta V = \frac{P_2^{1/3} - P_1^{1/3}}{K}$, where P_1 is the initial intraocular pressure, P_2 is the final intraocular pressure after an alteration (AV) of the intraocular volume, and K is the ocular rigidity function [42].

The effect of compliance can be important post-buckling as eyes with higher compliance can have higher volumes of substances injected into the eye without increasing intraocular pressure. Additionally, measurements of intraocular pressure in these eyes, especially with indentation tonometry, may be falsely low.

Johnson et al. found in a cadaver eye model that scleral buckling with a silicone encircling band reduces ocular rigidity fourfold; they attributed the reduction in compliance to greater elasticity of the silicone encircling element as compared with sclera [43]. They further postulated that as volume is added to the eye, volume expansion occurs preferentially at the indentation of the buckle, decreasing buckle

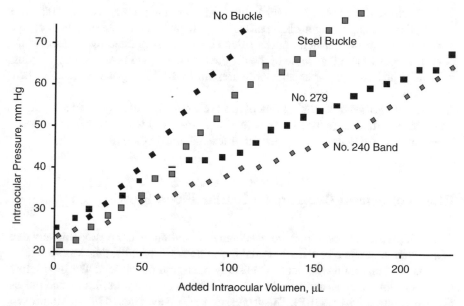

Fig. 23.4 Intraocular pressure vs. incremental volume added in unbuckled eyes, eyes buckled with a 360° 3-mm × 21.3-mm diameter stainless steel band, eyes buckled with a 360° No. 279 9-mm-wide symmetric silicone tire 68 mm in circumference, and eyes buckled with a 360° 2.5-mm No. 240 silicone band 64 mm in circumference. Ocular rigidity values, represented by the slope of the curves determined by linear regression, are 0.498 ± 0.012, 0.349 ± 0.009, 0.177 ± 0.003, and 0.174 ± 0.005 mmHg/μL, respectively. Reproduced with permission from Friberg and Fourman [12]

height at an area of least resistance. Additionally, as the volume expands, the eye can accommodate some of this volume by becoming more spheroid.

Friberg and Fourman disputed the explanation that the properties of the encircling buckle element were germane. In their experiments, Friberg and Fourman evaluated human donor eyes and noted that buckled eyes were less rigid than unbuckled eyes, with higher buckles being less rigid than shallower buckles. The authors also noted an increase in compliance with buckling using either a silicone or a rigid metal band (Fig. 23.4), underscoring that the increased compliance was due primarily to the change in eye shape and not the elasticity of the band [12]. They reasoned that in a normal spherical globe, fibers in the sclera are stretched uniformly with a rise in IOP, but in a buckled eye with an encircling band, the eye becomes more cylindrical causing more stress in the equatorial direction without change in the anteroposterior direction. The cylindrical eye therefore expands more easily along the radius instead of AP direction as these areas are under the greatest stress. Additionally, Friberg and Fourman suggested that indentation of the buckle into the vitreous cavity causes the force vectors of scleral tension and IOP to act together to push the sclera out against the indentation. These forces are counteracted by the circumferential tension in the encircling band and in the sutures. Additionally, they suggested that the alteration of scleral stress, with concentration of stresses within the sclera in the vicinity of the buckle, results in greater local deformation of the sclera near the buckle, affecting eye pressure.

Whitacre et al. performed a similar study, but conversely noted a greater increase in compliance using a silicone band instead of a metal band, attributing the increase in compliance to the elasticity of the silicone band as suggested by Johnson et al. [44]. They postulated that some of the differences may have been seen by keeping the eye at physiologic intraocular pressures up to 40 mmHg while making their PV curves.

In Aldhafeeri's model, the rigidity of the eye similarly was decreased after buckling. This was further reduced with reduction in the band width, positioning closer to the limbus, and decreasing the extent of a segmental buckle [9].

Effects of Scleral Buckling on Ocular Blood Flow

As previously discussed, ciliary body edema is thought to occur postoperatively due to a reduction in uveal or retrochoroidal blood flow. Classically, this was seen after placement of encircling elements. One study measured pulsatile ocular blood flow after encircling buckles and noted a reduction in ocular pulse amplitude and pulsatile ocular blood flow (POBF). The decrease in POBF averaged 43% and improved to 85.6% after cutting the band [45]. While they noted that venous obstruction or kinking of long posterior ciliary arteries may be factors, Lincoff et al. suggested that the elastic band blocks compliance of the globe and limits the volume of systolic pulse that the eye will accept, as they noted that the reduction is independent of the amount of constriction or the location of the band. Sugawara et al. also looked at choroidal blood blow in the foveal region using laser doppler flowmetry to compare buckled eye to fellow eye and noted decrease in flow at 2 and 4 weeks with a return to baseline at 12 weeks [46]. Furthermore, increased choroidal thickness has been found following buckling surgery, potentially from restriction of choroidal blood flow. Some studies have reported this was transient, normalizing within 4 weeks or 3 months [47, 48], while another demonstrated a persistent increase at 22 months [49]. Band size, location, height, and small sample size all may play a role in the discrepancies that currently exist in the literature.

For segmental buckling, Kimura et al. noted an increase in choroidal thickness of 13% following segmental buckling up to 1 month that normalized at 3 months and suggested both restriction of blood flow and post-operative inflammation contributed to these transient changes [50]. Iwase et al. looked at choroidal blood flow following segmental buckling with laser speckle flowgraphy and noted a reduction in choroidal blood flow at the buckle and unbuckled side choroid, but not the macular choroid [51]. Subfoveal choroidal thickness was transiently increased for 1 week after surgery.

In case reports, authors have suggested cutting encircling bands has led to improved blood flow. Yoshida et al. described a constricted visual field in an eye with an encircling band and recovery after the band was cut [52]. Kimura et al. reported a patient who had a visual field defect after buckling surgery and noted delayed ICG filling and improved blood flow following cutting the encircling band as well [53]. Despite these isolated reports, the practice of loosening or removing encircling elements is now rare.

Conclusions

Scleral buckling has numerable effects on eye physiology, affecting axial length, corneal topography, anterior chamber depth, ocular blood flow, ocular rigidity, which may differ depending on surgical selection and technique as well as the pre-existing biomechanical properties of a patient's eye. A vitreoretinal surgeon should carefully weigh these factors during surgical evaluation and selection of patients for potential buckling.

References

1. Okada Y, Nakamura S, Kubo E, Oishi N, Takahashi Y, Akagi Y. Analysis of changes in corneal shape and refraction following scleral buckling surgery. Jpn J Ophthalmol. 2000;44(2):132–8.
2. Smiddy WE, Loupe DN, Michels RG, Enger C, Glaser BM, de Bustros S. Refractive changes after scleral buckling surgery. Arch Ophthalmol. 1989;107(10):1469–71.
3. Wong CW, Ang M, Tsai A, Phua V, Lee SY. A prospective study of biometric stability after scleral buckling surgery. Am J Ophthalmol. 2016;165:47–53.
4. Huang C, Zhang T, Liu J, Ji Q, Tan R. Changes in axial length, central cornea thickness, and anterior chamber depth after rhegmatogenous retinal detachment repair. BMC Ophthalmol. 2016;16:121.
5. Wang HZ, Chen MT, Chang CH, Tsai MC, Wu WC, Chung CB. The changes of ocular axial length and corneal curvatures after scleral buckling for retinal detachment. Gaoxiong Yi Xue Ke Xue Za Zhi. 1994;10(2):77–83.
6. Bedarkar A, Ranjan R, Khan P, Gupta RC, Kushwaha R, Mohan S. Scleral buckling-induced ocular parameter changes in different age group patients of rhegmatogenous retinal detachment. Taiwan J Ophthalmol. 2017;7(2):94–9.
7. Rubin ML. The induction of refractive errors by retinal detachment surgery. Trans Am Ophthalmol Soc. 1975;73:452–90.
8. Harris MJ, Blumenkranz MS, Wittpenn J, Levada A, Brown R, Frazier-Byrne S. Geometric alterations produced by encircling scleral buckles. Biometric and clinical considerations. Retina. 1987;7(1):14–9.
9. Aldhafeeri R. Analysis of scleral buckling surgery: biomechanical model. Pittsburgh, PA: Mechanical Engineering, Swanson School of Engineering, University of Pittsburgh; 2017. Ph.D thesis, University of Pittsburgh.
10. Malukiewicz-Wisniewska G, Stafiej J. Changes in axial length after retinal detachment surgery. Eur J Ophthalmol. 1999;9(2):115–9.
11. Hinrichsen G, Eberhardt A, Springer H. Mechanical behaviour of cerclage material consisting of silicon rubber. Albrecht Von Graefes Arch Klin Exp Ophthalmol. 1979;211(3):251–8.
12. Friberg TR, Fourman SB. Scleral buckling and ocular rigidity. Clinical ramifications. Arch Ophthalmol. 1990;108(11):1622–7.
13. Larsen JS, Syrdalen P. Ultrasonographic study on changes in axial eye dimensions after encircling procedure in retinal detachment surgery. Acta Ophthalmol. 1979;57(3):337–43.

14. Toyota K, Yamakura Y, Hommura S. Ultrasonographic evaluation of axial length changes following scleral buckling surgery. In: Ultrasonography in ophthalmology, vol. 14. Cham: Springer; 1995. p. 100–3.
15. Hayashi H, Hayashi K, Nakao F, Hayashi F. Corneal shape changes after scleral buckling surgery. Ophthalmology. 1997;104(5):831–7.
16. Burton TC, Herron BE, Ossoinig KC. Axial length changes after retinal detachment surgery. Am J Ophthalmol. 1977;83(1):59–62.
17. Kinoshita M, Tanihara H, Negi A, et al. Vector analysis of corneal astigmatism after scleral buckling surgery. Ophthalmologica. 1994;208(5):250–3.
18. Ornek K, Yalcindag FN, Kanpolat A, Gunalp I. Corneal topographic changes after retinal detachment surgery. Cornea. 2002;21(8):803–6.
19. Karimian F, Moradian S, Yazdani S, Mashayekhy A, Anisian A, Kouhestani N. Corneal topographic changes after scleral buckling. Eur J Ophthalmol. 2006;16(4):536–41.
20. Weinberger D, Lichter H, Loya N, et al. Corneal topographic changes after retinal and vitreous surgery. Ophthalmology. 1999;106(8):1521–4.
21. Cetin E, Ozbek Z, Saatci AO, Durak I. The effect of scleral buckling surgery on corneal astigmatism, corneal thickness, and anterior chamber depth. J Refract Surg. 2006;22(5):494–9.
22. Goel R, Crewdson J, Chignell AH. Astigmatism following retinal detachment surgery. Br J Ophthalmol. 1983;67(5):327–9.
23. Domniz YY, Cahana M, Avni I. Corneal surface changes after pars plana vitrectomy and scleral buckling surgery. J Cataract Refract Surg. 2001;27(6):868–72.
24. Okamoto F, Yamane N, Okamoto C, Hiraoka T, Oshika T. Changes in higher-order aberrations after scleral buckling surgery for rhegmatogenous retinal detachment. Ophthalmology. 2008;115(7):1216–21.
25. Panozzo G, Parolini B. Relationships between vitreoretinal and refractive surgery. Ophthalmology. 2001;108(9):1663–8.
26. Belda JI, Ruiz-Moreno JM, Perez-Santonja JJ, Alio JL. Scleral buckle and corneal ectasia after LASIK. Ophthalmology. 2002;109(11):1950–1. disscussion 1951
27. Esfahani MR, Hashemi H, Ghaffari E. Evaluation of corneal biomechanical properties following scleral buckling using the ocular response analyzer. Iran J Ophthalmol. 2013;25(2):151.
28. Kotecha A. What biomechanical properties of the cornea are relevant for the clinician? Surv Ophthalmol. 2007;52(6):S109–14.
29. Ansem RP, Bastiaensen LA. Glaucoma following retinal detachment operations. Doc Ophthalmol. 1987;67(1–2):19–24.
30. Perez R, Phelps C, Burton T. Angel-closure glaucoma following scleral buckling operations. Trans Sect Ophthalmol Acad Ophthalmol Otolaryngol. 1976;81(2):247–52.
31. Kawana K, Okamoto F, Hiraoka T, Oshika T. Ciliary body edema after scleral buckling surgery for rhegmatogenous retinal detachment. Ophthalmology. 2006;113(1):36–41.
32. Kawahara S, Nagai Y, Kawakami E, Ida RYN, Takeuchi M, Uyama M. Ciliochoroidal detachment following scleral buckling surgery for rhegmatogenous retinal detachment. Jpn J Ophthalmol. 2000;44(6):692–3.
33. Goezinne F, La Heij EC, Berendschot TT, et al. Anterior chamber depth is significantly decreased after scleral buckling surgery. Ophthalmology. 2010;117(1):79–85.
34. Fiore JV, Newton JC. Anterior segment changes following the scleral buckling procedure. Arch Ophthalmol. 1970;84(3):284–7.
35. Khanduja S, Bansal N, Arora V, Sobti A, Garg S, Dada T. Evaluation of the effect of scleral buckling on the anterior chamber angle using ASOCT. J Glaucoma. 2015;24(4):267–71.
36. Pavlin CJ, Rutnin SS, Devenyi R, Wand M, Foster FS. Supraciliary effusions and ciliary body thickening after scleral buckling procedures. Ophthalmology. 1997;104(3):433–8.
37. Thompson JT, Michels RG. Volume displacement of scleral buckles. Arch Ophthalmol. 1985;103(12):1822–4.
38. Shi M, Qiao B, Zhou Y. The volume and dimensions of eyeball analyzed by MRI following encircling scleral buckles. [Zhonghua Yan Ke Za zhi] Chin J Ophthalmol. 2006;42(2):150–4.

39. Thompson JT. The biomechanics of scleral buckles in the treatment of retinal detachment. In: Schachat AP, Wilkinson CP, Hinton DR, Sadda SVR, Wiedemann P, editors. Ryan's retina, vol. 3. 6th ed. London: Elsevier; 2018. p. 1875–88.
40. Friberg TR, Lace JW. A comparison of the elastic properties of human choroid and sclera. Exp Eye Res. 1988;47(3):429–36.
41. Friedenwald JS. Contribution to the theory and practice of tonometry. Am J Ophthalmol. 1937;20(10):985–1024.
42. Van Der Werff TJ. A new single-parameter ocular rigidity function. Am J Ophthalmol. 1981;92(3):391–5.
43. Johnson MW, Han DP, Hoffman KE. The effect of scleral buckling on ocular rigidity. Ophthalmology. 1990;97(2):190–5.
44. Whitacre MM, Emig MD, Hassanein K. Effect of buckling material on ocular rigidity. Ophthalmology. 1992;99(4):498–502.
45. Lincoff H, Stopa M, Kreissig I, et al. Cutting the encircling band. Retina. 2006;26(6):650–4.
46. Sugawara R, Nagaoka T, Kitaya N, et al. Choroidal blood flow in the foveal region in eyes with rhegmatogenous retinal detachment and scleral buckling procedures. Br J Ophthalmol. 2006;90(11):1363–5.
47. Miura M, Arimoto G, Tsukahara R, Nemoto R, Iwasaki T, Goto H. Choroidal thickness after scleral buckling. Ophthalmology. 2012;119(7):1497–8.
48. Montezuma SR, Tang PH, Miller CJ, et al. The effect of scleral buckling surgery on choroidal thickness measured by enhanced depth optical coherence tomography: a cross-sectional study. Ophthalmol Therapy. 2016;5(2):215–22.
49. Odrobina D, Laudańska-Olszewska I, Gozdek P, Maroszyński M, Amon M. Influence of scleral buckling surgery with encircling band on subfoveal choroidal thickness in long-term observations. Biomed Res Int. 2013;2013:586894.
50. Kimura M, Nishimura A, Yokogawa H, et al. Subfoveal choroidal thickness change following segmental scleral buckling for rhegmatogenous retinal detachment. Am J Ophthalmol. 2012;154(5):893–900.
51. Iwase T, Kobayashi M, Yamamoto K, Yanagida K, Ra E, Terasaki H. Change in choroidal blood flow and choroidal morphology due to segmental scleral buckling in eyes with rhegmatogenous retinal detachment. Sci Rep. 2017;7(1):5997.
52. Yoshida A, Feke GT, Green GJ, et al. Retinal circulatory changes after scleral buckling procedures. Am J Ophthalmol. 1983;95(2):182–8.
53. Kimura I, Shinoda K, Eshita T, Inoue M, Mashima Y. Relaxation of encircling buckle improved choroidal blood flow in a patient with visual field defect following encircling procedure. Jpn J Ophthalmol. 2006;50(6):554–6.

Chapter 24
Ocular Rigidity and Drugs

Andreas Katsanos, Anna I. Dastiridou, and Anastasios G. P. Konstas

Introduction

Ocular rigidity is an old concept, that was introduced to characterize the pressure-volume relationship in the eye [1]. Since then, limited data are available in the literature concerning the effects that drugs can have on ocular rigidity and eye biomechanics. This may at least in part be attributed to the difficulties in measuring ocular rigidity and the biomechanical properties of the ocular tissues in vivo. In this chapter, the evidence available on the topic is reviewed.

Most of the drugs studied are used in glaucoma treatment. Differences in ocular rigidity reported in studies in glaucoma using paired Schiotz (or other indentation) tonometry could be attributed to an effect of the drug, the IOP and the accuracy of the calibration tables [2]. In addition, biomechanics have already been shown to be clinically relevant in the course of glaucoma (see section "ocular rigidity and glaucoma" of Chap. 17) [3]. Patients with seemingly well-controlled intraocular pressure (IOP) that progress faster are more likely to have thin corneas and low corneal hysteresis. Therefore, despite the inherent difficulties, there is clinical need to gain insight into the biomechanics of the eye.

Friedenwald has reported his findings in a limited set of eyes and reported that pilocarpine and epinephrine can differentially influence ocular rigidity [1]. In another study, the effects of orally administered propranolol on IOP and ocular

A. Katsanos
Ophthalmology Department, University of Ioannina, Ioannina, Greece

A. I. Dastiridou (✉)
2nd Ophthalmology Department, Aristotle University of Thessaloniki, Thessaloniki, Greece

School of Medicine, University of Thessalia, Larissa, Greece

A. G. P. Konstas
1st and 3rd University Departments of Ophthalmology, Aristotle University of Thessaloniki, Thessaloniki, Greece

© Springer Nature Switzerland AG 2021
I. Pallikaris et al. (eds.), *Ocular Rigidity, Biomechanics and Hydrodynamics of the Eye*, https://doi.org/10.1007/978-3-030-64422-2_24

rigidity were evaluated in 22 patients [4]. Propanolol was reported to effectively lower the IOP, without inducing changes in the rigidity of the eye [4]. Rigidity was measured with a combination of applanation and indentation tonometry. In another study, Ebneter et al. used acetazolamide to pharmacologically modulate the IOP [5]. They measured the IOP reduction due to acetazolamide, and the change in axial length in order to estimate a surrogate parameter for rigidity. They assumed that the drug itself does not induce any short-term change in the rigidity coefficient. The authors identified differences between glaucoma and controls, with increased rigidity observed in the glaucoma group.

Other studies on ocular rigidity and the biomechanics of the eye have focused on pilocarpine and prostaglandin analogues and are discussed below.

Pilocarpine

Pilocarpine is a parasympathomimetic drug and its actions in the eye include increase in trabecular outflow and ciliary muscle contraction, accommodation of the ciliary body and crystalline lens complex, miosis, shallowing of the anterior chamber, ciliary and conjunctival vessel congestion and breakdown of the blood aqueous barrier [6]. Manometric experiments in cynomolgous monkeys revealed an increase in outflow facility with pilocarpine [7]. In fact, there is now evidence from enhanced depthoptical coherence tomography imaging that Schlemm's canal expands after instillation of pilocarpine both in glaucoma and in normal eyes [8].

In a study in rabbits, pilocarpine was used to induce contraction of the ciliary body and the elastic modulus of both the cornea and the sclera was tested to inquire whether there was a detectable change [9].While the elastic modulus of cornea and anterior sclera strips showed no difference, sclera strips from the equatorial and posterior regions revealed changes in the diameter of collagen fibrils, the collagen content and finally the elastic modulus. Therefore, there is evidence in animals that the elasticity of the sclera changes with pilocarpine.

Very limited data is available in the literature on the effects of pilocarpine on ocular rigidity. In the report by Friedenwald, the drug was shown to decrease ocular rigidity initially, followed by a return to normal in glaucoma eyes [1].

Prostaglandins

Prostaglandin analogues are a widely used, first-line therapeutic option for patients with glaucoma, due to their safety, efficacy and convenient dosage Scheme [10]. Interestingly, IOP and aqueous dynamics in the course of uveitis led to further research on the role of prostaglandins release and the introduction of prostaglandin analogues in the treatment of glaucoma [11]. Prostaglandin analogues work by enhancing the uveoscleral pathway, while some studies have also suggested improved conventional outflow [12]. Studies have shown that matrix metallopro-teinases are upregulated, keratocyte cell density decreases and extracellular matrix undergoes significant remodeling with prostaglandin use, leading to the effects seen in uveoscleral outflow [13–15].These changes along with changes in IOP could pos-sibly affect the pressure-volume relationship and ocular rigidity.

Prostaglandin analogues use has been associated with breakdown of the blood aqueous barrier. There is also some evidence that ocular blood flow may increase with prostaglandin use [16]. However, these changes are probably of small magni-tude, with no change in optical coherence tomography subfoveal choroidal thick-ness measurements noted after a 1-month course of latanoprost treatment [17].

While there is a paucity of data in the literature on the effects of prostaglandin analogue use on ocular rigidity, several studies have investigated the link between their use and changes in the biomechanical properties of the eye. Laboratory evi-dence on the biomechanical effects induced by travoprost has been reported in rab-bit corneas post mortem [18]. The authors identified significant reductions in the stiffness of the corneal tissue with travoprost treatment. Therefore, similar effects in human corneas in vivo could have important clinical implications.

Detorakis et al. tested the hypothesis that if latanoprost produces a change in the biomechanics of the cornea, then this may result in a difference between the tonom-etry reading with applanation and dynamic contour tonometry [19]. In that study, the difference between applanation and dynamic contour tonometry was larger in latanoprost-treated eyes. However, this difference was very small and did not reach significance in another study analyzing contralateral eyes, with one eye receiving bimatoprost or travoprost and the fellow eye serving as control [20].

The majority of clinical studies that attempted to characterize the effects of pros-taglandin analogues on eye biomechanics used the Ocular Response Analyzer (ORA, Reichert Inc.). In an initial study that aimed to assess the biomechanical properties with the ORA in glaucoma, the authors found no change in corneal hys-teresis (CH), while corneal resistance factor (CRF) was lower in eyes treated with topical prostaglandin analogues [21]. However, the results of the study by Bolivar et al. suggest that CH increases with topical prostaglandin analogues [22]. Newly diagnosed treatment naïve open angle glaucoma or ocular hypertension patients were enrolled in that study and CH at 6 months post prostaglandin analogue treat-ment initiation was increased compared to that at baseline. However, no correlation was found between the change in IOP and the change in CH, suggesting that latano-prost directly affects the biomechanics of the cornea. Whether these changes are at least in part related to a possible change in central cornea thickness (CCT) remains unknown [23, 24]. Interestingly, there are conflicting studies in the literature that point to an effect of prostaglandins on CCT [25, 26]. Meda et al. used different methods to investigate the effects of prostaglandins on ORA measurements [27]. They recruited primary open angle glaucoma patients on chronic prostaglandin ana-logues and used one eye as a control, while stopping treatment in the other and then re-introducing the same treatment. They measured CH and CRF with the ORA and also quantified cornea thickness and IOP. They reported that topical prostaglandins led to a reduction in CH, CRF and CCT. These changes could result in error in the measurement of IOP with applanation tonometry and underestimation of true IOP.

Corneal hysteresis measurements have been suggested to provide information regarding the magnitude of IOP-lowering effect that can be anticipated in an eye. Agarwal et al. reported that CH at baseline was an independent significant predictor for the observed IOP-lowering effect of prostaglandin therapy [28]. The authors suggested that patients in the lowest quartile of CH had their IOP lowered by 29% while those in the highest CH quartile experienced a 8% IOP decrease. This finding can have direct clinical implications, suggesting that some patients have an increased likelihood of a favorable IOP-lowering effect on prostaglandins and this can in some cases be predicted with the measurement of CH at baseline.

Other studies used the Corvis ST to characterize the effects of prostaglandin F2a use on the biomechanics of the eye. Amano et al. used the Corvis-ST and the Casia 1 or 2 tomography device to compare between primary open angle glaucoma eyes that were treated with either prostaglandin or beta-blockers and the fellow untreated contralateral eye [29]. Their results showed that although the dimensions of the cornea remain stable and the shape does not change with prostaglandin treatment, there are several changes in numerous biomechanical parameters in prostaglandin-treated eyes. It remains however unknown which of these parameters are more clinically relevant.

In a cross-sectional study, Tejwani et al. compared corneal biomechanical parameters measured with the Corvis ST [30]. They enrolled primary open angle and primary angle closure patients that were under topical treatment and others than had undergone glaucoma surgery. No difference was found in that study in eyes with and without glaucoma. In their model, the authors also tested for the effect of filtration surgery and medication (prostaglandins versus beta-blockers versus both) and found that antiglaucoma drugs were not associated with an effect in eye biomechanics [30]. Variables such as CCT, IOP and anterior chamber depth were found to strongly influence corneal biomechanical properties in that study.

Sánchez-Barahona et al. prospectively examined how latanoprost affects IOP measurements with three tonometers: Goldmann applanation tonometer, ORA and Corvis ST [31]. The authors reported that the change in IOP with latanoprost measured with the Corvis ST tonometer was smaller compared to that measured with the other two modalities [31]. Biomechanical corneal properties were also significantly different at 3 months of latanoprost use. Importantly, this study may suggest that the IOP lowering effect of latanoprost may be overestimated with applanation tonometry.

Finally, Wu et al. reported that the changes observed after topical prostaglandin use are not short-lived [32]. Their findings with the Corvis ST were present in eyes on at least 2 years of prostaglandin use.

New drug delivery methods may also have an effect on the observed changes in ocular biomechanics. It is currently unknown if the ocular biomechanical effects caused by prostaglandin analogues are similar in eyes treated with topical versus intracameral formulations [33]. Interestingly, intracameral delivery of bimatoprost has been associated with a sustained decrease in episcleral venous pressure which may be associated with blood flow changes and also biomechanical implications [34].

New drugs have recently been introduced in glaucoma treatment. Latanoprostenebunod and netasurdilare increasingly being used in glaucoma treatment and represent new classes of antiglaucoma medications [35]. The possible biomechanical effects of these drugs in the eye are currently unknown [36].

References

1. Friedenwald J. Contribution to the theory and practice of tonometry. Am J Ophthalmol. 1937;20(10):985–1024.
2. Marlow SB. Tonometry: the variation of ocular rigidity in chronic glaucoma and an adaptation of the Souter tonometer. Trans Am Ophthalmol Soc. 1949;47:349–64.
3. Susanna BN, Ogata NG, Jammal AA, Susanna CN, Berchuck SI, Medeiros FA. Corneal biomechanics and visual field progression in eyes with seemingly well-controlled intraocular pressure. Ophthalmology. 2019;126(12):1640–6.
4. Borthne A. The treatment of glaucoma with propranolol (Inderal). A clinical trial. Acta Ophthalmol. 1976;54(3):291–300.
5. Ebneter A, Wagels B, Zinkernagel MS. Non-invasive biometric assessment of ocular rigidity in glaucoma patients and controls. Eye (Lond). 2009;23(3):606–11.
6. Zimmerman TJ. Pilocarpine. Ophthalmology. 1981;88(1):85–8.
7. Barany EH. The mode of action of pilocarpine on outflow resistance in the eye of a primate (Cercopithecus ethiops). Investig Ophthalmol. 1962;1:712–27.
8. Skaat A, Rosman MS, Chien JL, Mogil RS, Ren R, Liebmann JM, et al. Effect of pilocarpine hydrochloride on the Schlemm canal in healthy eyes and eyes with open-angle glaucoma. JAMA Ophthalmol. 2016;134(9):976–81.
9. Xie Y, Wang M, Cong Y, Cheng M, Wang S, Wang G. The pilocarpine-induced ciliary body contraction affects the elastic modulus and collagen of cornea and sclera in early development. Biomed Pharmacother. 2018;108:1816–24.
10. Prum BE, Rosenberg LF, Gedde SJ, Mansberger SL, Stein JD, Moroi SE, et al. Primary open-angle glaucoma preferred practice pattern(®) guidelines. Ophthalmology. 2016;123(1):P41–111.
11. Camras CB, Alm A. Initial clinical studies with prostaglandins and their analogues. Surv Ophthalmol. 1997;41(Suppl 2):S61–8.
12. Winkler NS, Fautsch MP. Effects of prostaglandin analogues on aqueous humor outflow pathways. J Ocul Pharmacol Ther. 2014;30(2–3):102–9.
13. Toris CB, Gabelt BT, Kaufman PL. Update on the mechanism of action of topical prostaglandins for intraocular pressure reduction. Surv Ophthalmol. 2008;53(Suppl 1):S107–20.
14. Weinreb RN, Kashiwagi K, Kashiwagi F, Tsukahara S, Lindsey JD. Prostaglandins increase matrix metalloproteinase release from human ciliary smooth muscle cells. Invest Ophthalmol Vis Sci. 1997;38(13):2772–80.
15. Trier K, Ribel-Madsen SM. Latanoprost eye drops increase concentration of glycosaminoglycans in posterior rabbit sclera. J Ocul Pharmacol Ther. 2004;20(3):185–8.
16. Georgopoulos GT, Diestelhorst M, Fisher R, Ruokonen P, Krieglstein GK. The short-term effect of latanoprost on intraocular pressure and pulsatile ocular blood flow. Acta Ophthalmol Scand. 2002;80(1):54–8.
17. Sahinoglu-Keskck N, Canan H. Effect of latanoprost on choroidal thickness. J Glaucoma. 2018;27(7):635–7.

18. Zheng X, Wang Y, Zhao Y, Cao S, Zhu R, Huang W, et al. Experimental evaluation of travoprost-induced changes in biomechanical behavior of ex-vivo rabbit corneas. Curr Eye Res. 2019;44(1):19–24.

19. Detorakis ET, Arvanitaki V, Pallikaris IG, Kymionis G, Tsilimbaris MK. Applanation tonometry versus dynamic contour tonometry in eyes treated with latanoprost. J Glaucoma. 2010;19(3):194–8.

20. Ang GS, Wells AP. Goldmann applanation tonometry and dynamic contour tonometry after treatment with prostaglandin analog/prostamide. J Glaucoma. 2010;19(5):346. author reply 347

21. Detry-Morel M, Jamart J, Pourjavan S. Evaluation of corneal biomechanical properties with the Reichert ocular response analyzer. Eur J Ophthalmol. 2011;21(2):138–48.

22. Bolívar G, Sánchez-Barahona C, Teus M, Castejón MA, Paz-Moreno-Arrones J, Gutiérrez-Ortiz C, et al. Effect of topical prostaglandin analogues on corneal hysteresis. Acta Ophthalmol. 2015 Sep;93(6):e495–8.

23. Yolcu U, Civan DY. Effect of topical prostaglandin analogues on corneal hysteresis. Acta Ophthalmol. 2016;94(1):e80.

24. Bolívar G, Sánchez-Barahona C, Teus M, Castejón MA, Paz Moreno-Arrones J, Gutiérrez-Ortiz C, et al. Effect of topical prostaglandin analogues on corneal hysteresis: author's reply. Acta Ophthalmol. 2017;95(2):e152.

25. Bafa M, Georgopoulos G, Mihas C, Stavrakas P, Papaconstantinou D, Vergados I. The effect of prostaglandin analogues on central corneal thickness of patients with chronic open-angle glaucoma: a 2-year study on 129 eyes. Acta Ophthalmol. 2011;89(5):448–51.

26. Maruyama Y, Mori K, Ikeda Y, Ueno M, Kinoshita S. Effects of long-term topical prostaglandin therapy on central corneal thickness. J Ocul Pharmacol Ther. 2014;30(5):440–4.

27. Meda R, Wang Q, Paoloni D, Harasymowycz P, Brunette I. The impact of chronic use of prostaglandin analogues on the biomechanical properties of the cornea in patients with primary open-angle glaucoma. Br J Ophthalmol. 2017;101(2):120–5.

28. Agarwal DR, Ehrlich JR, Shimmyo M, Radcliffe NM. The relationship between corneal hysteresis and the magnitude of intraocular pressure reduction with topical prostaglandin therapy. Br J Ophthalmol. 2012;96(2):254–7.

29. Amano S, Nejima R, Inoue K, Miyata K. Effect of topical prostaglandins on the biomechanics and shape of the cornea. Graefes Arch Clin Exp Ophthalmol. 2019;257(10):2213–9.

30. Tejwani S, Francis M, Dinakaran S, Kamath V, Tilva B, Das RK, et al. Influence of anterior biometry on corneal biomechanical stiffness of glaucomatous eyes treated with chronic medication or filtration surgery. J Glaucoma. 2019;28(7):626–32.

31. Sánchez-Barahona C, Bolívar G, Katsanos A, Teus MA. Latanoprost treatment differentially affects intraocular pressure readings obtained with three different tonometers. Acta Ophthalmol. 2019;97(8):e1112–5.

32. Wu N, Chen Y, Yu X, Li M, Wen W, Sun X. Changes in corneal biomechanical properties after long-term topical prostaglandin therapy. PLoS One. 2016;11(5):e0155527.

33. Craven ER, Walters T, Christie WC, Day DG, Lewis RA, Goodkin ML, et al. 24-month phase I/II clinical trial of bimatoprost sustained-release implant (Bimatoprost SR) in Glaucoma patients. Drugs. 2020 Feb;80(2):167–79.

34. Lee SS, Robinson MR, Weinreb RN. Episcleral venous pressure and the ocular hypotensive effects of topical and intracameral prostaglandin analogs. J Glaucoma. 2019;28(9):846–57.

35. Schehlein EM, Novack GD, Robin AL. New classes of glaucoma medications. Curr Opin Ophthalmol. 2017;28(2):161–8.

36. Katsanos A, Dastiridou AI. Pharmacotherapy of glaucoma: new opportunities, old challenges. Expert Opin Pharmacother. 2017;18(13):1289–90.

Chapter 25
Ocular Rigidity and Surgery

Yann Bouremel, Christin Henein, and Peng Tee Khaw

Introduction

Definition of Ocular Rigidity

Ocular rigidity is a parameter describing the elasticity of the ocular shell, and is defined as the ratio of the log change in intraocular pressure (ΔIOP) over change in volume (ΔV). In other terms, ocular rigidity characterises the resistance of the eye to deform when its shape changes with intraocular pressure (IOP). An ocular rigidity coefficient was first described by Friedenwald [1] in 1937, where he specified that above 5 mmHg:

$$K = \frac{\log IOP_2 - \log IOP_1}{V_2 - V_1} \tag{25.1}$$

where IOP_2 is the intraocular pressure for the volume injected V_2, IOP_1, the intraocular pressure for the volume injected V_1, and K, the ocular rigidity coefficient. Friedenwald believed that there was no change in the ocular rigidity coefficient with variation in pressure above 5 mmHg [1]. However, two decades later, a series of authors proved that the ocular rigidity both varies with ocular pressure and differs from one animal species to another [2–6]. It is crucial to understand how the rigidity of the eye affects surgery. To measure ocular rigidity, different methods have been proposed: from inflating the anterior chamber in an invasive way to, more recently, looking at the variation of the choroidal thickness [7, 8]. It remains a topic for debate which ocular rigidity equation or measurement most accurately describes the rigidity of the eye [9–11]. More recently, parameters such as corneal hysteresis

Y. Bouremel · C. Henein · P. T. Khaw (✉)
National Institute for Health Research (NIHR) Biomedical Research Centre, Moorfields Eye Hospital NHS Foundation Trust and UCL Institute of Ophthalmology, London, UK
e-mail: y.bouremel@ucl.ac.uk; c.henein@ucl.ac.uk; p.khaw@ucl.ac.uk

© Springer Nature Switzerland AG 2021
I. Pallikaris et al. (eds.), *Ocular Rigidity, Biomechanics and Hydrodynamics of the Eye*, https://doi.org/10.1007/978-3-030-64422-2_25

factor or corneal resistance factor have been introduced to improve on IOP measurements. These parameters have also been used as risk factors for the development of glaucoma and used as a proxy for ocular rigidity.

Definition of Corneal Hysteresis and Corneal Resistance Factor

The cornea is a complex tissue which exhibits age-dependent non-linear viscoelastic properties. It exhibits anisotropia in terms of strain, deformation and elastic strength. Biomechanical changes in the cornea can arise from surgery-related modification and post-operative corneal oedema. Surgeries which alter the IOP, corneal viscosity, elasticity and thickness also impact the corneal response to deformation i.e. corneal hysteresis and corneal resistance factor. Until now, there was no theoretical concept that considered the impact and interaction of independent factors such as IOP, geometric and structural biomechanical parameters of the cornea on ocular rigidity.

The corneal hysteresis (CH) parameter is the calculation of the difference between the inward (P_1) and outward applanation (P_2) pressures derived from the measuring device e.g. the Ocular Response Analyzer® (ORA) (Reichert Technologies) during its dynamic bidirectional applanation process. ORA is a non-invasive device used to measure corneal biomechanical properties such as CH and CRF. ORA also measures corneal compensated IOP (IOPcc) and Goldmann-correlated IOP (IOPg). These IOP estimates are less affected by corneal elasticity, hydration, rigidity or hysteresis, and provide improved accuracy. The CH factor is a dynamic measure of the viscous damping in the corneal tissue and represents the energy absorption capability of the cornea. The corneal resistance factor (CRF) is also derived from these two pressure values but in a more complex calculation (see Eq. 25.2). The CRF parameter is an indicator of the total corneal response, including the elastic resistance of the corneal tissue. CRF is correlated with IOP and central corneal thickness (CCT) and therefore corneal elasticity. CRF is defined as:

$$CRF = k_1 \times \left(P_1 - 0.7 \times P_2 \right) + k_2 \tag{25.2}$$

where the constants k_1 and k_2 have been empirically determined [12]. As the cornea is more accessible than the sclera for measurement, CH and CRF may offer useful surrogate markers to ocular rigidity.

Previous studies have shown a positive correlation between CH and CCT [13–15]. In a large population cohort over 90,000 participants, CH was significantly associated with age, sex, and ethnicity, which should be taken into account when interpreting CH values [16]. There is scarce evidence linking CH and CRF (ORA parameters) and the standard mechanical properties (Young's modulus and ocular rigidity) used to describe elastic materials [17]. CH and CRF are entirely empirical parameters, each of which characterises the response of the cornea to deformation by an air impulse. As there is considerable research in understanding the rigidity of the eye, we have proposed defining ocular rigidity using engineering parameters; to facilitate surgeons' understanding of the impact of surgery on ocular rigidity. By rewriting the equations using engineering and geometrical parameters, we are able to assess the impact of ocular rigidity on different types of ocular surgical situations.

Rewriting Ocular Rigidity Using Engineering Parameters

A series of different ocular rigidities have been proposed based on Friendenwald's work. All the definitions of ocular rigidity are different expressions of $\Delta IOP/\Delta V$, with one of the latest equations being the work of Van Der Werff [18]:

$$K = \frac{IOP_2^{1/3} - IOP_1^{1/3}}{V} \tag{25.3}$$

This one parameter expression is insensitive to changes in intraocular pressure and is called cube root ocular rigidity. It is equal to approximately 0.03 mmHg$^{1/3}$µl^{-1} for enucleated human eyes. The eye can be seen as being divided into two different compartments, the front of the eye made up of the anterior segment delimited by the lens-iris diaphragm, and the posterior segment of the eye. Injecting volume into the anterior chamber will increase the volume of the anterior segment but not necessarily of the posterior segment (for relatively small quantity of fluid). We can therefore rewrite the cube root ocular rigidity equation using the pursing of elastic pocket equation developed by Bouremel et al. [19]. Firstly, there are two different types of pursing according to the height of the anterior chamber: If the maximum height of the anterior chamber is less than the thickness of the cornea, the anterior chamber is said to be *bending* (flat anterior chamber). If the maximum height of the anterior chamber is greater than the thickness of the cornea, the anterior chamber is said to be *stretching*. We assumed in the latter scenario, the anterior chamber height is approximately 3 mm and the average cornea thickness 0.55 mm. We can rewrite this function by analysing the way it is measured. In order to measure the ocular rigidity in living patients, Pallikaris [62] performed studies to measure ocular rigidity in vivo by recording the change in intraocular pressure change (ΔIOP) after injecting repeated boluses of balanced salt solution into the anterior chamber (ΔV), as shown

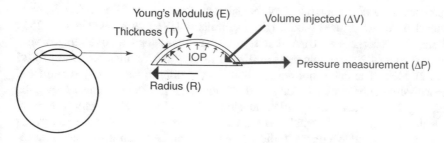

Fig. 25.1 Schematic diagram illustrating the method to measure ocular rigidity following Friendenwald's Equation (brown) and relevant geometrical parameters (blue)

in Fig. 25.1. From the work of Bouremel et al. [19] on pursing of elastic pockets, we can rewrite the cube root ocular rigidity from Van Der Werff as shown in Eq. (25.4):

$$K \approx 1.06 \left(\frac{ET}{R^{10}} \right)^{1/3} \tag{25.4}$$

where E, is the average Young's Modulus of the cornea which is approximately 0.29 MPa or 2175.2 mmHg [20]; T, the average thickness of the central cornea approximately 0.55 mm, and R, the average corneal radius approximately 5.85 mm [21]. The respective physiological values replace each parameter in Eq. (25.4), giving a cube root ocular rigidity, **k = 0.031 mmHg$^{1/3}$ µl^{-1}** (with 1 m^3 = 10^{9}µl), within 3.8% of Van Der Werff results [18]. The expression of the ocular rigidity function in Eq. (25.4) combining corneal geometrical parameters (corneal thickness and averaged radius) as well as material elastic properties of the cornea (Young's Modulus).

Modelling Corneal Incisions

By redefining ocular rigidity using engineering parameters for the anterior segment compartment, we can model the impact of corneal incisions on ocular rigidity in different scenarios. For this purpose, we developed an experimental and numerical model for incisions. The experimental modelling consists of simulating different anterior chamber depths, sizes, intraocular pressures and cornea thicknesses using elastic materials such as silicone. We then create incisions through the models and measure the pressure at which they leak and the flow rate of the leak. Each incision is self-sealed at the start of each experiment before increasing the pressure ultimately resulting in a leak from the incision. We used the numerical models to understand the stress along different cornea geometries and rigidities and to understand the stresses obtained at the pressure at which the incision leaks in the experimental model.

Experimental Modelling

Experimental corneas constructed of thin silicone sheets (from Silex Ltd., UK) were clamped on a 3D printed model (from Formlabs, USA) as shown in Fig. 25.2. Different sized corneas were simulated from a very small diameter of 5 mm to a very large diameter of 20 mm, thickness of 0.25 to 1.6 mm and Young's Modulus of 1.25 and 4.21 MPa. The cube root ocular rigidity according to Eq. (25.5) varied from extremely low cube ocular rigidity of 0.007 mmHg$^{1/3}$ µl^{-1} to extremely high cube ocular rigidity of 1.24 mmHg$^{1/3}$µl^{-1}. Incision of 1 mm long and 0.2 mm wide were made through the experimental corneas using a micro feather blade. The corneas were then connected to a microfluidic set-up (Fluigent, Le Kremlin-Bicêtre, France) varying automatically the pressure within the experimental corneas and recording

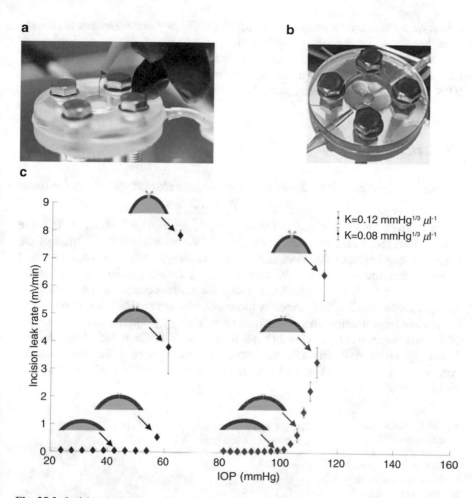

Fig. 25.2 Incision (**a**) into experimental silicone corneas clamped to 3D printed models followed by the experimental cornea leaking at the site of incision (**b**) and (**c**) the flow rate associated across the incision using two experimental corneas of different ocular rigidity when the pressure within the experimental anterior chamber increases. In (**c**), the incision leak rate is shown with black diamonds for lower ocular rigidity, and with red diamonds for higher ocular rigidity. This diagram shows that experimental corneas with lower ocular rigidity (K = 0.08 mmHg$^{1/3}$μl^{-1}) leak at a lower IOP compared to those with a higher ocular rigidity (K = 0.12 mmHg$^{1/3}$μl^{-1}). Ocular rigidity, K is defined using Eq. (25.4)

the flow rate through the incision. If the incision was self-sealed, the flow rate through the incision was zero. The pressure was increased automatically in steps as low as 1 mmHg every hour to ensure that the system had time to stabilize between each recording. Typical examples of incision leak rate are shown in Fig. 25.2c for two experimental corneas of two different ocular rigidities. Once the incision started to leak, increasing IOP led to higher flow rate through the incision. Interestingly, all experimental corneas started to leak with a flow rate of 0.4 ± 0.2μl/min [22].

Lower ocular rigidity corneas started to leak at lower pressure compared to corneas of higher ocular rigidity. Below, we investigate the reasons for lower ocular rigidity eye to leak at lower pressure by simulating corneas of different ocular rigidity and mapping the stresses and strains along the corneas associated to the experimental IOPs obtained when the incision started to leak.

Numerical Modelling

Commonly, the cornea is modelled as a homogenous elastic sphere with the stress along it given by the Laplace Equation:
$$\sigma = \frac{IOP \times d}{4 \times T}$$
with σ, stress within the stroma, IOP, intraocular pressure, d, diameter of the cornea and T, thickness of the cornea. While Laplace's equation only gives an averaged value for a fixed corneal diameter and thickness, a simplified model of the cornea can be presented using finite element modelling (Fig. 25.3) using the finite element analysis software Abaqus version 6.12.3. The cornea is modelled as a hyper-elastic membrane with the strain energy density function derived from Mooney [23]. The change in height of the experimental anterior chamber is linked to the IOP. The model shows the different regions of strain/stress of the cornea. An example of a simulated healthy cornea model is shown in Fig. 25.3 with an ocular rigidity of K = 0.036 mmHg$^{1/3}$μl^{-1} and an IOP of 10 mmHg.

Fig. 25.3 Simulation generated with Abaqus software showing the pursing of an experimental healthy cornea with the isocontours of stresses for an ocular rigidity using Eq. (25.4) of K = 0.036 mmHg$^{1/3}$μl^{-1} and IOP = 10 mmHg

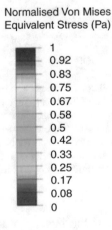

Normalised Von Mises Equivalent Stress (Pa)

1
0.92
0.83
0.75
0.67
0.58
0.5
0.42
0.33
0.25
0.17
0.08
0

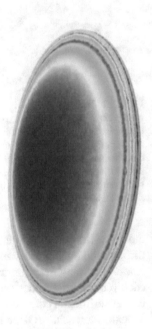

Ocular Rigidity Affects Corneal Stress Zones

Using our numerical modelling, experimental corneas of different ocular rigidities were simulated to understand how stress affects them. We varied three parameters (E is Young's modulus, T is thickness and R is radius) defined in Eq. (25.4) and studied the stress distribution across the cornea. Figure 25.4 summarises our findings. When increasing the Young's Modulus (E) of the cornea, the ocular rigidity increases as shown by Eq. (25.4) at a power of $E^{1/3}$, this results in lower stress at a constant IOP compared to a cornea of a lower ocular rigidity. Lower iso-contour stresses are represented by green-blue plotted data. Conversely, if the thickness (T) is decreased or the size of the cornea increased (R), the ocular rigidity decreases following $T^{1/3}$ and $R^{-10/3}$. This leads to higher stress along the corneas at constant IOP. When creating incisions into the cornea, we have shown recently that lower ocular rigidity corneas leak at lower pressure compared to corneas of higher ocular rigidity [22]. This is explained by relating the higher stresses of low ocular rigidity corneas to higher corneal strains compared to higher ocular rigidity corneas. In this experimental model, corneas of ocular rigidity ranging from 0.007 to 1.25 mmHg$^{1/3}\mu$l^{-1} were found to leak when the strain at the point of incision is 2.8 ± 0.5% with a flow rate of 0.4 ± 0.2μl/min in all cases. Therefore, lower ocular rigidity corneas achieved this type of low strain at lower IOP compared to higher ocular rigidity corneas [22]. Keeping this principle in mind, we will now review the different surgeries and the impact ocular rigidity may have on them.

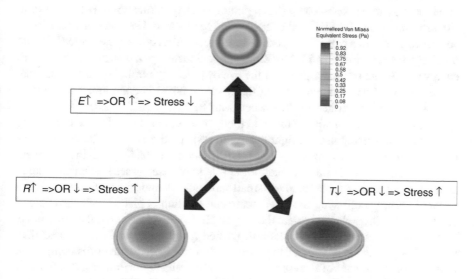

Fig. 25.4 Simulation demonstrating how ocular rigidity affects the stress along the experimental corneas at a constant IOP. When Young's Modulus (E), corneal thickness (T) and radius (R) from the ocular rigidity Eq. (25.4) are modified, the other parameters are kept constant

Ocular Rigidity and Surgery

Globe Rupture

Globe rupture occurs when there is a defect in the cornea, the sclera, or both structures. Most often, globe rupture occurs after direct penetrating trauma; however, if sufficient blunt force is applied to the eye, the intraocular pressure can increase enough to rupture the sclera where it is the thinnest and the weakest. The sclera is thinnest, 0.3 mm thick, posterior to the rectus muscle insertions. It is 0.4 mm thick at the equator and 0.6 mm thick anterior to the muscle insertions. The sclera may rupture open from blunt trauma at structural weak points, especially at the corneal limbus bordering the sclera, the rectus muscle insertion of the optic nerve and sites of prior eye surgery such as glaucoma or cataract surgery [24, 25]. However, phacoemulsification through a self-sealing corneoscleral tunnel is associated with significantly less risk of traumatic wound dehiscence [26]. The risk of eye injury increases with age; as a result, the eyes of elderly patients may be more susceptible to ciliary body related eye injuries in traumatic impact situations [27]. Peak deformation of the lens decreases with increasing lens stiffness.

Refractive Surgery

Refractive surgery was developed for the correction of myopia, hyperopia, and astigmatism with the aim of achieving spectacle independence. The different surgeries namely radial keratotomy (RK), photorefractive keratectomy (PRK), laser in situ keratomileusis (LASIK) and laser-assisted subepithelial keratectomy (LASEK), consist of removing part of the cornea to correct the vision of the patients. More precisely, LASIK, PRK, and LASEK are surgical techniques that use excimer laser energy to alter the refractive status of the eye by precisely removing corneal stromal tissue. The primary difference is that the tissue removal is done under a flap with LASIK and on the surface of the cornea with PRK/LASEK. In PRK, the corneal epithelium is mechanically removed, then an excimer laser is used to apply computer-controlled pulses of light energy to reshape the cornea. The corneal epithelial layer grows back over 3–4 days. LASIK consists of first making a corneal flap with a device called a microkeratome (blade or laser based). After the flap is created, the excimer laser removes small amounts of underlying tissue from the exposed cornea. Following the laser treatment, the flap is placed over the eye and carefully repositioned to complete the surgery. In LASEK, the corneal epithelium is soaked in a dilute solution of alcohol, pushed aside as a single sheet, and then pushed back over the surface of the cornea after the laser treatment is completed. Maximal displacement of the cornea occurs in the mid-peripheral cornea after PK, in the central cornea after PRK, and paracentrally after LASIK and SMILE procedures [28]. By removing part of the corneal stroma, refractive surgeries reduce the thickness of the cornea, which will therefore decrease the rigidity of the eye

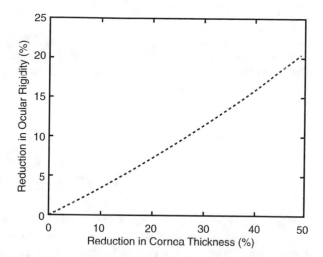

Fig. 25.5 Reduction in ocular rigidity following Eq. (25.4) with reduction in cornea thickness

following Eq. (25.4). A decrease in thickness (*T*) will decrease the ocular rigidity following $T^{1/3}$, as shown in Fig. 25.5. This has been shown by Cronemberger et al. where they showed that ocular rigidity decreases after LASIK, up to 24 months post-operatively [29].

CH and CRF are also reduced after LASIK, LASEK and PRK compared to controls [30]. Similar reductions occurred following LASIK and LASEK procedures with similar amounts of corneal ablation. Post-operative CH at 3 months were not significantly different between LASIK and LASEK, indicating that LASIK involving a thin 120-mm flap did not induce additional biomechanical change [30]. A relatively new refractive procedure, small incision lenticule extraction (SMILE) used to treat a magnitude of refractive errors, utilises femtosecond laser to create a corneal lenticule, which is extracted whole through a small corneal incision. A systematic review of three RCTs found no statistically significant differences between SMILE or flap-based procedures concerning corneal hysteresis (CH) or corneal resistance factor (CRF), as measured with the Ocular Response Analyzer [31]. Corneal thinning surgeries that change the rigidity of the cornea will affect IOP measurements which rely on corneal rigidity and could lead to underestimation of IOP. Pressure rises can be missed if they occur after corneal thinning surgery and other evidence of raised pressure such as corneal oedema or increased cupping must be detected.

Phacoemulsification Surgery

Peripheral corneal incisions avoid the visual axis and produce less astigmatic effects and are therefore preferred to more central corneal incisions. Peripheral corneal incisions self-seal better compared to central corneal incisions (where the cornea is thinner) at the same intraocular pressure. This is related to the stress strain zones of the cornea (see Fig. 25.4). The central corneal zone is under greater stress.

Fig. 25.6 Self-sealing
incision for thick and thin
corneas. A longer stromal
tunnel is created to
improve sealing in
thin corneas

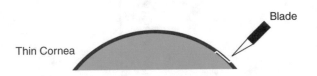

Symmetrical corneal incisions are better at self-sealing, where the roof of the incision is the same thickness as the floor. In the case of thinner corneas and therefore lower ocular rigidity eye, incisions leak at lower pressure, as shown in Figs. 25.2 and 25.4, therefore longer tunnelling of the incision are created to improve self-sealing and reduces an astigmatic effect but at the expense of restrictive manoeuvring of surgical instruments and greater optical distortion. Schematic of incisions for thick and thin corneas are shown in Fig. 25.6.

Surgical adjustments need to be made when operating on myopic eyes and other large eyes such as those in patients with congenital glaucoma. Eyes with abnormal extracellular matrix such as Ehler Danlos syndrome and Marfans may also behave similarly. Myopic eyes tend to have larger anterior chambers and thinner corneas. CCT is known to be correlated with the degree of myopia in adults. Highly myopic eyes have a lower ocular rigidity based on Eq. (25.4) where the thickness and the radius of the anterior chamber appear respectively at a power (1/3) and (−10/3) and are more susceptible to intraoperative anterior chamber instability (shallowing) and wound leakages. To mitigate against these risks, an understanding of intra-operative fluidics and wound construction is needed. The aim of phacoemulsification surgery in these eyes is to maintain a stable anterior chamber. This can be achieved by keeping the anterior chamber pressurised by elevating the irrigation bottle height of phacoemulsification machine. Approximately 11 mmHg is produced intraocularly for every 15 cm of height above the level of the patient's eye. Keeping the anterior chamber adequately pressurised is particularly important while performing capsulorrhexis. Newer phacoemulsification machines generate a pre-set intraocular pressure during surgery by utilising forced infusion pumps that constantly adjusts irrigation fluid inflow to maintain anterior chamber stability. Creating a longer intrastromal incision allows for greater contact surface area of opposing sides of the wound for closure. Alternatively, a superiorly placed scleral tunnel incision with an internal corneal lip can be used. Small, posteriorly placed superior stepped scleral tunnel incisions reduce the incidence of both early and late surgically induced astigmatism. The initial scleral step incision should be made perpendicular to the scleral surface, at a depth of approximately 0.3 mm and placed 1.0–3.0 mm posterior to the surgical limbus. The initial incision length should be 2.75–7.00 mm, depending on the style of IOL to be implanted. When operating on paediatric eyes which have

K (mmHg$^{-1/3}$μl^{-1})

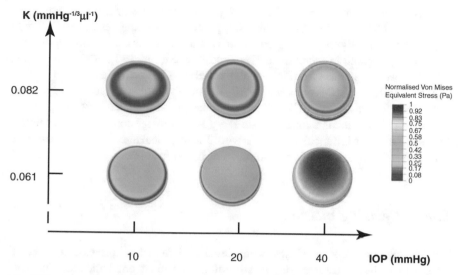

Fig. 25.7 Experimental model showing the impact of ocular rigidity (K) on corneal stress at IOPs of 10, 20 and 40 mmHg

more elastic tissues and softer eyes compared to adult eyes, a longer scleral tunnel is warranted. Re-approximation of the surfaces of the tunnel allows for wound closure. However, thin soft, less rigid cornea or sclera (low ocular rigidity) often does not self-seal well and may require suturing for closure unlike a normal adult eye.

Our experimental model demonstrates that corneas of lower ocular rigidity, e.g. thin corneas, consistently leak at lower pressures compared to thick corneas (higher ocular rigidity), as expected. Lower ocular rigidity of experimental corneas was associated to higher corneal stress compared to higher ocular rigidity corneas at the same intra-ocular pressure. Higher stresses lead to higher strain, and therefore, larger wound gaps. Figure 25.7 shows the stress distribution of two experimental corneas of different ocular rigidities against increasing IOP. It can be seen that the higher ocular rigidity cornea is consistently associated with lower stress for the same intraocular pressure compared to the lower ocular rigidity cornea. Lower stress means lower strain and a reduction in size of any corneal wound gaping.

Clear corneal incisions used in phacoemulsification surgery offers the benefit of a suture-less, self-sealing, easy to construct incision. Earlier use of phacoemulsification with self-sealing incisions was associated with increased national rates of endophthalmitis, hence the importance of good wound closure without leaks. To avoid wound leakage, postoperative hypotony or the ingress of fluid and bacteria from the ocular surface, many surgeons hydrate the stroma with a balanced salt solution at the end of a cataract operation. Hydration of the corneal incisions result in temporary increase in central corneal thickness (CCT). At day 1 after clear corneal cataract surgery, CH is diminished whereas CCT is increased significantly. Postoperative corneal oedema leads to a change of corneal viscoelastic properties, resulting in a lower damping capacity of the cornea when compared to a control group of 48 pseudophakic eyes (surgery >3 months previously) [32]. Structural differences and changes in the viscoelastic properties of the cornea are better measured using CH instead of CCT. However, postoperative changes in the CCT will impact the ocular rigidity if only temporarily. Increased corneal thickness through hydration will result in increased ocular rigidity according to Eq. (25.4) following $T^{1/3}$. A lower baseline CH (but not the baseline CCT) was associated with a larger magnitude of IOP reduction at 10–12 months after cataract surgery, when controlling for patient age [33]. If the intraocular pressure falls after surgery to low levels seen after glaucoma filtrations surgery (5–10 mmHg) combined with cataract surgery, the lower intraocular pressure would lead to leakage. Therefore, suturing would be safer in situations where intraocular pressure is lower.

Limbal Relaxing Incisions

Limbal relaxing incisions (LRIs) were developed to reduce pre-existing corneal astigmatism during cataract surgery. Simultaneous phacoemulsification and LRI procedures require a clear corneal or sclero-corneal incision of approximately 2.0–3.0 mm as well as paired arcuate incisions on the limbus. In a study by Kamiya et al., two paired arcuate incisions were created with a guarded micrometre diamond blade set at 500µm [34]. The CH and CRF values decreased 1 day after simultaneous cataract surgery with LRIs but soon recovered to preoperative levels [34]. The CCT also increased 1 day after surgery and soon recovered to preoperative levels. No studies assessing ocular rigidity and LRIs could be identified but one could speculate that LRIs alone is unlikely to impact overall ocular rigidity beyond 1 week postoperatively.

Corneal Transplantation Surgery

Current principles of corneal transplantation involve selective replacement of the diseased corneal layer in order to avoid complications associated with full thickness corneal replacement, penetrating keratoplasty (PK). Deep anterior lamellar keratoplasty (DALK) is performed for corneal pathologies not affecting the endothelium and Descemet's membrane. Descemet stripping automated endothelial keratoplasty (DSAEK) and Descemet's Membrane Endothelial Keratoplasty (DMEK) are performed for patients with only endothelial dysfunction. The different corneal transplantation surgeries are summarised in Fig. 25.8.

PK and DALK surgeries in keratoconic eyes restore the corneal biomechanical parameters to a normal range [35]. Changes in corneal biomechanics after these surgeries may have implications for interpreting intraocular pressure or planning graft refractive surgery after keratoplasty. However, after PK in a heterogenous cohort of non-keratoconic patients (with herpetic corneal scar, corneal stromal dystrophy, Fuchs endothelial dystrophy, traumatic and chemical corneal opacity), graft

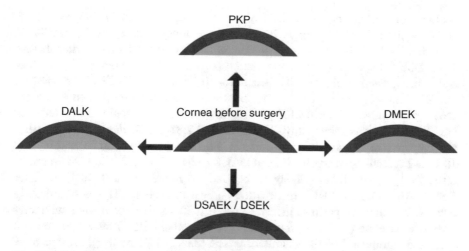

Fig. 25.8 Schematic of the different corneal transplantation surgeries. Recipient cornea shown in dark blue and donor cornea shown in red

biomechanics did not return to average values even at 2-year follow up [36]. In 2017, Jiang et al. conducted a meta-analysis on corneal biomechanical properties after penetrating keratoplasty (PK) or deep anterior lamellar keratoplasty (DALK) in a heterogenous cohort using the ORA; they suggested that both CH and CRF had better recovery after corneal transplantation with DALK than PK [37]. This may be due to discontinuity of Descemet's membrane after PK. Descemet's membrane has a greater stiffness than Bowman's membrane. The thickness of Descemet's membrane increases with age from ~3µm at birth to >10µm in old age [38].

After keratoplasty, the ocular rigidity will be affected. Looking at Eq. (25.4), two parameters may be potentially affected, i.e. the thickness of the transplanted cornea (T) as well as its elasticity or Young's modulus (E). They both appear as numerators in the equation with a power of (1/3). If the cornea is thinner or more elastic, this will reduce the ocular rigidity. Conversely, if the cornea is thicker or stiffer, it will increase the ocular rigidity. The stiffness of the human cornea can increase by a factor of approximately two between the ages of 20 and 100 years [39]. The Young's modulus of the donor cornea may vary depending on the age of the donor. Long-term follow longitudinal studies have shown an increase in corneal thickness after PK at 20 years compared to 2 years after transplantation [40]. Corneal thickness > 600µm at 1 year has been shown to be a predictor of graft failure [41]. The increase in corneal thickness in the postoperative period was found to be higher for corneas preserved in McCarey-Kaufman medium compared with the corneas preserved in organ culture [40].

Endothelial keratoplasty is a corneal transplant technique that is the preferred way to restore vision in endothelial layer disorders such as Fuchs' dystrophy, bullous keratopathy, and iridocorneal endothelial syndrome. Descemet's Membrane Endothelial Keratoplasty (DMEK) and Descemet's Stripping Endothelial Keratoplasty (DSEK) are types of endothelial keratoplasties that selectively replace the diseased endothelial layer and Descemet's membrane, leaving the remaining healthy corneal layers intact. In DSEK, transplanted tissue is approximately 100–200 microns thick which is 20–30% of the donor cornea, and in DMEK, an ultra-thin 5% endothelium/Descemet's membrane of donor cornea is transplanted. Thus, DSEK results in an overall increased corneal thickness compared to DMEK and hence greater ocular rigidity, according to Eq. (25.4). Studies have shown a long-term increase in recipient corneal thickness in DSEK patients up to 36 months post-transplant [42]. CH and CRF were significantly lower in patients who received DSAEK for bullous keratopathy (7.79 ± 2.0 and 7.88 ± 1.74 mmHg, respectively) as compared to the keratoconus patients who received PK (10.23 ± 2.07 and 10.13 ± 2.22 mmHg, respectively) and DALK (9.64 ± 2.07 and 9.36 ± 2.09 mmHg, respectively) [35]. This is likely to be due to greater corneal thickness after DSEK. After DMEK, which reduces the corneal thickness, CH was significantly increased 6 months postoperatively (8.66 ± 2.50 mmHg) compared with pre-operative baseline (7.43 ± 1.56 mmHg). Pre-operative CRF (7.89 ± 1.68 mmHg) increased significantly 6 months after DMEK (8.49 ± 1.71 mmHg). Pre-operative central corneal thickness showed a significant decrease from 629 ± 58μm to 550 ± 40μm after 3 months and 535 ± 40μm after 6 months post-operatively [43].

Eyes with low scleral rigidity, such as paediatric or enlarged thinned eyes such as myopia cases, are predisposed to globe collapse during penetrating keratoplasty. A scleral fixation ring such as a Flieringa ring (or a double Flieringa ring) or the Goldman scleral fixation ring and blepharostat should be used to stabilise the globe. The younger the child, the more pliable and less rigid the tissue, the more difficult it is to handle the tissue and suture. Furthermore, higher posterior pressure can cause forward displacement of the lens-iris diaphragm, increasing the risk of iris prolapse, lens extrusion, and suprachoroidal haemorrhage. Positioning of the patient with the head higher than the rest of the body can help to reduce this pressure. Pre-operative ocular massage or use of the Honan balloon can reduce the risk of high posterior pressure and retrobulbar blocks should be avoided where possible.

Glaucoma Surgery

Glaucomatous eyes have thinner CCT, lower CH and CRF than in healthy eyes, and the reduction of CH and CRF is associated with an increased severity of glaucomatous damage. Thinner corneas were associated with glaucomatous damage in terms of cup disc ratio [44]. Studies suggest central corneal thickness should be considered in determining the risk of glaucoma conversion in patients with ocular hypertension [45]. However, CH was associated with glaucomatous visual field progression [44] and a CH cut off value of less than 10.1 mmHg has been suggested as part of the clinical assessment for glaucoma [16]. The CH has a significant effect on rates of visual field progression over time. Each 1 mmHg lower CH was associated with a 0.25% per year faster rate of visual field indices decline over time. A multivariable model showed that the effect of IOP on rates of progression depended on CH. Eyes with high IOP and low CH were at increased risk for having fast rates

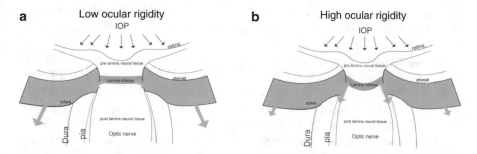

Fig. 25.9 Theoretical effect of high intraocular pressure (IOP) on deflection of sclera and lamina cribosa in the case of low scleral rigidity (**a**) and experimentally crosslinked sclera with high scleral rigidity (**b**)

of disease progression [46]. Low CH may be associated with less rigidity of the eye coat including the lamina cribosa, and thus more damage to the lamina cribosa for a given intraocular pressure. In the case of differential ocular rigidity, with sclera more compliant under high IOP than the lamina cribosa, the sclera expands which would stretch the lamina cribosa.

For higher scleral ocular rigidity with a less rigid lamina, the sclera is stiffer with little deformation under IOP allowing the less rigid lamina cribosa to displace posteriorly under the effect of high IOP (see Fig. 25.9) [47]. Experimental cross-linking of just the sclera to strengthen it, without cross-linking the lamina cribosa (the cross linking process is potentially toxic to the lamina cells and axons), results in more damage to the lamina cribosa and retinal ganglion axons for a set of intraocular pressure [48].

Trabeculectomy is a glaucoma filtering surgical procedure that aims to lower the intraocular pressure by creating an ostium into the anterior chamber from underneath a partial thickness scleral flap. Important considerations to control aqueous outflow from the scleral flap are flap construction, suture placement and type of suture. Partial thickness rectangular flaps can be difficult to achieve in myopic or paediatric eyes due to thin and more elastic sclera respectively. Titration of IOP can be achieved with use of releasable sutures. There is the possible weakening of ocular walls reducing ocular rigidity however this may be counteracted by the healing process and degree of fibrotic tissue deposition. CH is dynamic and may increase in eyes after IOP-lowering surgical interventions. In a prospective comparative case series, CH was assessed before and 3 months after trabeculectomy, phacotrabeculectomy and Ahmed glaucoma value implantation [49]. Corneal hysteresis significantly increased after 3 months following all three types of glaucoma surgeries ($P < 0.001$). Postoperative corneal hysteresis increase in glaucomatous eyes was more significant when IOP was reduced by >10mmHg [49].

Following augmented trabeculectomy with mitomycin-C (MMC), CH and CRF increased in patients with primary open angle glaucoma (POAG) and pseudoexfoliation (PXG) [50]. Corneal structural tissue properties may be altered in the immediate post-operative period and, therefore, the accuracy of IOP measurements is changed. However, after 6 months follow-up there does not appear to be changes in corneal biomechanical properties that cannot be explained by the reduction in IOP [51]. The increase observed in corneal hysteresis is due to the IOP-lowering effect of the surgery.

Glaucoma often is asymmetrical and in paediatric eyes changes in corneal diameter can differ between the two eyes. The change in corneal diameter will lead to eyes of different ocular rigidity equation following Eq. (25.4) with larger corneal diameter being associated with lower ocular rigidity. In congenital glaucoma when changes are unilateral the eye can enlarge front to back but in megalocornea (large corneas only), enlargement of the corneas is symmetrical and bilateral. Challenges are encountered when operating in paediatric cases due to differences in ocular biomechanics when compared to adults. Children have lower scleral rigidity and are therefore at risk of intraoperative positive vitreous pressure which results in the forward movement of the lens-iris diaphragm. Large eyes in children with congenital glaucoma (called Buphthalmic eyes after the size of cows eyes) have low scleral rigidity and are predisposed to surgical complications related to low IOP, such as anterior chamber collapse, maculopathy, choroidal effusion, suprachoroidal haemorrhage, and phthisis. Procedure-specific difficulties may also be encountered. Modifications to the surgical procedure can be taken to mitigate against these risks. When fashioning a scleral flap in elastic, myopic or buphthalmic eyes, care is taken to avoid overly thin flaps which can cause early hypotony. The trabeculectomy flap needs to be correctly positioned. A rectangular flap with small side incisions to ensure posterior outflow and prevent deleterious reduction in ocular rigidity, and a more corneal component would reduce the dependence on the softer scleral tissues. An excessively large sclerostomy should also be avoided as it reduces the rigidity of the surrounding tissues, and hence increases the potential risk of leaks. When suturing the scleral flap, care is taken to avoid cheese-wiring through the delicate thin tissue and to adequately seal the aqueous outflow of the trabeculectomy. An anterior chamber maintainer is used to minimise intraoperative hypotony and also to facilitate the accurate judgement of flow through the scleral flap, by in part maintaining overall globe rigidity. In very soft or thin eyes tissue flaps may need to be avoided and tubes with flow control inserted instead which avoids reliance on tissue rigidity to maintain controlled flow.

The impact of ocular rigidity on the geometrical construction of the scleral flap is shown in Fig. 25.10. Schematic of scleral flaps are shown in Fig. 25.10a and deflections of scleral flap associated to increasing ocular rigidity simulated at a constant pressure in Fig. 25.10b. Deflections of the flap have been normalised by the same value across all simulations. It can be shown that for higher ocular rigidity, the scleral flap deflection is reduced compared to lower ocular rigidity. To mitigate against large scleral flap deflection and excessive leakage in cases of low ocular rigidity shortening the length of the side incision should be considered to reduce the deflection of the scleral flap.

In very soft on thin eyes tissue flaps may need to avoided altogether and a glaucoma drainage device used (typcially a microtube usually attached to a spacer plate to keep tissues open). This avoids the relaince on a soft tissue flap to maintain resistance. However other problems related to rigidity may occur. During early childhood, the elastic nature of the eye and low ocular rigidity makes glaucoma drainage

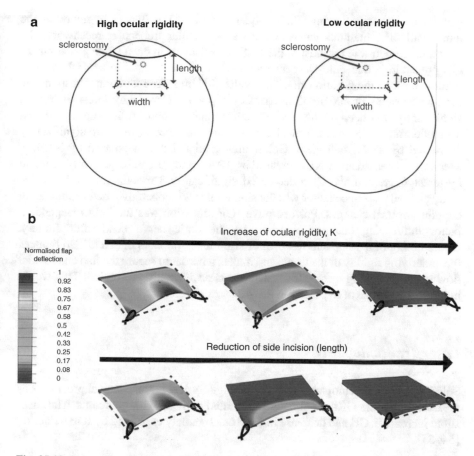

Fig. 25.10 Schematic of trabeculectomy flap in high and low ocular rigidities. The length of the side incisions is shortened to prevent gaping of the flap in less rigid eyes. Simulations showing scleral flap deflections for different ocular rigidities (**a**) and length of flap side incisions depicted by dotted red line (**b**). All simulations have been obtained at the same pressure

device (GDD) positioning problematic. Low ocular rigidity shown in Fig. 25.7 is associated with higher stress and therefore higher tissue strain. In such cases patients are more predisposed to tube migration as the tissue is under more stress and leakage around the scleral tunnel of a glaucoma drainage device tube. Despite restriction of aqueous flow through the GDD, hypotony may still occur unless a watertight tunnel into the anterior chamber is achieved. A tight tunnel with tube sizes used with the Molteno, Ahmed and Baerveldt tube can be achieved with a 25-gauge needle (orange in UK) rather than larger needle sizes. Myopic eyes with low ocular rigidity and thinner sclera are at risk of tube exposure. Like in paediatric cases this risk can be reduced by constructing a long tunnel or a tunnel at least 1–2 mm from the limbus and covering the tube with a patch graft. Patch graft material that can be used include sclera, cornea, pericardium, thick amniotic membrane or dura mater.

Deep Sclerectomy (DS) is a non-penetrating surgical procedure for the treatment of open angle glaucoma. The technique was developed to improve the safety of glaucoma surgery. Following DS, the aqueous outflow is enhanced by removing the inner wall of Schlemm's canal and juxta-canalicular trabecular meshwork, the structures responsible for most of the outflow resistance in open angle glaucoma. In this procedure a trabeculo-Descemet's membrane is left intact to control aqueous outflow through the filtration site. This controlled pressure reduction is responsible for a better safety profile of DS in terms of hypotony. Corneal hysteresis increased significantly after deep sclerotomy at 3 months and 6 months follow-up [52, 53]. At 3 months follow-up, mean corneal compensated intraocular pressure significantly decreased by 27.9% and mean Goldmann-correlated IOP decreased by 30.52%. Mean CH increased and CRF decreased by 18.4% and 10.1%, respectively. Corneal hysteresis increased and CRF decreased significantly 3 months after DS. In this study corneal resistance factor was the single largest preoperative factor influencing cupping reversal changes. Postoperative IOP reduction was the only independent factor influencing changes observed in the optic nerve head after surgery. Undermining of the flap and removal of significant amounts of sclera also reduces the underlying rigidity of the tissue and makes it harder to secure the flap and restrict flow if the remaining meshwork resistance is accidentally perforated. This would increase the chance of hypotony in this circumstance.

Laser Trabeculoplasty

Selective laser trabeculoplasty does not change corneal biomechanical properties as measured with the ORA in already pre-treated patients with glaucoma. The measured increase in CH and decrease in CRF can be solely explained by IOP reduction [54, 55].

Strabismus Surgery

Extraocular muscle surgery in patients in their second to third decade, increased the postoperative CH and CRF [56]. Since the stiffness of the tissue (Young's Modulus) increases with age and hence the ocular rigidity following Eq. (25.4), the effect of strabismus surgery on ocular structures may be variable between paediatric and adult patients. Weakening muscle procedures such as recti recession or inferior oblique muscle weakening had a greater effect on overall corneal biomechanics. Weakening muscle procedures were associated with a mean CH increase up to 4 weeks post-operatively. The release of forces from the yielding effect of weakening procedures could propagate along the ocular wall to the corneal tissue. It remains unclear if the change in CH is only temporary.

Scleral Buckling

Scleral buckles help in several ways to counteract the forces that tend to detach the retina. Indentation of the eye wall produced by the scleral buckle can decrease vitreous traction on the retinal tear in rhegmatogenous retinal detachment. Absorbable and nonabsorbable materials has been used to manufacture the scleral buckles. Absorbable buckles suffer from the problem that reabsorption of the implant reduces the buckling effect. Historically, polyethylene tubing was commonly used for nonabsorbable encircling scleral implants. However, such devices tend to erode the underlying sclera and choroid with time. The use of softer silicones and silicone sponges has overcome the problems of erosion, and offers the advantage of the formation of a tough fibrous capsule around the implant, which both strengthens the sclera.

Buckled eyes were significantly less rigid than unbuckled eyes, and eyes with higher buckles were significantly less rigid (lower ocular rigidity) than those with shallower buckles. Changes in rigidity are secondary to changes in the shape and the distribution of stress in the scleral shell; they are related to the elasticity of the encircling element only partially [57]. Greater volumes of vitreous substitutes, gases, or antibiotics may be injected into buckled eyes compared with unbuckled eyes before excessive intraocular pressures are reached [57]. In a different study of enucleated human eyes, a marked reduction in ocular rigidity during buckling was achieved by encircling silicone elements, permitting buckled eyes to tolerate volume changes several times greater than those tolerated by nonbuckled eyes [58]. While this may be counter-intuitive as the eye diameter is locally reduced that ocular rigidity decreases, it may follow Eq. (25.4). Indeed, if the one part of the eye is locally reduced with the buckling, the other part of the eye should be increased as shown in Fig. 25.11. According to Eq. (25.4), the ocular rigidity changes as $R^{-10/3}$, indeed a small increase of the radius as shown in Fig. 25.11 will decrease the ocular rigidity.

Riazi et al. measured mean CRF and CH after scleral buckling with an ocular response analyser. CRF and CH measurements were significantly lower after scleral buckling with segmental sponge, but there was no significant change with encircling band [59]. Also, no significant change in IOPg and IOPcc postoperatively was observed. Lower CH measurements observed in the scleral sponge group could be due to localised scleral fibrosis at the site of the device. However, the time at

Fig. 25.11 Schematic of scleral buckling showing globe before (**a**) and after (**b**) buckling. After buckling, the eye elongates with an increase axial length and wider radius on either side of the buckle

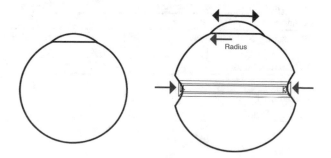

measurements were taken in relation to the surgery was not reported. It is in keeping with the sentiment that CH and CRF may measure different biomechanical aspects of *anterior segment* ocular rigidity and are likely to be useful additional measurements in the assessment of ocular rigidity when measuring IOP. Corneal hysteresis may actually act more like a surrogate marker for the biomechanical properties of tissues in the back of the eye. Thus, a buckled eye may be less sensitive to optic nerve damage to IOP fluctuations because it is less rigid (lower ocular rigidity). This observation may be concordant with the protective effects of high CH and explain why no significant change in CH in the encircling band group compared to the control group, while the scleral sponge group demonstrated a significant reduction in CH after surgery which can be attributed to the absence of the buffering effect of the encircling element [59].

Corneal biomechanical changes are observed after scleral buckling. CH decreased significantly at 1 month after combined PPV and encircling scleral buckle and CH did not change after PPV alone [60]. No change in corneal viscoelastic properties after 23G transconjunctival suture-less vitrectomy [61]. CRF did not change significantly after surgery in both groups. IOPg and IOPcc increased significantly in the PPV/SB group (p = 0.019 and p = 0.010, respectively) but not in PPV group

Table 25.1 Summary of patient, medication and surgical factors likely to impact overall ocular rigidity and engineering parameters defined in Eq. (25.4)

Patient factors	Likely change of engineering parameter	Potential effect on ocular rigidity	Reference(s)
Older age	$E\uparrow$	$\uparrow$	[62, 63]
Ethnicity of African ancestry	$?\,E\uparrow$	$?\uparrow$	[63]
Increasing axial length	$R\uparrow$	$\downarrow$	[64]
Megalocornea	$R\uparrow$	$\downarrow$	[65]
Buphthalmos	$R\uparrow$	$\downarrow$	[66]
Aphakia	–	$\downarrow$	[67]
Connective tissue disorders e.g. osteogenesis imperfecta, Marfan's syndrome	$E\downarrow$	$\downarrow$	[68]
Longstanding primary open angle glaucoma	$E\uparrow$	$\uparrow$	[62, 69]
Age-related macular degeneration	–	$?\leftrightarrow$	[70]
Keratoconus	$T\downarrow$	$\downarrow$	[71]
Penetrating ocular trauma	$R\downarrow$	$\downarrow$ due to loss of volume	[72]
Medication factors			
Pilocarpine	$E\downarrow$	$\downarrow$	[73]
Latanoprost	$E\downarrow$	$\downarrow$	[74]
Surgical factors			

Table 25.1 (continued)

Patient factors	Likely change of engineering parameter	Potential effect on ocular rigidity	Reference(s)
Corneal hydration	$T\uparrow$	↑	[75]
Corneal cross-linking	$E\uparrow$	↑	[76]
Refractive surgery	$T\downarrow$	↓	[77]
Descemet stripping automated endothelial keratoplasty	$T\uparrow$	↑	[78]
Descemet's membrane endothelial Keratoplasty	$T\downarrow$	↓	[79]
Trabeculectomy	–	↓	[80]
Buckled eye with encircling band	$R\uparrow$	↓	[57, 59, 81, 82]
Injection of intravitreal agent	–	↑ due to transient increase in volume	[83]

E = average Young's modulus, T = average corneal thickness, R = average corneal radius, ? = uncertainty

(p = 0.715 and p = 0.273, respectively). Unlike the PPV group, values were significantly higher than IOPg values before (p = 0.001) and after surgery (p = 0.003) in the PPV/SB group IOPcc. Neither the PPV/SB group nor the PPV group showed any significant changes in the corneal morphological parameters after surgery (p > 0.05) [60]. Encircling scleral buckling surgery leads to a change in corneal biomechanics. It may cause an underestimation error in IOP measurement. Table 25.1 below summarises the potential effect of various patient factors on engineering parameters and ocular rigidity (OR).

References

1. Friedenwald JS. Contribution to the theory and practice of tonometry. Am J Opthalmol. 1937;20:985–1024.
2. Perkins ES, Gloster J. Further studies on the distensibility of the eye. Br J Ophthalmol. 1957;41(8):475–86.
3. Gloster J, Perkins ES. Distensibility of the eye. Br J Ophthalmol. 1957;41(2):93–102.
4. Gloster J, Perkins ES, Pommier ML. Extensibility of strips of sclera and cornea. Br J Ophthalmol. 1957;41(2):103–10.
5. Macri FJ, Wanko T, Grimes PA, Von Sallmann L. The elasticity of the eye. AMA Arch Ophthalmol. 1957;58(4):513–9.
6. Ytteborg J. Further investigations of factors influencing size of rigidity coefficient. Acta Ophthalmol. 1960;38:643–57.
7. Detorakis ET, Pallikaris IG. Ocular rigidity: biomechanical role, in vivo measurements and clinical significance. Clin Exp Ophthalmol. 2013;41(1):73–81.

8. Beaton L, Mazzaferri J, Lalonde F, Hidalgo-Aguirre M, Descovich D, Lesk MR, et al. Non-invasive measurement of choroidal volume change and ocular rigidity through automated segmentation of high-speed OCT imaging. Biomed Opt Express. 2015;6(5):1694–706.

9. White OW. Ocular elasticity? Ophthalmology. 1990;97(9):1092–4.

10. Kalenak JW. More ocular elasticity? Ophthalmology. 1991;98(4):411–2.

11. Purslow PP, Karwatowski WS. Ocular elasticity. Is engineering stiffness a more useful characterization parameter than ocular rigidity? Ophthalmology. 1996;103(10):1686–92.

12. Terai N, Raiskup F, Haustein M, Pillunat LE, Spoerl E. Identification of biomechanical properties of the cornea: the ocular response analyzer. Curr Eye Res. 2012;37(7):553–62.

13. Kida T, Liu JHK, Weinreb RN. Effects of aging on corneal biomechanical properties and their impact on 24-hour measurement of intraocular pressure. Am J Ophthalmol. 2008;146(4):567–72.

14. Mangouritsas G, Morphis G, Mourtzoukos S, Feretis E. Association between corneal hysteresis and central corneal thickness in glaucomatous and non-glaucomatous eyes. Acta Ophthalmol. 2009;87(8):901–5.

15. Shah S, Laiquzzaman M, Cunliffe I, Mantry S. The use of the Reichert ocular response analyser to establish the relationship between ocular hysteresis, corneal resistance factor and central corneal thickness in normal eyes. Cont Lens Anterior Eye. 2006;29(5):257–62.

16. Zhang B, Shweikh Y, Khawaja AP, Gallacher J, Bauermeister S, Foster PJ, et al. Associations with corneal hysteresis in a population cohort: results from 96 010 UK biobank participants. Ophthalmology. 2019;126(11):1500–10.

17. Lau W, Pye D. A clinical description of Ocular Response Analyzer measurements. Invest Ophthalmol Vis Sci. 2011;52(6):2911–6.

18. van der Werff TJ. A new single-parameter ocular rigidity function. Am J Ophthalmol. 1981;92(3):391–5.

19. Bouremel Y, Madaan S, Lee R, Eames I, Wojcik A, Khaw PT. Pursing of planar elastic pockets. J Fluids Struct. 2017;70:261–75.

20. Hamilton KE, Pye DC. Young's modulus in normal corneas and the effect on applanation tonometry. Optom Vis Sci. 2008;85(6):445–50.

21. Sridhar MS. Anatomy of cornea and ocular surface. Indian J Ophthalmol. 2018;66(2):190–4.

22. Bouremel Y, Henein C, Brocchini S, Khaw PT. Intraocular pressure (IOP) effects on self-sealing clear corneal incisions using 3D printed anterior segment model. Invest Ophthalmol Vis Sci. 2019;60(9):1016.

23. Mooney M. A theory of large deformation. J Appl Phys. 1940;11:582–92.

24. Zeiter JH, Shin DH. Traumatic rupture of the globe after glaucoma surgery. Am J Ophthalmol. 1990;109(6):732–3.

25. Lambrou FH, Kozarsky A. Wound dehiscence following cataract surgery. Ophthalmic Surg. 1987;18(10):738–40.

26. Ball JL, McLeod BK. Traumatic wound dehiscence following cataract surgery: a thing of the past? Eye (Lond). 2001;15(Pt 1):42–4.

27. Stitzel JD, Hansen GA, Herring IP, Duma SM. Blunt trauma of the aging eye: injury mechanisms and increasing lens stiffness. Arch Ophthalmol. 2005;123(6):789–94.

28. Shih PJ, Wang IJ, Cai WF, Yen JY. Biomechanical simulation of stress concentration and intraocular pressure in corneas subjected to myopic refractive surgical procedures. Sci Rep. 2017;7(1):13906.

29. Cronemberger S, Guimaraes CS, Calixto N, Calixto JM. Intraocular pressure and ocular rigidity after LASIK. Arq Bras Oftalmol. 2009;72(4):439–43.

30. Kirwan C, O'Keefe M. Corneal hysteresis using the Reichert ocular response analyser: findings pre- and post-LASIK and LASEK. Acta Ophthalmol. 2008;86(2):215–8.

31. Raevdal P, Grauslund J, Vestergaard AH. Comparison of corneal biomechanical changes after refractive surgery by noncontact tonometry: small-incision lenticule extraction versus flap-based refractive surgery—a systematic review. Acta Ophthalmol. 2019;97(2):127–36.

32. Hager A, Loge K, Fullhas MO, Schroeder B, Grossherr M, Wiegand W. Changes in corneal hysteresis after clear corneal cataract surgery. Am J Ophthalmol. 2007;144(3):341–6.
33. Deol M, Ehrlich JR, Shimmyo M, Radcliffe NM. Association between corneal hysteresis and the magnitude of intraocular pressure decrease after cataract surgery. J Cataract Refract Surg. 2015;41(6):1176–81.
34. Kamiya K, Shimizu K, Ohmoto F, Amano R. Evaluation of corneal biomechanical parameters after simultaneous phacoemulsification with intraocular lens implantation and limbal relaxing incisions. J Cataract Refract Surg. 2011;37(2):265–70.
35. Feizi S, Montahai T, Moein H. Graft biomechanics following three corneal transplantation techniques. J Ophthalmic Vis Res. 2015;10(3):238–42.
36. Abd Elaziz MS, Elsobky HM, Zaky AG, Hassan EAM, KhalafAllah MT. Corneal biomechanics and intraocular pressure assessment after penetrating keratoplasty for non keratoconic patients, long term results. BMC Ophthalmol. 2019;19(1):172.
37. Jiang MS, Zhu JY, Li X, Zhang NN, Zhang XD. Corneal biomechanical properties after penetrating keratoplasty or deep anterior lamellar keratoplasty using the ocular response analyzer: a meta-analysis. Cornea. 2017;36(3):310–6.
38. Ali M, Raghunathan V, Li JY, Murphy CJ, Thomasy SM. Biomechanical relationships between the corneal endothelium and Descemet's membrane. Exp Eye Res. 2016;152:57–70.
39. Knox Cartwright NE, Tyrer JR, Marshall J. Age-related differences in the elasticity of the human cornea. Invest Ophthalmol Vis Sci. 2011;52(7):4324–9.
40. Patel SV, Diehl NN, Hodge DO, Bourne WM. Donor risk factors for graft failure in a 20-year study of penetrating keratoplasty. Arch Ophthalmol. 2010;128(4):418–25.
41. Verdier DD, Sugar A, Baratz K, Beck R, Dontchev M, Dunn S, et al. Corneal thickness as a predictor of corneal transplant outcome. Cornea. 2013;32(6):729–36.
42. Ivarsen A, Hjortdal J. Recipient corneal thickness and visual outcome after Descemet's stripping automated endothelial keratoplasty. Br J Ophthalmol. 2014;98(1):30–4.
43. Siggel R, Christofi E, Giasoumi F, Adler W, Siebelmann S, Bachmann B, et al. Changes in corneal biomechanical properties after Descemet membrane endothelial keratoplasty. Cornea. 2019;38(8):964–9.
44. Congdon NG, Broman AT, Bandeen-Roche K, Grover D, Quigley HA. Central corneal thickness and corneal hysteresis associated with glaucoma damage. Am J Ophthalmol. 2006;141(5):868–75.
45. Mcdeiros FA, Sample PA, Weinreb RN. Corneal thickness measurements and visual function abnormalities in ocular hypertensive patients. Am J Ophthalmol. 2003;135(2):131–7.
46. Medeiros FA, Meira-Freitas D, Lisboa R, Kuang TM, Zangwill LM, Weinreb RN. Corneal hysteresis as a risk factor for glaucoma progression: a prospective longitudinal study. Ophthalmology. 2013;120(8):1533–40.
47. Sigal IA, Ethier CR. Biomechanics of the optic nerve head. Exp Eye Res. 2009;88(4):799–807.
48. Kimball EC, Nguyen C, Steinhart MR, Nguyen TD, Pease ME, Oglesby EN, et al. Experimental scleral cross-linking increases glaucoma damage in a mouse model. Exp Eye Res. 2014;128:129–40.
49. Pakravan M, Afroozifar M, Yazdani S. Corneal biomechanical changes following trabeculectomy, phaco-trabeculectomy, ahmed glaucoma valve implantation and phacoemulsification. J Ophthalmic Vis Res. 2014;9(1):7–13.
50. Sorkhabi R, Najafzadeh F, Sadeghi A, Ahoor M, Mahdavifard A. Corneal biomechanical changes after trabeculectomy with mitomycin C in primary open-angle glaucoma and pseudoexfoliation glaucoma. Int Ophthalmol. 2019;39(12):2741–8.
51. Pillunat KR, Spoerl E, Terai N, Pillunat LE. Corneal biomechanical changes after trabeculectomy and the impact on intraocular pressure measurement. J Glaucoma. 2017;26(3):278–82.
52. Diez-Alvarez L, Munoz-Negrete FJ, Casas-Llera P, Oblanca N, de Juan V, Rebolleda G. Relationship between corneal biomechanical properties and optic nerve head changes after deep sclerectomy. Eur J Ophthalmol. 2017;27(5):535–41.

53. Casado A, Cabarga C, Perez-Sarriegui A, Fuentemilla E. Differences in corneal biomechanics in nonpenetrating deep sclerectomy and deep sclerectomy reconverted into trabeculectomy. J Glaucoma. 2017;26(1):15–9.
54. Pillunat KR, Spoerl E, Terai N, Pillunat LE. Effect of selective laser trabeculoplasty on corneal biomechanics. Acta Ophthalmol. 2016;94(6):e501–4.
55. Hirneiss C, Sekura K, Brandlhuber U, Kampik A, Kernt M. Corneal biomechanics predict the outcome of selective laser trabeculoplasty in medically uncontrolled glaucoma. Graefes Arch Clin Exp Ophthalmol. 2013;251(10):2383–8.
56. El Gendy HA, Khalil NM, Eissa IM, Shousha SM. The effect of strabismus muscle surgery on corneal biomechanics. J Ophthalmol. 2018;2018:8072140.
57. Friberg TR, Fourman SB. Scleral buckling and ocular rigidity. Clinical ramifications. Arch Ophthalmol. 1990;108(11):1622–7.
58. Johnson MW, Han DP, Hoffman KE. The effect of scleral buckling on ocular rigidity. Ophthalmology. 1990;97(2):190–5.
59. Riazi EM, Jafarzadehpur E, Hashemi H, Ghaffari E. Evaluation of corneal biomechanical properties following scleral buckling using the ocular response analyzer. Iran J Ophthalmol. 2013;25(2):151–4.
60. Ruiz-De-Gopegui E, Ascaso FJ, Del Buey MA, Cristobal JA. [Effects of encircling scleral buckling on the morphology and biomechanical properties of the cornea]. Arch Soc Esp Oftalmol 2011;86(11):363–7.
61. Seymenoglu G, Uzun O, Baser E. Surgically induced changes in corneal viscoelastic properties after 23-gauge pars plana vitrectomy using ocular response analyzer. Curr Eye Res. 2013;38(1):35–40.
62. Pallikaris IG, Kymionis GD, Ginis HS, Kounis GA, Tsilimbaris MK. Ocular rigidity in living human eyes. Invest Ophthalmol Vis Sci. 2005;46(2):409–14.
63. Grytz R, Fazio MA, Libertiaux V, Bruno L, Gardiner S, Girkin CA, et al. Age- and race-related differences in human scleral material properties. Invest Ophthalmol Vis Sci. 2014;55(12):8163–72.
64. Dastiridou AI, Ginis H, Tsilimbaris M, Karyotakis N, Detorakis E, Siganos C, et al. Ocular rigidity, ocular pulse amplitude, and pulsatile ocular blood flow: the effect of axial length. Invest Ophthalmol Vis Sci. 2013;54(3):2087–92.
65. Moshirfar M, Hastings J, Ronquillo Y. Megalocornea. [Updated 2021 Jan 21]. In: StatPearls [Internet]. Treasure Island (FL): StatPearls Publishing; 2021 Jan-. Available from: https://www.ncbi.nlm.nih.gov/books/NBK554374/.
66. Feroze KB, Patel BC. Buphthalmos. [Updated 2021 Feb 17]. In: StatPearls [Internet]. Treasure Island (FL): StatPearls Publishing; 2021 Jan-. Available from: https://www.ncbi.nlm.nih.gov/books/NBK430887/.
67. Sampaolesi R, Sampaolesi JR, Zárate J. Ocular Rigidity or Resistance to Distension. In: The Glaucomas. Springer, Berlin, Heidelberg. 2014. https://doi.org/10.1007/978-3-642-35500-4_9.
68. Kaiser-Kupfer MI, McCain L, Shapiro JR, Podgor MJ, Kupfer C, Rowe D. Low ocular rigidity in patients with osteogenesis imperfecta. Invest Ophthalmol Vis Sci. 1981;20(6):807–9.
69. Wang J, Freeman EE, Descovich D, Harasymowycz PJ, Kamdeu Fansi A, Li G, et al. Estimation of ocular rigidity in glaucoma using ocular pulse amplitude and pulsatile choroidal blood flow. Invest Ophthalmol Vis Sci. 2013;54(3):1706–11.
70. Pallikaris IG, Kymionis GD, Ginis HS, Kounis GA, Christodoulakis E, Tsilimbaris MK. Ocular rigidity in patients with age-related macular degeneration. Am J Ophthalmol. 2006;141(4):611–5.
71. Brooks AM, Robertson IF, Mahoney AM. Ocular rigidity and intraocular pressure in keratoconus. Aust J Ophthalmol. 1984;12(4):317–24.
72. Sung EK, Nadgir RN, Fujita A, Siegel C, Ghafouri RH, Traband A, Sakai O. Injuries of the Globe: What Can the Radiologist Offer? RadioGraphics. 2014;34(3):764–6.

73. Roberts W, Rogers JW. Postural effects on pressure and ocular rigidity measurements. Am. J. Ophthal mol. 1964;57:111–118.
74. Tsikripis P, Papaconstantinou D, Koutsandrea C, Apostolopoulos M, Georgalas I. The effect of prostaglandin analogs on the biomechanical properties and central thickness of the cornea of patients with open-angle glaucoma: a 3-year study on 108 eyes. Drug Des Devel Ther. 2013;7:1149–56.
75. Ytteborg J, Dohlman CH. Corneal Edema and Intraocular Pressure: II. Clinical Results. Arch Ophthalmol. 1965;74(4):477–484.
76. Yuheng Zhou, Yuanyuan Wang, Meixiao Shen, Zi Jin, Yihong Chen, Yue Zhou, Jia Qu, Dexi Zhu, "In vivo evaluation of corneal biomechanical properties by optical coherence elastography at different cross-linking irradiances. J. Biomed. Opt. 2019;24(10):105001.
77. Zhao MH, Wu Q, Jia LL, Hu P. Changes in central corneal thickness and refractive error after thin-flap laser in situ keratomileusis in Chinese eyes. BMC Ophthalmol. 2015;15:86. Published 2015 Jul 29. https://doi.org/10.1186/s12886-015-0083-2.
78. Thasarat S. Vajaranant and Marianne O. Price and Francis W. Price and Jacob T. Wilensky and Deepak P. Edward, Intraocular Pressure Measurements Following Descemet Stripping Endothelial Keratoplasty. American Journal of Ophthalmology. 2008;145(5):780–6.e1.
79. Huang T, Ouyang C, Zhan J, Jiang L. [Descemet's membrane endothelial keratoplasty for treatment of patients with corneal endothelial decompensation]. Zhonghua Yan Ke Za Zhi. 2017;53(7):534–9.
80. Yang YC Hulbert MF. Effect of trabeculectomy on pulsatile ocular blood flow. Br J Ophthalmol. 1995;79: 507–508.
81. Syrdalen P. Intraocular pressure and ocular rigidity in patients with retinal detachment. II. Postoperative study. Acta Ophthalmol. 1970;48(5):1036–44.
82. Harbin TS Jr, Laikam SE, Lipsitt K, Jarrett WH 2nd, Hagler WS. Applanation-Schiotz disparity after retinal detachment surgery utilizing cryopexy. Ophthalmology. 1979;86(9):1609–12.
83. Kampougeris G, Spyropoulos D, Mitropoulou A. Intraocular Pressure rise after Anti-VEGF Treatment: Prevalence, Possible Mechanisms and Correlations. J Curr Glaucoma Pract. 2013;7(1):19-24. https://doi.org/10.5005/jp-journals-10008-1132.

Printed in the United States
by Baker & Taylor Publisher Services